Genome

Genome

Howard Grodman

GrodmanWright
Lynn, Massachusetts

This is a work of fiction. Names, characters, places, and incidents are a product of the author's imagination. Locales and public names are sometimes used for atmospheric purposes. Any resemblance to actual people, living or dead, or to businesses, companies, events, institutions, or locales is completely coincidental.

Published by GrodmanWright
Lynn, Massachusetts
grodmanh@gmail.com

Book Layout & Design by Booknook.biz

Ordering Information:
Quantity sales. Special discounts are available on quantity purchases by corporations, associations, and others. For details, contact the "Special Sales Department" at the address above.

First edition

ISBN:
979-8-9941371-0-9 (Paperback)
979-8-9941371-1-6 (Hardback)
979-8-9941371-2-3 (Ebook)

Dedicated to my wife and muse, Caresse, for her support and almost infinite patience.

And to the children and their families who may unfortunately find some of this story too familiar.

Bad things sometimes happen to good people.

I don't know why.

PROLOGUE

It was 2 AM. John Stevens walked the same circuit around the high-security lab hour after hour, week after week. It had become so routine that at any moment, even blindfolded, he would know which tile he stepped on, which overhead light hummed, and where every shadow was cast. He knew how far he had come by singing the same song in his head over and over, California Dreamin', every night, for seven years.

It was almost a perfect job. John didn't like people much, he preferred that he was by himself. He was glad to be alone at the lab, well except for the mice. He wasn't happy about the part of his route that took him through the animal room. John loved animals. But all those mice in cages, and their smell, it was disturbing. It bothered him to think about how Dr. Benzi and the others were performing experiments on those poor animals. The song in his head helped, but John was always glad to be past that section of his route.

The fact that nothing ever happened during his graveyard shift suited him just fine. Nothing ever happened for miles around. The half buried lab sat near a fault under the California desert. It could only be reached by locating a hidden turnoff, not marked on any GPS map, and then following a 3 mile long isolated road, surrounded by nothing but rolling tumbleweeds and jackrabbits. John had no idea how many people worked here during the day, they were all gone before he arrived. In seven years he'd never met anyone other than the daytime security guard at shift change.

Until tonight.

The phrase "got down on my knees" was in his head as he rounded the same corner at which he had sung those words each night before. This time was different, his attention was drawn to a flash of light beyond the double-thick plexiglass wall that stretched from floor to ceiling, clearly revealing the darkened lab space within.

There was never a flash of light.

Never a deviation from "all quiet."

John eased forward sideways and scanned the lab. The bio hoods that would have been busy with technicians during the day were dark and quiet. The automated cell processing units were shut down. All seemed eerily still, until out of the corner of his eye, he glimpsed a black clad figure scamper across the room and slip through the emergency exit. Alarms should have sounded. Red lights should have flashed. The entire subterranean building should have gone into lockdown when that door opened.

But not this time.

This wasn't good. His knew his night would soon become busy with people. John imagined difficult questions from his supervisor, someone he barely knew. Who was that black clad figure? What was he doing? How did he get away? He shook his head, it wouldn't go well.

1.

It wasn't until several hours after Richie arrived at school that he noticed the bruise.

Richard J. Samuelson (he had never told anyone what the J stood for; there were guesses and taunts, but they were all wrong) considered himself, at least until then, a perfectly average 17-year-old. He'd made the track team as a junior and surprised everyone by setting records in the 800-meter run and the 110-meter hurdle. It was no accident that he'd chosen track rather than a team sport. Richie was usually quiet, and rather shy. Making new friends had never been easy. There were no girlfriends, not yet, but hey, there was always hope.

Third period French class was not his favorite, but his high school required a language elective, and French had seemed more useful than Latin. He tried to follow what the teacher was saying during the immersive language course, but her words seemed to run together. She might as well have been speaking Martian.

That gave him an idea. Absentmindedly, he tugged at his left sleeve while he opened the notebook on his desk. He flipped through the spiral bound pages past moonscapes and detailed closeups of creatures, both real and imagined. Philip K. Dick and Ray Bradbury were among his favorite authors, their stories transported him to distant worlds. At night, as he drifted off to sleep, he would imagine himself somewhere out there, among the galaxies, where his life might be different.

He paused, staring down at his drawing of the Perseverance rover set among the scattered rocks in the foreground, the Ingenuity helicopter above, and a very small setting sun overlooking a Martian mountain range far in the distance. The scene needed something else, but until now, he hadn't been sure what. He sketched an astronaut on the ground beneath the hovering helicopter, and then he drew a creature that looked remarkably like an Earth turtle. It towered over the curious spacefarer, standing on its hind legs, seven feet tall, wearing round, gold rimmed glasses and dressed like Lawrence of Arabia. He added a bubble above the creature's head and filled it with arcane symbols depicting Martian dialogue.

Pleased, maybe he'd even develop the sketch into a comic strip, Richie looked up and caught a pair of green eyes in the next row quickly turning away. He grinned. Now *she* was much more interesting than the French class. They'd never talked, but Richie remembered seeing her the last time he used the Nautilus machines in the school gym. Their desks were so close that he could almost reach out and touch her. She had lovely red hair, braided and wrapped around her head. A dozen or more freckles dotted her face. He wondered if she worried about them as so many of the girls he knew might, but he thought she was beautiful.

Richie sighed, closing his eyes and imagining that they were magically transported to a dance floor, just the two of them, alone. The band is playing a slow dance, *I only have eyes for you*, and in that special place he's holding her closely, she responds, pressing against him. Her perfume is delicious. As they glide across the floor, they kiss. They're in love. He feels warm all over, alive, excited and he never wants it to end.

"Richard... Richard!"

The vision instantly dissolved and his eyes shot open. Richie stretched and rubbed his sore left arm, as he replayed the dance in his head. She was back in his arms, it felt real.

He wasn't focused on the teacher calling on him, but on those nearby green eyes peeking at him from above a quiet smile. There'd been a question from the teacher linked to his name, but he hadn't quite heard it.

"Je ne sais pas," he mumbled, ducking his head, one of the few phrases he knew, and which had often come in handy.

The teacher murmured something in French that sounded scathing. Why had he ever thought French was better than Latin? He started to breathe again when she quickly turned to find someone else to question.

Richie forced himself to focus on the lesson for the next twenty excruciatingly long minutes until the bell finally rang. By the time he'd shoved his notebook into his bag, his desk neighbor was gone. Oh, well. He slung his backpack over his shoulder, and that's when he noticed that his arm was throbbing.

He pulled his left sleeve up past the elbow. There was a bruise, dark and raised. Richie poked at it. It was tender. His arm felt funny as he flexed it. He figured that he must have irritated his already bruised elbow by leaning on it while he was drawing. Or was it dancing with that girl in his dream? It had seemed so real. For a moment, a sense of unease crept into his head. He remembered his mad scramble down the stairs that morning, jamming his left elbow against the newel post. He'd been in a rush. His mother had gone to work at the art gallery early, and he'd already hit the Snooze button several times trying desperately to eke out every possible second of sleep. Finally he had no choice but to get up or miss the bus.

And with that, his discomfort and unease flew out of his head as he followed the rest of his classmates out into the hallway. He was laser focused on finding out more about the girl with the red hair.

2.

His last class of the day was gym. The nasty New England pea soup fog, rolling in from the shore, as it often did, forced Richie to switch his usual outdoor track workout to an indoor run. Sprinting on the treadmill, it was soon clear that something was terribly wrong. He was short of breath. He slowed his pace but that didn't help. Sweat poured from his brow, dripping down his face and falling onto his shirt. Richie hit the red pause button. As the treadmill ground to a halt, he leaned over to grab the sports drink sitting on the floor by the machine. Reaching down, the blood drained from his head. He felt awful. The room began to spin. He tried to grab the rail, but everything was fuzzy. As he reached out, his hand waved through the air. He teetered and the room went black.

He lay there, face up, sprawled out on the floor, his eyes glazed over and breathing hard. He had no idea how long he'd been there. Finally color slowly began to return. Richie blinked several times as he became aware of his surroundings. All around eyes were staring down at him.

"Oh, shit," he said as he tried to sit up.

The gym teacher was kneeling over him, "just lay still for a moment, don't try to get up," she directed. "You passed out, Richie." The teacher shooed the other students away.

Slowly, over several minutes, the haze began to lift. The teacher tested him. "What's your name? What day is it? Where are you?" After some moments of hesitation, Richie could finally answer her questions. Satisfied, she helped him sit up. She offered the sports drink.

"Take a few sips, do it slowly."

The cool sweet fluids felt good. He started with a few tastes, but he was soon gulping down the rest of the bottled drink. He needed hydration.

"I guess, I skipped breakfast this morning, and I haven't had anything to drink," he said. "Kinda dumb. But I'm OK, now." He glanced around the gym and saw the students' surreptitious glances. Richie looked downward, he imagined there'd be talk. He looked back at the teacher, "thanks for helping. I'm really OK now."

She looked him over carefully. "I want you to get up slowly and we'll walk over to my office. You need to sit for a while. I'll bring you a container of orange juice and a protein bar. Take your time and we'll see how you feel."

As Richie sat alone in her office quietly sipping the juice and munching on a chocolate Clif bar, he tried to figure out what happened. He closed his eyes, picturing himself on the treadmill. It was like watching a doorbell video image, small and fuzzy. He saw someone collapse. But that guy couldn't really be him, could it? Something deep in the pit of his stomach churned.

3.

Going home, Richie sat on the left side of the clunky old yellow school bus as it traveled along the pothole littered road. Without warning, the left front bus wheel found a large pothole and his arm slammed against the side of the bus. A sharp pain shot up his left arm, exploding in the shoulder.

"Shit!" He pulled away. Did he really hit his arm that hard this morning? He couldn't remember.

When he arrived home, he was still worried, but now his hunger demanded attention. He put his backpack down, and with his junior varsity track jacket half on, he opened the fridge and peered inside. His mother, Betty, was aware of the need to keep the refrigerator stocked, making sure to avoid a hangry crisis, at least until she got home from work. He found the food bridge he needed, cold chicken leftovers, and a container of milk. That and a few chocolate chip cookies assuaged his hunger.

Feeling momentarily sated, Richie climbed the stairs to his room, passing that damned newel post. It was unexpectedly an effort. As he entered his room, he looked over the desk crowded with school papers. The pajamas from the morning were still there, crumpled across an unmade bed. The cream-colored walls were decorated with some of the avatars of his favorite video games. There were also two black and white movie posters. One with Boris Karloff as the 1931 Frankenstein's monster, and one had Bela Lugosi as Count Dracula from that same year. As the creatures hung on his wall, they seemed to be sizing each other up. They reminded him of some of his favorite movies. He's always liked the Godzilla movie, the original Japanese version from 1954, not the American one with Raymond Burr randomly edited in. And the first King Kong movie from 1933, he's not sure how many times he'd seen it, a lot. Godzilla was just a guy in a suit, but King Kong was a spectacle of stop action movie magic by Ray Harryhausen, way back then. All those creatures, Frankenstein's monster, Godzilla, King Kong and the Werewolf, found themselves thrown into situations they never asked to be in. They reacted in the only way they knew how, and they were hunted down and destroyed for it. Richie felt sorry for them, well except for Count Dracula, he got what he deserved.

He asked Siri to play some music, *study volume*, as he plopped down on his bed, seriously intending to get at least some of his homework done before his mother got home and the real dinner appeared. The room was his Fortress of Solitude, the Man of Steel was invulnerable inside. Richie had his mom to protect, she was everything. There was a father, of course, but not a dad, he had disappeared before Richie was born. Richie didn't think about him, not ever. Why should he?

All he needed was his mom, they managed together. If it weren't a school night, they'd sit with a bowl of buttered popcorn and enjoy a TCM movie together. He could almost always tell his mom what was on his mind. She would listen and nod and tell him to go figure it out. He worried about his mom, someday he'd find a girl, they would marry, he'd move out and have a family. What would happen to her then? Who would she have? He tried to put those thoughts on dim and get some work done.

It seemed only a moment later when he was awakened by Betty knocking on his door, "dinner's ready."

Surprised to find Richie asleep, she asked, "are you OK, didn't you sleep well last night?" She sounded worried. This wasn't her Richie.

"Oh, yeah, fine, I think... I don't remember any problems."

Down in the dining nook by the kitchen, Richie sat down. Betty would often cook enough for the week during the weekend before and keep the meals frozen but available to heat and serve. Betty Samuelson was practical and worked hard to avoid working too hard. Though she tried to be both mom and dad, that second role didn't come so easily.

As the mom of young Richie, Betty read whatever she could to help guide her parenting. She had no outside support, her parents had been mostly missing in action. Watching her son grow up, she expected him to be polite and respectful. When there was trouble at school, Betty presumed the teachers were right, as they usually were. Betty still remembered the time she had to leave the Gallery early because Richie had super glued Billy's locker shut. He was suspended for three days. Boys and their testosterone. She had grounded him for a week, though Betty was secretly glad that Richie fought back. She knew that Billy teased him mercilessly. "Hey, Richie, you skinny track bastard, whose chasing you now?" he would say. It was mean, but her son had to learn life was like that sometimes. With his budding maturity, she allowed him the freedom to make mistakes. When something went wrong, Richie needed to address it. He would have to find out how his choices worked out. Mistakes had consequences. How would he ever learn to navigate those storms if someone always polished the path? Betty understood that as an adolescent his job was to transition to an independent adult. Eventually he would move out and be on his own. Though she knew that to be the natural order, Betty hoped that time was still far away. Richie was her life.

At the table, Richie usually wolfed down his food, but not today. Betty shot him a worried look. "Not so hungry? First, you're sleeping in the afternoon, now you're not eating. Something's wrong."

"Ah Mom, I'm okay, I guess I ate a bunch of food when I got home. Don't worry, it's nothing. I gotta get to my homework. I guess I didn't get much of it done this afternoon. I have calculus problems, a unit in social and a French exam later this week. I've really got to bone up on the French."

"OK, go on," she answered. Betty usually had Richie help clean up after dinner, but she saw that this day wasn't going as planned, so she let it slide. She watched as he climbed the stairs. He seemed to struggle, not the typical two steps at a time scamper. Something was wrong, but she didn't know what it might be. She was anxious and worried, but she had things to do for her job tomorrow, all those invoices to review and clients' orders to process. Her assignments soon captured her attention.

Upstairs Richie went to work. He assigned two hours to do all his stuff and broke it down into smaller chunks of time. There were 30 minutes for math, 45 minutes to read the social studies unit and 45 minutes for the French, and that included practicing French dialogue using the app. Richie donned the headphones and mic. The app would correct his pronunciation. He would repeat the phrases several times before the bot would agree that it sounded like French.

"Bonjour madame, avez vous froid? Prenez ce plaid. Je suis très bien."

It wasn't great, he knew, but after spending some time with his French, he felt a bit more prepared for the upcoming exam. He had to work harder to get the French right than to manage his calculus problems. Oh well, vive la différence. Finally, done with his schoolwork, Richie went to take a shower before bed. That was his usual school night routine, there was no time in the morning. He took his time, enjoying the steamy hot shower. The soothing spray of water helped ease the soreness of his arm. He could bend it more easily now. It didn't hurt quite as much. Maybe it was getting better. The bruise turned from dark blue to a lighter green and yellow, all part of the natural healing process. Finishing up, he rinsed off and dried himself gingerly. Normally, he'd be on one of those multiplayer games before going to sleep, but not tonight. He was asleep five minutes later.

Betty came to check on him, not something she ordinarily did. She quietly opened his door and watched him. He seemed comfortable, breathing normally. Her anxiety eased a bit. She quietly withdrew, closing the door behind her. Across the hall, in her room, she got ready for bed. Ten minutes later, she too was sleeping.

Alarms went off in the morning, it was time to get ready for the new day. The sun was up, and it looked like it would be gorgeous. The skies were bright blue with scattered wisps of clouds. It was Tuesday, still lots of the week to go. Betty took her showers in the morning. All finished, she was dressed, minimal make up. Lips and eyes done, a bit of blush on her cheeks and she was set. Betty went across the hall to see how Richie was coming along. She checked his room and, not seeing him there, figured he was already downstairs getting something to eat before heading off to school.

Indeed, Richie was in front of the Amana fridge. He found a blueberry muffin that Betty had baked the weekend before and had stored in the freezer. All it required was a minute visit (hit the "add 30 second" button twice) to the microwave. A pat of butter sat melting in the shallow slice he made in its top. A glass of milk with a bit of coffee and sugar was downed in a jiff. He used the sleeve to wipe his mouth (save a tree). Grabbing his backpack and cell phone, a quick shout out to Betty, and he was out the door just as the bus horn announced its presence.

Betty called out her required "be careful and have a great day," as he danced down the walkway and disappeared into the bus. He had never mentioned the bruise or the event in the gym.

4.

The bus went over the same potholes in reverse order but this time he sat on the right side of the bus and his left arm never bothered him. As the bus approached his school, Richie could see the long queue of cars waiting to drop students off. The line inched forward slowly. A car stopped briefly at the designated area, a door shot open, a kid escaped, and the next one took his place. It easily took 20 minutes from the beginning to the end of the procession. The bus had its own space to discharge the students, bypassing the pokey motorcade. As soon as the bus stopped and the door opened, the troops promptly poured out with a bit of whoopin' and hollerin'. As Richie left the bus, he felt stiff and tired. He had to stretch his legs just to keep moving and though it was a warm late spring day, still, a chill shot up his spine. He shivered, it scared him. "It's nothing," Richie told himself, "just coming down with a bug." He tried to refocus. What he really wanted was to find out more about that red haired girl from French class.

When he saw Franny, the social butterfly, hanging out with her friends near the flag pole, he thought she ought to know.

Richie hesitated, but he was determined. He took a big breath, trying to work up his courage and walked over toward Franny and her clique of girls.

Franny, saw Richie approaching with that meek look on his face, "Hi, Richie."

"Uh, can we talk? I've got a question for you."

"Yeah, sure, Richie."

"I mean alone, just us."

Franny turned to her friends, "be back in a few." They all giggled, exchanging knowing looks as she and Richie found a little space apart.

As soon as they were alone Richie asked about the redhead with the braided pigtails in French class. Franny knew exactly who he was talking about.

"Nancy Peters is like new to the school, her family just moved to town over on Bennit Street, big gray brick house, with a pool in back. Used to be the Foster place. I heard that her dad had to relocate for work. I'm not sure what he does." Franny reported her news in one breath.

"Hey, do you think she's seeing anyone?" Richie wanted to know.

"I don't think so, they're new here. Of course, there could be someone from back before her move, dunno," she answered. Franny had that look, she tilted her head, "so, ah, you might be interested? Want me to find out more for you?"

"Ah, that's OK, thanks for that, see you later Franny," Richie certainly didn't want anyone snooping around school for him. Franny already knew too much. Richie was sure that his interest in Nancy would be shared throughout Franny's clique. Well that couldn't be helped. Thinking back, Richie thought Nancy might have been looking at him in French class yesterday. He dared to hope that she might be interested. As the homeroom bell sounded, he turned to enter the school. Richie resolved to find out.

His homework the night before prepared him for the first two classes, math, and social studies. French was third period. As he entered the class, Richie looked around for Nancy. He quickly spotted her toward the back of the room. He imagined she looked up at him, but maybe that was just what he had hoped to see. The moment passed. Richie walked toward the back, not far from where Nancy was seated. He wasn't ready to get too close too soon. He was nervous. He felt his heart racing. What to do now? He glanced toward the front of the room and the teacher had written A.L.I.C.E. in big block letters across the blackboard. He tried to remember from his homework the night before, but nothing about ALICE came to mind.

Curiously, and unusual for the immersive French class, Ms. Moreau began speaking in English. She had an accent, hinting at her Parisian upbringing.

"We're going to have an active shooter drill this period. As you know A.L.I.C.E. stands for Alert, Lockdown, Inform, Counter and Evacuate. Today, we will practice the second component of this acronym. You'll hear the announcement over the PA system in a few minutes." Ms. Moreau added some of her own thoughts: "we all see the news. We pray that we never need to do this for real, but sadly we also know that it happens far too often."

The teacher went on with the instructions. Richie had heard them all before. He barely paid attention as she droned on. It was a drill after all.

The announcement came through the PA system, interrupting Ms. Moreau: "this is a drill for an active shooter. Begin to implement Lockdown. This is a drill. GO!"

The roles for the different groups had been assigned. Richie's group would block the classroom door. The teacher locked the door and pulled down its shade, while two other students and Richie pushed the heavy desk against the door. They piled on anything they could find that would help fortify the barricade. Other students hurried to pull down the window shades around the room and turn off the lights. All their cell phones were switched to vibrate. They crouched down and hid behind the overturned long tables, backpacks hugged to their chests, as they tried to make their profiles appear as small as possible. It was eerily quiet, and it was all done in less than three minutes.

It was after Richie hunkered down and hid behind one of the overturned long desk tables, that he peeked to his side and realized that he had huddled right next to Nancy. Up until then the exercise had been routine. Normally he wouldn't have been excited, but now he could feel his heart pounding. It was unexpected and delightful. Richie ran through his options. What to do now? He didn't want to fuck it up by saying or doing the wrong thing. That was when Nancy turned to him, she was very close. Richie could smell her perfume, it was intoxicating. He gazed into her beautiful green eyes, just a touch of makeup on her cheeks. Everything else faded away, it was just Richie and the red-headed girl, the rest of the world had vanished.

She leaned in closer. Her mouth nearly touching his cheek. He felt her sweet breath gently waft across his face. Softly, seductively, she whispered, "meet me after school at the track." She didn't wait for a response. She knew he'd be there.

Outwardly the moment passed. Anyone watching right then would have seen two students hiding in place behind an overturned table, nothing would've seemed to connect them. But inside Richie's brain, the picture was very different, chemistry was playing havoc with his neurons. His head was ablaze, and he could think of nothing else. The drill was over, the classroom returned to normal, but not so much inside his head. The hours left until the end of school took like forever, time passed like cold molasses.

Richie could barely contain himself. He wondered how he could possibly wait all those hours until they'd meet again. He found a way to make the last class go faster, he fell asleep. No one seemed to notice. The final bell pulled him from his reverie. It took a minute to get oriented. "I need more sleep," he thought. But he was definitely awake now and a smile broke across his face as he thought about Nancy. Off to the track field he went. As he approached, Richie saw her turn toward him. No one else was nearby, they'd be alone.

"Hi Nancy." He wanted to say something witty but couldn't think of anything. The feelings were new.

"Yes, you can" she said as she looked up.

"Uh, what?"

"You were wondering if you could kiss me," she smiled, invitingly.

And he did, lips touching, slightly open, hesitant at first, but then tongues exploring, bodies held tightly.

"That was nice," she said.

Nancy and Richie didn't say very much. They went to sit down together on the bench by the track. They leaned against each other, holding hands, savoring the moment.

"I saw you in class and I was trying to find out more about you," Richie said.

"I knew you were, and I was hoping we would meet soon. When the drill started, that was the chance I was looking for."

They both smiled and giggled a bit, each replaying the moment in their heads.

Richie watched Nancy as she sat and smiled. The cool salty New England breeze played with her hair, which she gently pushed back behind her right ear. Something about her excited him. She wasn't like the other girls he knew. She sat quietly and composed. And when she looked away, into the distance, the look on her face suggested a girl with a past. Something hidden, he wondered about that. But they didn't talk. Comfortable with the silence, he reached out to hold her hand, which she accepted.

Nancy glanced at her phone and realized it was getting late. "My dad will be here soon to pick me up at the front of the school. Will you walk down with me?"

"Sure," he was still delightfully overwhelmed by everything.

She held his arm, linked in hers as they walked down the hill. Her face changed a bit, "I see a big bruise on your arm, what happened?"

Richie glanced over at his left elbow, touching it, "I think I bumped it on the stair post the other day."

"Gee, Richie, I'm not looking at your elbow, this bruise here on your right forearm looks kind of nasty."

He looked at his right arm and couldn't remember hitting it on anything, "maybe something happened during the drill."

"Hey, I gotta go, that's my dad pulling in right now." She reached up and kissed him on the cheek, and then ran towards the car and her waiting father.

Richie watched her hop in the front, the door closed, and their car sped off. He wondered if she would say anything to her dad. What would he say to his mother?

Richie took off too, seeing the school bus pull in, there'd be another ride in an hour, but he needed to get on this one, lots to do at home, lots to think about. Richie started to jog down to the pickup site, but very quickly he became short of breath. Soon he was gasping for air. Richie's heart raced, and his chest ached. He reached up with his hand and felt his heart pounding. That's weird, he thought. It forced him to slow down and stop. Richie bent forward. He grabbed his knees, leaning on them as he worked to catch his breath. This wasn't right. Dark thoughts passed through his head. The unexplained bruise, the gym and now this. Something was definitely wrong. It took a full minute before he felt well enough to start in again toward the bus. Richie kept to a brisk walk and made it there just as the bus was ready to leave.

5.

Richie arrived home just as his mom did. Betty was smiling and humming to herself as she pranced up to the house. "Hey, Richie, we don't usually get home at the same time. How was your day? Mine was good." She seemed happy. Richie noticed the twinkle in her eyes, and the way the edges of her smile turned up. "The boss said some nice things about my last project. Did I already ask how your day was?" They were inside now.

Richie smiled, thinking about Nancy, "yeah I had a good day too." He was about to say more about Nancy, but Betty looked at him and frowned.

"How do you feel, Richie? You look worn out. I don't like what I'm seeing. Your color is off." She did the mom thing and placed her hand on his forehead. It wasn't warm. Giving him that Sherlock Holmes scan, she noticed the bruise on his right arm, near the wrist. "How'd you do that?"

"I dunno, we had an active shooter drill at school today and I helped move the desk. Maybe that was it, but I don't remember hitting it, I just pushed with my hands, two other guys helped."

Betty was still inspecting, and then she found the bruise on his left elbow. "And that one? How'd you do that?"

Richie tried to think back, it happened yesterday. He had no answer. He almost told her about the incident in the school gym but decided it would really freak her out. He wasn't ready for that.

"Anything else?" now it was a full-blown inquiry.

"Well, there was this girl," he paused "and I fell asleep in my last class, I guess that was kind of strange."

Betty examined Richie carefully. Most any other time she would have asked about the girl, but not now. "I don't like what I'm seeing." She quickly added, "I'm going to call Dr. Pipkin."

Those dark thoughts came screaming back, the bruise, the gym, the exhaustion climbing down the hill. Richie had been worried and now he saw that his mom was worried too. It wasn't his imagination, his fear confirmed, his stomach knotted up. He felt nauseous. Richie closed his eyes and slowed his breathing, trying to control his frantic mind. He was anxious as he watched his mom pick up the phone.

She dialed the number of Richie's pediatrician and got the bot, of course. She punched in the appropriate responses to the voice prompts and listened to the pleasantly voiced robot report that her message would be delivered to the on-call physician.

They sat down to eat something while they waited for the callback. Neither seemed hungry. They pushed the food around the plate mostly avoiding their mouths, and barely speaking. After about 45 minutes, Betty's phone played the Chopin ring chime. She saw the service number on the screen and answered. It was Dr. Chang, covering for Dr. Pipkin, as the after-hours doctor.

Richie could only hear Betty's side of the call. He heard her describe the symptoms, the tiredness, the two bruises. She offered that she was usually pretty cavalier about this stuff, but this seemed different.

"No," she responded, "he hasn't vomited, he's been alert, he has been able to eat and drink, some, not his usual all you can eat meals, most definitely a change. No headache or dizziness. He's not feeling faint." Betty looked at Richie and told the doctor that "he was peeing normally." Richie nodded in verification. Betty said she had touched his forehead, and he didn't feel feverish, though she hadn't dug out the digital thermometer that usually hid in the bathroom medicine cabinet. She said "OK" and the call ended.

"What did Dr. Chang say? Did she seem worried?

"Well, she said there's an early summer virus going around and that might be what you have. But she'll let Dr. Pipkin know in the morning, and he'll follow up, that's all."

They both relaxed after not getting the order to march into the ER. Their appetites returned, at least somewhat. After a few minutes of quiet eating, Betty looked up again, this time with a little twinkle and a grin, she asked, "so, what's this about a girl? Mr. Valentino."

"Ah, Mom, I dunno, she's really cute, and I like her. I also know for sure she likes me too. She has red hair and she just moved here with her dad. We connected, you know. I'm not sure how to explain it, but we could be quiet together, not saying anything, and we're communicating. There's something we share, I feel it, but it's hard to explain."

"Wow," said mom, "in about ten seconds, you strung six sentences in a row about her. That's about the most I've ever heard you say about anyone. Well, well. What's this redhead girl's name?"

"Nancy, she's really nice, I'm pretty sure you'd like her," Richie answered.

"Whoa, that's intriguing, are you setting up a meeting with your parent already?" Betty asked.

"Gee, Mom, sorry. No, no meeting yet. I just like her is all."

Betty's tone changed a bit, "Well, I can see that young man. Ahem, you do remember the talks we've had about the female persuasion."

"Aw, gee Mom, really, are you going there?" he responded. "I gotta go upstairs and get to my homework."

"OK, go on up. Make sure you stay hydrated, bring your water flask. And try to get to sleep early, you need your rest young man. First come over and give me a kiss goodnight."

As he climbed the steps, she watched carefully. He was a young man. Oh, he was still her baby, but there were changes. Betty was definitely worried, her spidey-senses were tingling, and it was not about Nancy. No, something wasn't right, and she would not let it rest.

Upstairs, Richie had every intention of getting to his homework as he sat at his desk and signed on to his laptop. But as he stared at his assignment page, all he could think about was the bruising, the fainting and his weakness running down the hill. And of course, Nancy.

After some time he texted Nancy, "I'm thinking about you."

The reply showed up almost immediately, "me too, you're in my head!"

Richie sent an emoji, with a smiley beating heart.

Nancy smiled and sent back two of those.

Richie breathed deeply, looking at his screen, focused on the Google page he'd brought up. He tried to decide if he was ready to share what he had just learned online. Finally he texted, "I'm worried about the bruises."

"I'm sure it's nothing to worry about," she texted back.

"Well, it's not just bruises, there's fainting and weakness too."

There was a pause for a few minutes, and then Richie heard her gasp. "Richie, I just looked at ChatGPT for your symptoms. Have you looked online?"

"I, did," tears fell down his cheeks.

"Fuck! Richie, that can't be what you have."

By the time Dr. Pipkin called at 7 AM, Betty had been up, showered and dressed, ready for the new day. She'd gone in to check on Richie, who had just begun to stir. She gave him the first wake-up notice and closed his door as she answered the doctor's call.

Dr. Pipkin had been Richie's pediatrician since his birth. He'd been there for those late-night ear infections, and all those well checks. There were the early morning calls when Betty wasn't sure if she could just treat the fever at home or if she needed to come to the ER. Betty would struggle with those decisions, hashing it over in her head three or more times before calling the doctor. Dr. Pipkin was always there to provide the guidance she needed.

"How's Richie feeling this morning?" Dr. Pipkin asked.

"Thanks for calling back Dr. Pipkin," Betty answered. "I think he's OK, he's just waking up, so I'm not quite sure yet."

"Dr. Chang signed out to me this morning. She reported your conversation," Dr. Pipkin said. "Dr. Chang didn't think it was an emergency, but she was a bit concerned after hearing your description. Frankly, it has me a bit worried as well. According to her report he's been tired, has a couple of new bruises and his color isn't good. Is that about right?"

"Yes, that's about it, this isn't my Richie." Betty tried to be factual, but she was concerned.

"Well, there is a bug going around, but I don't think that fits with what you're telling me. I would like you to bring him in this morning. Can you do that?" Dr. Pipkin asked.

"Yes, of course, we can be there in about 45 minutes, will that work?"

"Perfect, I'll make sure the office knows to expect you," Dr. Pipkin ended the call.

Betty was still worried, but glad that the doctor had made time for Richie. She called upstairs to make sure Richard was getting ready. While she waited, Betty notified her work and his school that they'd be late. She then went upstairs, to see how Richie was doing. Betty knocked on the bathroom door, "are you nearly ready? Hurry up, we're going to see Dr. Pipkin, now, before school."

The bathroom door sprung open immediately in response to that news. He had a towel draped around his waist and a toothbrush dangling from his mouth.

"Ah, Mom, really, is that necessary? I've got stuff to do at school," and he garbled something that sounded like "Nancy."

Despite the toothbrush in his mouth Betty understood what he was saying.

Betty had a one-word answer, "yes."

They were out of the house 20 minutes later, driving to the pediatrician's office. Betty tried to pay attention to the road. Traffic was particularly awful at this time of day and the drivers were always crazy, but what bothered her most was what might be going on with her son. Betty would always imagine worst-case scenarios. Just thinking of those, not even daring to say them out loud, produced a knot in her stomach. It physically hurt. Not knowing, it ate at her. She tried to convince herself that the awful images in her head were just her, things imagined. Once the doctor saw him, she hoped he would smile at her concerns and declare him fine. But try as hard as she could, those black thoughts wouldn't go away.

Richie had been quiet during the ride. Betty didn't know what he was thinking, and she couldn't bring herself to ask. She was afraid of where that conversation might go.

Just then Richie turned to her, Betty watched him, anxious about what he was about to say. They'd had to manage everything together. Cutting the cord, 17 years ago, hadn't separated them. But she couldn't read his thoughts. She held her breath as he turned to speak.

"Mom," Richie began, "I know you're worried, and I can't say you shouldn't be, but we we'll get through this, we always have, and we always will." And then, those rarely spoken words, "I love you, Mom." And he reached over to lay his hand on hers.

Betty smiled, "I love you too, baby." His words had calmed her some. Betty could scarcely recognize how grown up he'd become. The anxiety eased a bit, the worries were still there, but Mom now had confidence that together, they could face whatever lay ahead.

6.

Soon they were pulling into the pediatric office lot. It was full and Betty tried to calculate how long they might need to wait. Sure enough, as they got inside, it was packed with people, mostly moms and their kids, and one or two dads. The kids seemed healthy, active and noisy.

Betty walked over to the counter to let the receptionist know that they'd arrived.

She went through the standard questions. Date of birth, insurance, any address or phone number changes. No allergies, no recent fevers, cough, chills, vomiting or exposure to known illnesses. When they were done with the formalities, the receptionist asked them to have a seat. The nurse would soon be out for them.

Betty didn't know what *soon* meant and the wait began.

Sooner than expected the nurse came out and called for "Richard Samuelson." They stood up, and followed her. Betty wondered if there was some sort of triage system, and the shorter waiting time was a measure of Dr. Pipkin's concern. She was able to find the downside of being called quickly.

The nurse pointed to one of the rooms, "Please go into room 3, the doctor will be with you shortly."

Within a few minutes, Dr. Pipkin knocked. Without waiting for a response, he opened the door and entered.

Dr. Pipkin looked older, it had been a while since Richie had been to see him. Betty thought that it was probably the stress of his job that aged him faster. He was as tall as Richie, thin, but not too thin. It looked like he kept in shape, not bulky muscle but sinewy. He had thinning white hair with a small round bald spot on top. Dr. Pipkin wore the long white clinic coat typical of doctors of his generation. He had a bow tie, the kind he had to knot himself. As required, it had an image of Snoopy. The bow tie was out of reach for the very young curious hands, and it carried less germs than those long dangly ones. One might imagine him stepping out of a Norman Rockwell painting, the one with the child about to receive a vaccine. Dr. Pipkin wore old-fashioned steel-rimmed spectacles, with round frames and hooked temples that snuggled around his ears. He pulled his glasses forward looking over the top when he spoke.

"We've talked a bit on the phone," Dr. Pipkin started, "is there anything new to add from this morning?"

"Well," Richie began after a slight hesitation and a glance at his mom, "yesterday, after school, when I saw the school bus waiting, I started running to catch it, and, well you know I'm on the track team and all, but after taking just a few steps I felt winded, and that worried me."

Betty looked at Richie, he hadn't mentioned that.

"OK, anything else?" the doctor asked.

"Uh, yes," he looked down at his feet, he knew his mom would be upset. "I was on the treadmill at school, and I guess I fainted."

"What! You never said. Richard Samuelson, how could you not tell me that?"

"Sorry, I was going to."

Dr. Pipkin looked at them both. He paused. "Is that all?"

Betty watched and waited to hear what else he might not have said. She was annoyed.

"No, that's all. I guess I'm worried."

"Any pain or aches in your arms, hips or legs?"

"Now that you mention it, I guess, yeah, I feel something in my hips and legs. It's sort of a dull ache."

Betty looked at him again, apparently there were things that he'd been hiding.

"I see," said the doctor. "In medicine, when investigating a set of symptoms, we have what's called a *differential*, a list of the usual suspect diseases that fit the symptoms. We must winnow the list down to come up with the correct diagnosis." Dr. Pipkin, as a doctor, was also a teacher. He believed that the more his families understood, the easier it was to work with them. He preferred a parent asking lots of questions to one who just sat there, showing little interest. "So," Dr. Pipkin continued, "I will do a complete physical exam, head to toe and everything in between. I'll then have the medical assistant come in and draw some blood samples. Any questions?"

Betty asked, "When will you have the results?"

Dr. Pipkin answered, "Later today. The test orders will be sent *stat* and I'll call you when they're ready."

The doctor continued, "OK, Richie, you stay here, and Mom will go out to the waiting room. You'll take off your clothes, there's a bag for them, and then put on the gown laid out on the exam bed. I'll be back in a few minutes."

Dr. Pipkin and Betty left the room together, as the door closed, Betty briefly glanced back, then turned and made her way to the waiting area. She couldn't help noticing the creeping, disquieting feeling that was growing inside her.

When Dr. Pipkin came back into room 3, Richie was ready, sitting on the exam bed. "Richie, what's bothering you the most?" the doctor asked.

"Well, I'm OK, just a bit tired is all, I don't feel as strong as I usually do," he replied.

"For people your age, I always ask a few more questions after the parent leaves the room. That gives you an opportunity to say anything to me that you might be reluctant to say in front of your mom. Your answers are completely confidential, except if you tell me that you're thinking about hurting yourself, or someone else. Otherwise, it stays between you and me." Dr. Pipkin was looking for any new clues, and Richie's state of mind.

"Tell me about your mood. How are you feeling? Have you been sad?" Dr. Pipkin was probing, he needed to know what Richie was thinking.

"Well, I'm worried. I know there's something wrong. I don't feel depressed or that I would hurt myself."

"You said you know something's wrong, what do you think it is?" Dr. Pipkin asked. He was sure Richie had ideas, no doubt he had gone online to search his symptoms. Keeping his thoughts hidden would not be good, not now and not for what Dr. Pipkin thought he would need in the coming months.

"Like, well, I have these bruises. I can't even run normally, I got short of breath. There's Google and I have done some reading, you know. There's so much stuff online, but I'm pretty good at sorting out what's just crap. Oh, sorry."

Dr. Pipkin said, "it's OK, go on."

"So," Richie continued, "I guess, one of the things that came up, one that scared me, is that I could have leukemia. It seems to fit, I think." Richie's voice was quiet, and the worry was evident.

Dr. Pipkin, who was standing in front of Richie, pulled up a chair and sat down.

"Richie," he began, "right now I don't know what you have, we should know more after the blood results are back. Leukemia is very rare in youngsters, but some of your symptoms, the bruising, and the pallor, the bony aches, make me concerned about that, at least it would be part of the *differential*. Listen to me Richie, this is very important, if it is leukemia, it can be treated. It's important to keep that in mind."

"Yes," he replied, "is that really true?"

"Absolutely. Richie, if it's OK with you, when your mom comes back after I examine you, I'd like to share what we've talked about with her. Would that be OK?"

"Yes, I want her to know. I think she may be worried and is afraid to say anything. My mom can be a little superstitious, you know, if she says it out loud, it might make it true."

"Good, I'm going to start the exam now. I will start at the top and work down to the feet, and everything in between, do you understand?"

"I'm ready."

Dr. Pipkin would do a standard physical exam, but he would be paying special attention to several areas, the eyes, lymph nodes, his skin, abdomen and the genital region.

He began with the head exam, looking carefully and feeling around the scalp. He searched for any enlarged lymph nodes around the neck, behind the ears and in the triangles above the clavicles. He pushed deeply into the axillae, the upper arms, the groin and behind the knees. He was exploring areas where abnormal lymph nodes might be hiding. He carefully examined the eyes. Pulling down the lower lids, he looked for pale conjunctivae. He darkened the room, to encourage his pupils to dilate. Using the ophthalmoscope, he could see the retina and the optic disk at the back of the eye. The disk was the beginning of the optic nerve that carried visual information to the brain, it was in fact the only part of the brain that could be seen without a knife. Any swelling of the optic disk or change in the retinal blood vessels could be ominous. Dr. Pipkin examined the tongue, and the back of his mouth including the uvula and tonsils. He rested his open hand on Richie's back and tapped against it with the other, carefully listening to the sounds as he percussed first his back and then his chest. He would hear an abnormal sound if there was anything lurking inside. He took the stethoscope from around his neck and listened to his heart and lungs. After finishing, he draped the stethoscope back around his neck, and asked Richie to lie down on the exam table with his knees drawn up. He pushed on his abdomen searching for evidence of an enlarged liver or spleen. He carefully examined his skin, looking at the bruises and for any rashes. Lastly, he asked Richie to stand up. Dr. Pipkin put on exam gloves, telling Richie that he was going to exam his testicles.

Richie nodded, "I'm ready."

With that the doctor completed his physical examination.

"OK, that's finished. I'll leave you to get dressed. The medical assistant will come in and draw the blood samples I've ordered. There will be a few tubes. After that, we'll get your mom back in, spend a few more minutes and then you'll be off, until I call later." With that Dr. Pipkin left the room.

Richie quickly got dressed, the M.A. came in and drew the labs, and Richie got a nice pedi band-aid, with an image of Mickey on it. He was feeling a bit better. Just having the discussion with Dr. Pipkin and talking about what was on his mind had helped. A few minutes later, Betty was back in the room.

"Dr. Pipkin, said he would be here in a few minutes and then we can go," Richie said.

They sat and waited. Both were quiet with their thoughts.

Soon, Dr. Pipkin was back. "I want to tell you about Richie's exam. There was some good news, but I also have some concerns. I carefully looked for but did not find any enlarged lymph nodes. His liver and spleen were not enlarged, and a careful examination of his testicles did not reveal any enlargement or hardening. His eye exam, except for a bit of pallor, was also OK. That's all the good stuff. The concerns I had was finding that his heart was beating fast, and it was loud. I could feel his heart working hard when I touched his chest. That's likely because he's anemic. He has a subtle rash, composed of tiny red dots. Those are *petechiae* and appear when the platelet count is very low. The dots are caused by small leaks of blood from the capillaries into the outer layers of skin. The likely anemia and the rash from a low platelet count imply that at least two elements of his blood are not normal."

Dr. Pipkin went on, "Richie and I had a short talk after you left and before the exam. I typically try to do that with all adolescents, but today I had a particular goal with Richie. These talks are typically confidential, but Richie gave me permission to speak with you about what we discussed."

"OK, Dr. Pipkin." Betty was quiet, she glanced at Richie and waited.

"Richie has been worried. He feels there's something wrong. He also knows that you've been worried too. He has been online, of course, and he's done some digging. Based on this, he's concerned that he might have leukemia. He thinks that you may be worried about the same thing, but you two haven't broached the subject with each other. In my experience, most of the time that people search for medical information on the internet, they come up with a lot of nonsense. But in this case, I share Richie's concern. We'll know more in a few hours when the blood test results are back. I want to be very clear, if it does turn out that he has leukemia, there are options for treatment. The reason I'm telling you this now, going into some detail, is because I know that you are *both* thinking about this, but you've been afraid to talk to each other about it. The concern is out now. Go home and talk to each other. You're not protecting each other by avoiding the subject."

Dr. Pipkin had one more thing to add. "I've been in practice, caring for children for more than 30 years. In all that time, I've had only one young child diagnosed with that disease, it is so rare in kids. I've had a lot of time since then to think about what I would have said differently if I ever had another child with that concern. And so I add now that there is hope." Dr. Pipkin was finished.

7.

Betty and Richie left the office, they'd not yet spoken. As they headed away from Dr. Pipkin's office, Betty turned toward Richie, "let's go to Sally's Diner, we can sit in one of the booths, it will be private, and we can get some breakfast, OK with you?"

Richie responded, "Ya know Mom, I am kind of hungry, first time in a few days, I think I'll order some pancakes."

Betty smiled at that, "me too, I'm hungry, and I need some coffee." Betty felt a little better hearing that Richie was hungry.

Sally's Diner was one of those old-fashioned diners built to look like a railroad car, shiny, silvery and ribbed on the outside. Inside, booths lined the walls, across the aisle counter tops were surrounded by round barstools. There were big old coffee urns sitting in the back (regular and decaf), near the cook's window. You could see the check orders hanging at the window, and watch him back there working the flat top. There were plenty of empty seats at this hour and the waitress behind the counter shouted out, "sit anywhere you want," so they did.

She soon sauntered over, "I'm Mildred, I'll be serving you, can I get you anything right away?"

Betty said, "I'll need a few minutes, but can I get a black coffee, and some ice water to start. Richie?"

"I'd like a small glass of fresh squeezed orange juice, and a cup of about two thirds milk and one third coffee. Could I also have a stack of pancakes, please?"

Betty's eyebrows rose, "that's quite a brew you've concocted. I'm worried that you might still taste the coffee, Richie. Maybe you need a little more milk in your cup?" Betty smiled, and then turned to Mildred, "I guess I'm ready, two eggs, easy over, some hash browns and whole wheat toast, oh, please don't butter the toast. Thanks."

Mildred had the orders, "be back with the drinks in a minute." and she hustled behind the counter to put in the orders and get the beverages ready. Still, Betty and Richie hadn't said anything about the doctor's visit, but that changed as soon as the drinks arrived.

"Mom," Richie started, "we can say anything to each other, right? I think Dr. Pipkin thought it would be better if we talk."

"Of course, Richie, you can say anything at all."

"Yes, I know, Mom, but you can say anything to me too, I'm not a kid anymore and I know there's something wrong." Richie wanted to hear what his mom was thinking. He had to be able to trust that his mom wouldn't hold secrets. "I need you to tell me what you're thinking."

"OK, I am sick with worry about you, Dr. Pipkin seemed very concerned too."

"Mom, he said *leukemia.*" replied Richie. "He was concerned it might be leukemia, you haven't even said that word," he fidgeted a bit on the bench, "and I'm scared, really scared."

Betty looked at him again, he was right. Richie needed her to be honest and open. She needed to say what she was thinking. Her son wasn't a child, and any attempt to hide what she was feeling could put up a wall and shut down any conversation before it began. Betty took a deep breath, "OK, honey, you're right, I'm scared too, but we will get through this, I promise."

"I hope the treatments will work. I've read about the shit they give you and I'm worried about how those medications will make me feel. It could be awful. I know I'll be sick." Richie said. He paused and looked at her, "Mom, I worry about you too, all you've got to do, and what will happen to you if the treatments don't work?"

For the first time since this all started, tears rolled down Betty's face, and a few barely stifled sobs emerged. "Oh, my Richard, you are quite the young man. You are my life, and we will get through this together.

But Richie, we don't know what it is yet. We've got to wait for the test results. Whatever it is, we'll take care of it. OK?" Betty got up, walked around the table, and sat down next to Richie. They hugged and cried together.

"I need you, Mom," Richie said, wiping his eyes. They sat quietly, holding on.

After a little while, Mildred was back, carrying the food.

Betty leaned over, kissed Richie, gave him one more squeeze and then went back to her side of the table, "time to eat."

After everything that happened, they were hungry and for the first time in a couple of days, able to enjoy their food. Within fifteen minutes both plates were empty. Mildred came over, "Looks like everything was good, it's all gone. Anything else I can get you now?"

"No," Betty said, "just the check when you get a chance." Mildred cleared the table.

"What should we do now? Anything you want Richie."

"Well, I'd like to go to school, I think I may have just missed a couple of periods, and I can make up what I've missed. Is that OK with you?" Richie could often be surprising.

"Sure, I guess, I could go to work for a few hours. I'll take you to school and sign your late excuse." Betty paid the check, and they were soon driving over to Horace Mann.

In the office, Betty told the secretary that Richie was late because of an urgent doctor's visit. The secretary told Richie that the third period would be starting soon and if he hurried, he could make the start of his French class. Richie started down the hall. Betty watched him for a minute and then she left for work.

As Richie approached the classroom, his head was a mess. He couldn't shake all that just happened at his visit with Dr. Pipkin, but he also wanted to see Nancy. Nancy and Dr. Pipkin, how could something so wonderful and so awful be happening at the same time? His brain swirled with conflicting emotions. With a deep breath and a brief hesitation he opened the classroom door and stepped inside. He quickly spotted the only girl with red hair. He smiled at her, and she smiled back. Their desks were catty corner, just a row apart. As he sat down, she whispered his name. When he turned toward her, she reached out to pass a pink folded paper. He reached for it. Their fingers touched, and lingered a moment.

The note had no words. Nancy had drawn a heart. He looked back at her. Richie took pen to paper and in a minute or two, snuck the refolded paper back to her. Nancy opened it and saw the second heart that Richie had drawn next to hers. Each heart now had a pair of arms, and they were holding hands. Nancy looked up at him. She giggled. Nancy scribbled again. Richie watched her write. This time there were words: "Meet me after school, same place, XOXOXO." Richie smiled back and mouthed "yes" to her. He could feel his heart flutter, but it wasn't because there was anything wrong with him, no, this was Nancy's fault.

The rest of the day's classes took like forever, but finally it was 2:30 and the last period was over. His thoughts were jumbled. He wanted to hold her, to feel her lips against his, to chase away those dark visions. Richie made his way up to the track. They had chosen a secluded area that didn't see much traffic, and as he got to the rendezvous spot, he was happy, again, they'd be alone.

She stood at the top of the rise. As Richie approached, she turned toward him, her red hair was down around her shoulders. He hadn't noticed that before, she must have let it down while she waited for him. Richie thought she was beautiful. There was a pleasant New England breeze that played with her hair. She brought her hand up and gently pulled a few strands away from her eyes and pushed them back behind her right ear. She smiled at him. And then he was there, face to face, for a few seconds they just looked at each other. They embraced, holding each other tightly. They pulled away just a bit, looking at each other longingly, and then their lips met. Softly at first, then a bit harder, their mouths open and tongues exploring. They leaned against each other.

"Ooh, Richie," she murmured, her lips touching his ear "I can tell that you like this, it's like that with me too." Still holding close, arms wrapped around each other.

"My head is spinning," he answered. I need to sit down."

They walked over to the nearby bench, hand in hand. It was a beautiful May day, the flowers were blooming, the bees were busy, and a lovely floral scent wafted through the New England air. They sat down as close together as they possibly could. She tilted her head, resting against his shoulder. After a few quiet minutes, she picked her head up and looked at Richie.

"You can touch me," she said. Richie didn't move, he just looked at her. Nancy reached for his hand and guided it to her breast. His hand gently embraced her, softly caressing where she had directed him.

"Ooh, that's nice, just like that," she whispered. Nancy let her hand drop down, for a moment resting along the inside of his knee. And then, slowly, she began to bring her hand up higher on his leg. Richie held his breath. She looked up at him, eyes locked on each other. They were alone in the universe.

Richie's heart raced, his head was on fire.

But even with all those wondrous feelings, darker thoughts tugged at him. He removed her hand, and slowly disentangled himself from Nancy. Richie stood up in front of her, looking down at her. His face torn with mixed emotions.

"What's wrong Richie? Is it something I did?" She looked at him.

"No, you didn't do anything wrong. I think you're perfect. He sat down again, slowly. "There's something wrong with me. I can feel it. I saw my doctor this morning and he was concerned too. Dr. Pipkin took some blood samples. I should know something soon. I expect he'll be calling my mom any minute."

"Richie, what are you telling me?"

"Maybe it's nothing, I hope that's what it turns out to be, but I have a bad feeling about this," he said. He looked down, shaking his head slowly. Then he picked up her hand and looked into her eyes, "Nancy, I'm really scared." Richie was very quiet. He had to look away. Before it had been easy, but suddenly it was different. When he looked at her, he saw fear looking back at him.

"Richie, say it, what's going on?" She reached out to him, trying to bring him close again, but something had changed.

He sighed and was quiet. Neither spoke.

Richie's phone rang, he looked down at the screen, "it's my mom," he said, "I've got to answer." He listened for a few minutes.

"Nancy, I'm sorry, my mom is coming to get me. She said Dr. Pipkin wants me to come back right now." Richie suddenly felt weak and unsteady.

Nancy said, "come on. Richie, I'll walk down the hill with you."

Together, they walked down to the school parking lot. As they approached Richie saw their green Subaru Forester with his mom inside.

Betty opened her door, got out and stood there, watching her son and a girl walking toward her.

"You must be Nancy," Betty said. "It's very nice to meet you, Richie told me that he has a new friend."

"Hi, Ms. Samuelson, very nice to meet you too," said Nancy. "Um, Richie told me that he needs to see Dr. Pipkin now. The way Richie talked about it, well, I can see that he's worried."

"Nancy," Betty began, she hesitated, and seemed unsure of what to say to Richie's new friend. Finally all she said was that "we really have to go now." Betty got back in the car and sat down behind the wheel.

Nancy looked at Richie, she walked with him a few more steps to the front passenger door. He stopped for a second, Nancy squeezed his hand, she got up on tiptoes and kissed him on the cheek, "call me when you can, any time, I'll be thinking of you," she said. With that Richie got in the car, put his seat belt on, and they were off.

8.

In the car, Betty looked at Richie, another time, there most certainly would have been a conversation about his new friend, but right now, she had other concerns. For a few minutes there was silence in the car.

Richie started, “Mom, first off, I like her, OK?”

Mom said, “OK.”

Richie continued, “I guess we can talk about her another time, right now, can you please tell me what Dr. Pipkin said?”

“He just said, come down to the office, he’ll discuss the results.”

“Oh,” Richie, paused, “I’m thinking that if everything was fine, he would have just said that over the phone.”

Mom looked at him, “Well, we’ll soon find out,” as they pulled into the doctor’s parking lot. “Dr. Pipkin told me that we’d be his last visit of the day.”

As they entered the office, the waiting room was empty. Jean, the receptionist stood up, and said the doctor would be with them shortly. She led them into the patient conference room. It was a quiet room. The walls were painted with muted colors. There were several oil paintings on the walls, picturesque landscapes, and water scenes, meant to be calming. There were three chairs in the room, nicer than the ones out in the waiting room. Betty noted that there were open tissue boxes on the small round side tables. They sat down and waited only a few minutes before Dr. Pipkin opened the door. Betty and Richie reflexively stood up, but Dr. Pipkin motioned for them to sit. He had a folder in one hand, and he wasn't smiling. Dr. Pipkin sat down in the third chair, facing them.

Betty looked at her son, she reached over to take his hand. She nodded at Richie, and he responded.

"We're ready, Dr. Pipkin," said Betty.

"I am sorry to say that it's not good news," Dr. Pipkin began, "the results of Richie's blood tests are consistent with leukemia." The doctor paused, he waited for it to sink in, he watched them carefully before going on.

Betty had known deep down that the doctor would say that word, even so, the confirmation, hearing it out loud from his lips, cut into her like a dagger plunging into her heart. Her world instantly collapsed. All she loved was now in danger. Betty clutched at her chest, a huge weight crushing her. She tried to breathe, but it hurt. Her vision went dark. Nothing made sense. It wasn't real, she thought, a bad dream and she would wake up. Tears rolled down her cheeks, the blood drained from her face. She felt weak and shaky. Leaning forward, she tried to catch her breath.

A guttural, primitive groan erupted from somewhere deep inside her, "Oh, Richie," was all she could say.

Richie was assaulted on both sides. That word he feared, but knew would come. A tsunami of bad news, crashed over him, knocking him down. If there had been any hope, it was rapidly extinguished. And then his mother, the sight of her clutching her chest and that groan. That groan, he had never heard anything like that. Like a bad movie. He felt his guts tighten and that acidy, nasty reflux flow up and catch in his mouth. Richie fell to his knees, trying to get a grip. Nothing had prepared him for this moment.

He crawled on his knees over to his mom and held her. For a while, there were no words, only raw emotion.

"It's OK," he said. Richie took a deep breath, very softly but deliberately he said, "we will get through this, I am going to be OK. Mom, look at me, I am going to be OK."

Betty nodded back. She could find no words.

Richie stood up and handed her the box of tissues. He took one for himself. He looked at his mom again, and then at Dr. Pipkin, he took a deep breath. "We're ready to hear the rest," Richie was talking to his doctor, but he was looking at his mom, "right, Mom?" He pulled his chair closer to his mom and they were both seated again.

Dr. Pipkin continued, "I know this is hard. Leukemia is very rare in young people. While most people know adults with cancer, few people know children with that disease. Much of what I'm going to say, you will not remember, but you'll hear it again from the other doctors. If you remember nothing else, remember this, leukemia, especially in young people is treatable and there is every expectation that your disease will respond to therapy."

Dr. Pipkin waited, he saw them nod. He went on, "Your white blood cell count was 43,000, that's very high, it should be no more than about 8,000. Those white blood cells are his leukemia. They are immature, malignant cells, called blasts. They do nothing but grow and divide. They're no longer providing the normal functions of your immune system, so you're at risk for infection. The cells have taken over the bone marrow space and crowded out normal blood cell production. That's why your red blood cell and platelet counts are so low."

There would be much more information, but not right now.

Silence for some moments.

Betty found her voice, "what do we do now?" she asked.

"Memorial Medical Center has an excellent pediatric oncology program," the doctor answered. "Richie is at that in-between age when he could go to an adult program or to a pediatric cancer program. I strongly recommend that he's treated in a pediatric program. It turns out that people like Richie have better outcomes when they're treated by pediatric oncologists. His care will be guided by a protocol, a thoroughly studied, step by step recipe for treating his leukemia." He paused and continued, "I've already talked to the doctor there, Dr. Stanner, and he will have a team ready, they are expecting Richie tonight."

"Tonight?" Betty was not ready for that. "Can't we go home? We can be ready to go in the morning."

"I believe you should go now," Dr. Pipkin was very firm in his recommendation. "It's about a 35-minute ride to the university medical center. There are some things that should be done for Richie tonight, and they'll be preparing for more testing in the morning. The sooner this gets done, the sooner treatment can start, and that's very important. They'll provide what you need for the night. Tomorrow, Betty can go home and get anything else that might be needed." Dr. Pipkin left little room to argue the plan.

Richie looked at his mom. He was scared. Richie had read a bit about leukemia, but there was so much he didn't know. Was there really hope, or was Dr. Pipkin just feeding him some bullshit to keep him calm? Hospitals in all the movies he had ever seen were always bad news. He would try to be strong enough for the two of them.

"Let's go do this, Mom, I want to start. I really don't want to be laying in my bed at home thinking about this."

Betty looked at Richie, she was worried, but she also saw someone who had recently been a young boy and who was growing up fast, very fast, "OK, Richie, let's go," she said.

9.

They were deep into their usual sign-out as the day doctor reported everything that the oncoming doctor would need during his overnight shift to manage the children on the pediatric oncology unit. Dr. Sandra Gardner, the day doctor this week and Dr. Paul Belkin, soon to be taking coverage for the night, were the two first-year pediatric fellows at Memorial Medical Center. They were in training to become attending physicians in pediatric cancer therapy. Now, halfway through May, they were nearly done with the first of three years of their fellowship program.

Sandra had grown up on a cattle farm in the rural mid-West. She was a typical middle child with two older brothers, an older sister and two younger sisters. By the time Sandra was born, her mom and dad were experienced parents, so although there were lots of pictures of the first two sons and the older sister, well, search as she might, there weren't so many of young Sandra. The novelty of babies had apparently worn off. Whenever Sandra looked through the family picture albums, she was reminded of that oversight. She was determined to make sure that would not happen when she someday had her own family.

Early on, Sandra had definite plans about how her family would be different. But it wasn't until she had been hospitalized as a young girl that the idea of becoming a doctor began to take shape in her head. She'd come down with infectious mononucleosis. It was going around in her middle school. Most of the kids just had a bit of a fever and didn't feel well for a few days. But Sandra turned a golden yellow, her liver was inflamed, and her blood counts were very abnormal. For a few days, the doctors thought she might have leukemia, but then her viral tests came back positive for the Epstein Barr Virus, and they knew she had mono. She remained in the hospital for a week, until her color started to return to normal, her liver had calmed down, and she could eat and drink without puking. Spending time in the pediatric department with all those who helped her made a lasting impression. She knew each person by name and would cheerfully greet them, the nurses, the child life specialists, the physical therapist, the medical aides, the staff who brought her meals (kind of yucky food, and always cold) and the doctors. She chatted up the doctors whenever they stopped long enough to listen. As she thought of them, she came to see her future self as a pediatrician.

Paul had a very different start. A city boy, he had one younger brother. Both parents were doctors, his father's father was a doctor and there were several more doctors among the close relatives. When he was four years old, he already had a doctor play kit and was caring for his toy bear. Within a few weeks he graduated to making sure that his baby brother was OK. As far back as Paul could remember, he was planning to be a doctor. His interest in pediatric oncology would come later, after a particularly poignant case his group managed during his third year of medical school. He was the junior member of a team that diagnosed a young girl with a brain tumor. As a student, he didn't have a direct role in the care of Mary, but he remembered her. The diagnosis had come after the neuroradiologist reviewed Mary's brain MRI. She was soon transferred to a pediatric neuro-oncology unit at another center. He continued to follow her even after she was no longer one of their patients. She underwent surgery, had radiation to her tumor bed and later endured several cycles of chemotherapy. Unfortunately, she didn't make it. Six months later he learned that she had passed. The tumor had grown back. Paul still had memories of when he first met her, when she was still smiling and playful. He remembered her parents. The way they looked at her was heart-wrenching. He could picture her mother. Her look was etched in his mind. It had been a mix of love, hope and angst, all at once. Paul could not shake that indelible image. Brain tumors continued to stubbornly resist effective treatment. It was the saddest diagnosis in pediatric oncology.

There they were together, Drs. Gardner and Belkin, two very different beginnings, now traveling along the same path. Their shared experiences over the last 10 months had knit them together, creating a bond that would last a lifetime. It was hard to explain this to anyone who'd never been on that road. Words were inadequate to convey what they'd been through, and they had stopped trying to explain it to others. When people found out what they did, their usual response, was "pediatric oncology, oh that must be so sad." But Sandra and Paul knew that although there were still some very sad cases like Mary's, many children did well, and it was a rewarding profession, like no other.

In six weeks, a new pair of graduating pediatric residents would take over as the newbie fellows. For Paul and Sandra, much of the following two years in the program would involve research in one of the medical laboratories. While they would still have intermittent coverage of inpatient children, most of that would be handled by the new incoming fellows and their attending physicians.

It would be a big change. In preparation for the next two years, they had started to visit various labs and met with the Ph.D. laboratory directors. Sandra was considering a month of research in gene therapy in Dr. Benzi's lab across the country. She had tried to interest Paul, but so far he hadn't been ready to commit. As part of a research laboratory team, their colleagues would be doctoral students completing their projects and then authoring a thesis to defend their work. Both Drs. Gardner and Belkin had a good idea of the demands their research would require during the next two years. They were prepared for long hours in the lab, and for even more time drafting their papers. But after graduating, they were determined to pursue a career in clinical medicine, caring for children. They did not want to work to become physicians and then be cooped up in a laboratory.

Now in the middle of May, they rarely had to call the attending physician to discuss any of the medical complexities their patients faced. They had managed treatments for children with leukemia and lymphoma, solid tumors of the organs, such as neuroblastoma and Wilms tumor, bone cancers and brain tumors and their consequent complications.

Sandra and Paul would usually conduct their sign-outs at Pat's Tavern, two blocks from the center. They sat at their usual table in an isolated dark corner, where their conversation would be private. In the late afternoon, the tavern wasn't busy. And while reporting on the children, they would often enjoy a bowl of moderately hot Buffalo wings and a pitcher of Coke. They always carried their cell phones. If anything came up at the hospital, the operator would find them. Calls might come from any source: the ER, a nurse or resident taking care of the floor patients, a parent of one of the children at home, or the attending physician. All the important numbers were on speed-dial: the pediatric oncology floor, the labs, the radiology department, the pathology department, the admitting nurse, the pharmacy, the resident call rooms and of course their attending physician.

Sandra was mostly finished reporting on the children currently in the unit and what possible complications Paul might have to manage when her phone rang.

She picked it up and saw the screen indicating the attending was calling. "Hi, Dr. Stanner, it's Sandra, what can I do you for?" Sandra listened for just a minute. "OK, I understand that you want to tell me about a new patient coming in tonight, let me hand you over to Paul, he's right here and he'll be taking over soon." Sandra slid the phone over to Paul.

Paul picked up the phone, plugged in his wired earbuds, handed one to Sandra and positioned the other earbud in his own ear. "Hello, Dr. Stanner, what have you got for me?"

Dr. Stanner spoke, "the referring doctor is Dr. Pipkin, and he's sending in a 17-year-old male, Richard Samuelson, with a probable diagnosis of leukemia. The patient has bruises, oral and skin petechiae and he's quite pale. The doctor faxed over lab reports from a blood sample drawn this morning. All three cell lines are abnormal, he had a white cell count of 43,000, hemoglobin was 7 gm/dL, his platelet count was 17,000. The Coulter counter differential listed 90% blasts. The chemistry panel looked OK. Dr. Pipkin said he confirmed the blast count with the lab tech who had reviewed the slide. The doctor told me that despite all of this, he doesn't appear ill. He will be arriving soon with his mother. I've already spoken with the charge nurse, and they're ready for him. They also have all the faxed lab reports."

Dr. Stanner paused, "any questions?"

Paul answered, "OK, I got it. I'll tuck him in for the night and make sure that he's ready for tomorrow. I presume that you want him NPO after midnight so that he can undergo a bone marrow exam in the morning. Is there anything else?" Paul asked.

Dr. Stanner replied, "That's good." Dr. Stanner reviewed the standard admission procedure which Paul and Sandra knew very well by this time of the year.

Sandra spoke up, "Dr. Stanner, you'll see me tomorrow. I'll walk over to the unit with Paul before I go home for the night, so they'll have met me before tomorrow."

"Great idea, Sandra, I'll be in early to go over things before the bone marrow exam," Dr. Stanner paused for a moment, when there were no further comments, he said, "Goodnight."

Sandra looked at Paul, "Sorry, I guess you'll have a bit of work tonight."

"It's fine, Sandra," Paul answered, "we don't get new diagnoses that often and there's still a lot to learn. Should we go over?" Paul was already gathering his notes, his phone, and stood up to go.

"I'm coming," said Sandra, "split the bill?"

"I'll pay the bill this time, can you take care of the tip? Next time it's yours," Paul finished, and they were out the door just as the tavern was starting to get busy. They were a 5-minute walk from the medical center. The night was warm, stars filled the sky, and the short walk exercise was welcome.

10.

As Paul and Sandra arrived on the pediatric oncology floor, they saw that the patient exam room was occupied. Inquiring at the nurses' station, they learned that the new patient was already being seen by his nurse. The contact information and health insurance documents as well as the faxed lab reports were all now part of his newly created medical chart.

Sandra knocked on the exam door, and opened it, Paul was by her side. Using her doctor's eyes, she saw a scared looking adolescent with a fretful young mom. They sat close together, holding hands, looking lost. And indeed, as Dr. Stanner had mentioned, despite the diagnosis, and looking pale, he appeared otherwise well. She could imagine that those around him would never have suspected he had leukemia.

"Excuse me," Sandra said. The nurse stopped her intake for the moment, "I just wanted to take a minute to introduce myself and Dr. Belkin, then I'll let your nurse finish. I'm Dr. Gardner. We are the pediatric oncology fellows that will be helping with Richard's care. I have been here during the day, and I'm set to leave now but you'll see me again in the morning. Dr. Belkin will be with you tonight. Sorry for the interruption, when the nurse is finished, Dr. Belkin will come in." Sandra finished, backed out and closed the door.

"OK," Paul said, "go home and get some rest."

After Sandra left, Paul went to find the senior pediatric resident who was covering for the night, she would be part of the team caring for the new patient. He found Dr. Carrie Johnson, at the computer workstation in the call room, finishing up her day's notes.

"Hi, Carrie," Paul said. "Do you know anything about Richard Samuelson, the new patient?"

"Just that he's 17 and they think he has leukemia." Carrie answered.

"OK, I have more." Paul went on to give Carrie most of the information he had just learned from Dr. Stanner. "Do you have any questions about that?"

"What's the plan for tonight?"

"After the nurse is finished, I'll go in and meet Richard and his mom, you can come in with me if you have time. I'll do the admitting exam and note, so you don't have to. You should review any medications he's taking and any allergies, but it's better if you don't repeat all the history questions. If there's anything you want to know after reading my note, just ask me later, OK?

For tonight," Paul went on, "he'll need an IV start and blood sampling. Please order a CBC with a manual smear so that the lab will review the cells. Order a basic chemistry profile, liver function tests, calcium, uric acid and phosphorous. Request a type and cross, he will need several blood transfusions tonight, both red cells and platelets. Order flow cytometry to identify the type of leukemia. He'll need imaging, so request a chest X-ray, an ultrasound of his liver, spleen and kidneys and a baseline echocardiogram before he starts chemotherapy. Make him NPO after midnight, nothing to eat or drink. I will arrange for his bone marrow exam in the morning. He'll need sedation, so consult the Pediatric ICU. Ask pediatric surgery to place a percutaneous central line. He will likely be enrolled on a protocol, so extra bone marrow samples will be needed. Multiple consents will need to be signed, which I'll manage. I'll be around, so please call me with any problems, got that?" Paul waited.

Carrie had been scribbling notes, "OK, I think I have everything."

"Please read back what you have," said Paul. Carrie did and she hadn't missed anything.

"His fluids must run slowly, and contain no potassium. Do you know why?" Paul asked, medicine was always didactic, questions were part of the teaching.

"Tumor lysis syndrome. Giving IV fluids can trigger a breakdown of his leukemia cells. When those cells break down, the potassium that had been safely stored inside is released into his blood stream. That increase in potassium can trigger heart arrhythmias or cardiac arrest." Carrie had done her homework.

"Exactly right. There will be many potential dangers tonight and we've got to be vigilant. His renal function has likely been compromised by leukemia cells that have already spread to his kidneys. He'll need help excreting the extra potassium. We'll monitor his blood salts including uric acid, calcium and phosphorous, any one of which can rapidly become abnormal and cause cardiac or neurologic catastrophe. Please order allopurinol, to mitigate the development of high levels of uric acid, which can result in the formation of damaging crystals in his kidneys.

We can talk more about what to do if any of those levels become worrisome." Although Paul could see the reports in the medical record by accessing his iPad mini linked to the hospital intranet, he still asked Carrie to call him ASAP after receiving each of the results, regardless of whether they were marked abnormal or not. Paul was trying to think of anything else he needed to tell Carrie.

Richard's nurse came over to let them know that she was finished.

“OK, thanks, is there anything you found that we should know?” asked Paul.

“Well, it'll all be in my note, but he seems OK. His doctor told them he probably has leukemia, so they know that, but not much else about what's going to happen. He has no allergies, and he's not taking any medications, that's about it. As I said it will all be in my note.” The nurse turned and went back to her seat at the nurses' station.

“OK, Carrie, let's go meet the family,” said Paul. They walked over to the exam room, Paul knocked on the door, and without waiting for a response, he opened it and went in.

11.

Richie was alone with his mom in the exam room, waiting for the doctors. Yesterday seemed so long ago. Overnight he'd been transported into an alien world. Nothing was familiar. People dressed differently and talked differently. The smells were different, there were new rules and he didn't know any of them. Richie was terrified. As he paced the room, he could feel his heart pounding. Taking short deep breathes, he worked to focus on something, anything. A million thoughts raced through his head. Everything around him screamed trouble. He knew he was in deep shit, but he couldn't really tell how bad it was. Richie looked at his mom, seeing her blank stare. How would they manage?

Abruptly there was a knock on the door and without missing a beat, in walked the doctors.

"Hello, remember, I'm Dr. Belkin, the pediatric oncology fellow, and this is Dr. Johnson, she's the senior pediatric resident. Please sit down, I want to talk to you for a few minutes."

The doctor waited while Richie sat next to Betty. "We'll be taking care of you tonight along with the rest of the team. I know this can be overwhelming and scary. I'll try to explain everything that's going to happen. It's a lot to get at once, so ask questions.

Let me start by asking what you are thinking now?"

Richie was too scared to speak. Betty hesitated a moment, but then looking at Richie, she started, "it's like we walked into some bizarre universe," Betty said. "It's surreal and confusing. We were worried before, we knew there was something wrong but we weren't sure what it was. But now that we know, we're ready to fight." Betty had some tissues in her hand just to be ready, but so far, they were dry.

"I know that this is all very difficult," said Dr. Belkin, "after we talk I'll ask mom to step out so that I can examine Richard. I know you've already had a physical exam and blood testing this morning, but we need to have our own exam and blood samples. Some of the testing will repeat what your doctor did, but we'll also order new targeted testing to determine the type of leukemia he has, and what needs to be addressed tonight. A venipuncture team will draw his blood and place an IV tube in his arm.

My job tonight is to make sure Richard is safe. There will be some preliminary testing and imaging to make sure Richard is ready for further investigations tomorrow. I'm going to give you a brief introduction to help you understand what we'll be doing over the next several hours."

Paul continued, "As I said, I'm the fellow, that means I'm in training to become a pediatric oncologist. My first year of clinical training is nearly finished, so I have a bit of experience. You briefly saw Dr. Gardner. She is the other fellow in this year's program at Memorial. Dr. Johnson is the senior pediatric resident, finishing her training in general pediatrics. You'll meet Dr. Stanner tomorrow, he's the attending physician in charge of the team. You'll also meet nurses, social workers, child life specialists, and many others."

"That sounds like a lot of people," said Betty, "I'm beginning to wonder how long we'll be here."

"The entire treatment for Richard's leukemia will take about 3 years, but most of that will be done from home or in the outpatient clinic," said Dr. Belkin. "This first admission," he continued, "will be about four weeks long with the goal of achieving remission of his leukemia. The goal of the rest of the three years is to consolidate that remission, keeping him free of disease for the rest of his life."

"Are you telling me I'll be here for a month?" Richie asked. "I have school and lots of things to do." Richie's thoughts went straight to Nancy. He had only known her a few days but he already felt a connection. She was really the first girl he liked, well it was more than like, wasn't it? And now he was a boy with leukemia. She certainly wouldn't have counted on that. Three years of treatment, caged up in a hospital for a month, why would she stick with him? He would be sick, have no hair, what kind of boyfriend could he be? How could he hope to compete with the normal boys at school? Someone would ask her to the prom and that would be the end of Nancy. There was a dark black cloud for sure. His doctor was speaking, but all he could think about was how his first relationship with a girl was about over before it really had a chance.

"It's hard to say exactly, but that's about right," answered Dr. Belkin. "We have tutors here, who will link up with your teachers and help you complete your school work."

Betty looked at Richie, "It's OK, hon, let's not worry about school now, we'll work it out. Let's focus on getting you better." She smiled and held his hand. "So, Dr. Belkin, what can we expect tonight?"

Paul began, "I'll examine Richard. Then, as I said, an IV tube will be placed, and lab tests drawn. Among those samples will be a complete blood count. From the sample we'll make a microscope slide to review the cells, confirming that it's leukemia. We'll take a blood sample for a type and cross, so that we can match his blood type for compatible red blood cells and platelets. He'll need multiple red cell and platelet transfusions tonight. We'll also check his chemistries several times during the night. Some of his blood salts can become abnormal and we'll need to address those immediately. Dr. Stanner, the attending physician, will talk to you in more detail about that tomorrow. Richard will have a chest x-ray to make sure his heart and lungs are OK. He'll also have an abdominal ultrasound to look at his liver, spleen and kidneys." Paul waited again. He expected more questions.

Richard so far had been quiet, he was trying to take it in, but his mind was elsewhere, consumed with fears about losing Nancy. He counted on his mom to be looking out for him.

"Is that all for now? When will he start treatment?" Betty asked.

"It will be a day or so of preparation before the treatment can begin," he paused again. "There is more I need to tell you. Leukemia is a cancer of the white blood cells, that process starts in his bone marrow, and so in the morning, we'll have to take a sample from his bone marrow."

That got Richie's attention. He'd read about the god awful monster needle that would be jammed into his hip. He imagined the crunching sounds, and the pain from the hole it would make.

"From what I have heard that's an awful test," said Betty, she was upset again.

"It can be," said Dr. Belkin, "but we're much more compassionate in pediatrics than they are in the adult world of oncology. It will be done in our procedure room, and Richard will be sedated during the exam, so he won't feel anything. The sedation will be managed by our attending intensivist, Dr. Street, from the Pediatric Intensive Care Unit, the PICU. Dr. Gardner, who you met a little while ago, along with Dr. Stanner will be here in the morning to perform the procedure. The marrow samples will be used to make a definitive diagnosis of his leukemia and to give us an idea about how much of his marrow has been taken over by those cells. Some of those samples will be analyzed in a way that can be used later to monitor his treatment progress. When it's finished and Richard wakes up, he may be a little sore at the site, but not much different than if he had fallen on his butt."

Richie and Betty seemed to relax. They were grateful again for Dr. Pipkin's advice to be treated at a pediatric oncology unit.

"You need to know a couple of other things, I know this is a lot to take in," continued Paul. "As I mentioned the IV team will place an IV line tonight. That'll serve its purpose for the next day or so, but before he starts therapy, he will need a larger tube, a semi-permanent IV line. The tube will be inserted by a surgeon. The catheter will enter through his chest wall, slip under the clavicle, the collar bone, and will then be threaded into one of the large central blood vessels called the subclavian vein. Using this larger central catheter, Richard will be able to have blood samples taken, and receive chemotherapy, as well as transfusions, antibiotics, fluids and whatever else he needs."

Richie tried to wrap his head around the onslaught of new information. He pictured a synthetic tube poking out of his chest. In his imagination, he would become this creature, a cyborg, with human and plastic parts. It was like a bad sci-fi movie. He had to suppress an urge to find the exit door. Tears welled up, again, "I don't know if I can do this Mom. Maybe I should've gone home from Dr. Pipkin's office."

Betty reached over to hold Richie, "It does sound pretty scary. But I'll be with you, and you can do this. You're stronger than you think, baby. Right now it's just talk, OK? Nothing's happening. Let's just listen to the rest of what the doctor has to say. We'll manage this together. We will."

Richie tried to summon up all his strength. He remembered breaking his arm in middle school. He had hit a sewer grate in the road and flew over his bike's handle bars. He broke three ribs, and his right elbow. Boy did that hurt, and he needed wires to put his elbow back together. There was surgery and pain, and rehab. Didn't he have a piece of metal in his body back then? He wiped his tears, "I guess I've already been a cyborg once, I could do it again."

"What?" asked Betty.

Richie could sometimes manage a crisis by thinking of a scene from one of his favorite old movies. "It's OK, Mom. They're just monsters from the Id."

Dr. Belkin looked confused. But Betty said, "Forbidden Planet right?"

"Yeah, Mom, if Captain John J. Adams could face them, I guess I can too. I'm ready to hear the rest."

"OK, you're right, there's more." Paul responded. "Chemotherapy is strong, and there are many potential side effects. Those possible effects are listed in order of their likelihood, from most likely to very rare. Among those side effects is the possibility of infertility." Paul paused again. He waited.

Richie had some idea where this was going, but this was definitely not something he wanted to talk about with his mom in the room. And children, that hadn't been on his 'to do' list.

"For Richard, we recommend that he produces a sperm sample for banking before therapy starts." Paul looked at Betty and Richard, then continued, "I can explain that in a bit more detail to Richard in private, if he prefers. There's a dedicated room in the Reproductive Medicine Department, where that can be done."

Betty again looked at Richie. "It'll be OK, Richie, they'll help you. It's important that it gets done."

"I believe that I've covered most of what you'll need for tonight. I'll be here, so if something comes up and you feel that you want to speak with me, just ask Richard's nurse to page me. Look, this is very complicated, it's a lot of information. It'll be repeated many more times. You'll receive detailed written material about the disease and its treatment. No one could possibly remember all of this in one sitting. If you have no other questions, I'd like to examine Richard now. I'll leave for a few minutes, and mom should step out. Then Richard can get undressed and put on the medical gown from the drawer. There's also a bag in the drawer that you can use for your clothes."

Alone in the exam room he changed quickly and then sat waiting for the doctor. "Didn't this just happen?" thought Richie.

Richie had been deep in thought when the doctor knocked on the door and came in. He looked up at Paul. "I had a complete exam this morning from Dr. Pipkin, so I know what this will be. I'm ready," said Richie.

Indeed, Paul did a physical examination like the one that Dr. Pipkin did that morning. Paul found the same petechiae, and pallor, his heart sounded just as Dr. Pipkin had described earlier. The examination took about ten minutes. Dr. Belkin explained what he found to Richie.

Richie said, "I guess I haven't changed since the physical this morning, which as I think about it, seems like a very long time ago."

"After I leave, put on the hospital clothes that are laid out for you. When you're done, open the door so your mom can come back in and wait with you for the IV team."

12.

Sandra knocked three times on the fellow's call room and not getting a response, she opened the door and walked in. Paul was on the cot, curled up on his side, sleeping soundly and mostly quietly. She watched him for a while, a smile came to her face.

"Hey, sleeping beauty, rise and shine." Sandra walked around the call room hoping to make enough noise to get Paul moving. Opening the locker door, putting her bag away and then closing it forcefully, finally did the trick.

Paul, took about a half minute to sit up, and be wide awake. Years of being on call honed his ability to wake up quickly and be ready to coherently answer a page, no matter the hour. He rose to his feet and walked into the fellow's bathroom. Morning pee, simultaneously brushing the teeth, a splash of Old Spice aftershave and he was ready for anything.

"How was your night?" Sandra asked.

"It was OK, Carrie called me twice with lab results. The initial CBC was about the same as the one faxed over from the referring pediatrician and the chemistries remained stable throughout the night. Of course, the differential remained pending, but I saw lots of leukemia blasts when I went down to check his blood smear in the heme lab. I'm sure the hematopathologist will confirm that on review this morning. The second CBC showed an increase in the hemoglobin and platelet count, reflecting the transfusions. Carrie said the chest x-ray was normal. Flow cytometry should have been sent. I didn't hear about any problems with his IV."

"I'm sure Dr. Stanner will be here soon. Why don't you come out with me, we'll see how the new patient is, and then you can get outta here," Sandra was all business.

Paul and Sandra walked over to Richie's room and noted that the transfusion of the second unit of pRBCs was nearly complete. Richie was NPO for the upcoming procedure, he could have nothing to eat or drink. His mom had chosen to join in solidarity with her son by fasting as well. "How was your night?" Paul asked.

"It was OK, it took me a little while to fall asleep with the tube in my arm," Richie answered, "but I got used to it. The nurse woke me up twice for the blood tests. She was very good, and I fell back to sleep almost immediately."

Betty slept in a chair that reclined into a sleeper. "The chair was surprisingly comfortable, and I guess I slept through Richie's blood tests," Betty answered a bit guiltily.

"I'll be leaving now, but I'll be back tonight," Paul said, "Dr. Gardner will be here for the day." Paul turned to go.

"Thanks, for your help, Dr. Belkin," Richie said.

Paul turned back and smiled, and then left quickly. He had to get home and get some shut-eye.

Sandra spoke with Betty and Richie, quickly going over the day's plan. "There are two procedures scheduled and we'll try to get you to the Department of Reproductive Medicine. Both the bone marrow exam and the central line placement will be done while he's asleep," Sandra explained, "that means he can't eat or drink anything until they're both done. First up will be the bone marrow exam. We'll take Richie to the procedure room. There'll be several people in the room, a nurse, the pathology tech, the intensivist providing the sedation, myself and Dr. Stanner. You may see trays covered with the instruments we use to perform the procedure along with large syringes to collect the specimens. The PICU doctor will ask some questions and then administer the sedation. Mom can be there with you at the start, but once you're asleep we'll ask her to leave. The actual procedure will take less than fifteen minutes, but you'll be in the room for about an hour. That includes the prep and recovery times. Any questions?"

"So, I won't feel anything?" Richard checked to be sure.

"You'll receive a sedating medicine called propofol along with morphine to manage the pain. The doses can be adjusted during the procedure as needed. You won't be awake, and you won't remember any of the testing."

Just then, the medical student stuck her head in the room, "Dr. Gardner, we're starting rounds."

"OK, I'll be right out," Sandra answered. She turned back to Richie and Betty, "I'll be back for you in a bit, the nurses will get you ready." With that she left the room to join the team on rounds.

It was a large team. It included a medical student, one senior and two junior pediatric residents as well as the pharmacist, the charge nurse, the social worker, a child life specialist, and of course Drs. Gardner and Stanner. Following everyone, and pushed around by the junior resident, was the C.O.W., *Computer-On-Wheels*, affectionately named Elsie. The portable laptop was Bluetooth connected to the hospital intranet, essential for checking labs, visualizing imaging, reviewing previous notes and importantly for placing new orders on the fly. The senior resident led the rounds, Dr. Gardner was the referee, and Dr. Stanner, the 30 year veteran, overseeing the rounds, was the final arbiter.

"By the way, Dr. Gardner," Dr. Stanner was checking, "please make sure that our study data manager, Selma, knows that we're preparing for a '*Day One*' marrow. She'll need to be sure we get all the samples required for the protocols and an additional tube sent out to the Pharma Gene Lab in California to search for any unusual genetic mutations."

"Of course," said Sandra. She pulled out her phone and took a step away from the team. Selma was on her speed-dial list, and Sandra had her on the horn in a few seconds. She quietly spoke to Selma, who knew just what to do. A minute later Sandra informed Dr. Stanner, "it's all taken care of, she found our patient in medical records. She'll be up shortly with what we need."

Rounds continued, covering three other children before circling around to Richie, their newest patient. "OK, let's hear about Richard Samuelson," said Dr. Stanner as the team walked over and stopped outside of his room.

Carrie led the presentation, she explained about the bruises, becoming short of breath with minimal exertion, and the episode of syncope. The very latest update from Elsie included the pathologist's report showing 90% blasts on the peripheral smear. Carrie told the team that his chemistries and liver tests were mostly normal, and his flow cytometry was pending. He had received a single donor unit of platelets overnight, and a unit of pRBCs. His second unit of red cells was nearly finished. Fluids without potassium ran at half maintenance throughout the night. Two repeat chemistries were still mostly normal.

Sandra asked Carrie, "what's your differential?"

Carrie replied, "all three cell lines are abnormal, which leads to the presumption that he has a disease infiltrating his bone marrow. He has a high white blood cell count with blast cells on his differential, so this is most likely a leukemia."

"Good," Sandra said, "what types of leukemia could this be, and based on the evidence, which one is most likely?"

"Cancer of the white blood cells could be either from B or T lymphocytes, or possibly myelocytes. As an adolescent, T cell leukemia is quite possible, but typically we find changes on a chest x-ray. His image was normal, no widened mediastinum, that argues against T cell leukemia or lymphoma. So, it's probably AML, Acute Myelocytic Leukemia or ALL, Acute pre-B cell, Lymphocytic Leukemia," Carrie answered, "I'm not sure which one."

"Very good," said Sandra, "if I forget, please remind me to take you all down to the pathology lab where we can use the multiheaded microscope to view his marrow smear. Myeloblasts and lymphoblasts will look different under the scope. The flow cytometry, now pending, will show the antigen profile of the surface proteins on his blast cells, and that will give us information as to the type of leukemia he has.

Madelyn, as the social worker, what is your assessment of the family?" Dr. Gardner asked.

"I only met them briefly, last night. There's just Richard and the mother," Madelyn answered, "I haven't found out anything about the father or other family members. Mom and Richard seem very strong, and they ask appropriate questions. Mom will need some help with her job. I believe they have what it takes to get through this."

"OK, thank you Madelyn, let's go in and see them," said Sandra.

The team filed into Richie's room. They had to shuffle around to all fit into the space surrounding his bed. Sandra checked the bag hanging from the IV pole. She noted that the red cell transfusion was nearly finished. She reached up to check the label, verifying Richie's name, the blood type, that it was irradiated and CMV negative. "This looks good, your second RBC unit is almost done," she remarked. "I want to introduce the team, you already know Dr. Johnson, and the social worker, Madelyn. This is our esteemed Child life therapist, Carol."

Carol raised her hand, "I will come in to see you later, we have some neat virtual reality headsets, with some cool games, I think you'll like."

Sandra continued with the rest of the team. You'll see us push Elsie, the C.O.W., *Computer-On-Wheels*, and last but certainly not least, is our chief, Dr. Stanner, he will be speaking with you later."

Dr. Stanner said, "we'll have some time soon for a discussion about Richard's leukemia, and what the next few days will be like. You're in excellent hands with Drs. Gardner and Belkin, and our entire crew. They are dedicated and experienced, and you will get to know each of them."

Sandra asked, "Do either of you have any questions right now?"

Richard asked, "when is the bone marrow test?"

Sandra had already taken care of about a half dozen children with newly diagnosed leukemia during her first year as a fellow in training. Since the most common ages at diagnosis are 3 to 5 years old, this was Sandra's first opportunity to see how an adolescent reacted to the diagnosis. It was certainly different from the little ones, who didn't understand the implications of having cancer and so her discussions had mostly been geared to the parents. Working with a teen was strangely familiar, it wasn't all that long ago that she was one. She could imagine her adolescent self, reacting like Richie. Sandra knew that she shouldn't become emotionally involved with her patients. She needed to remain an objective professional, but that line was often difficult to keep.

What was his question?

Sandra refocused, "as soon as we're done here, the medical assistant will take you to the procedure room," Sandra answered. "Your mother will have a consent to sign, and you will need to sign an assent. There will be another consent from the PICU attending for the sedation."

Sandra explained, "the large bones of the body, the pelvis, and the femurs, would be too heavy if they were solid, and so, apparently by design they are hollow, and yet still strong. In order not to waste that hollow space, the bone marrow, the soft spongy tissue where the blood elements are made sits within that cavity. That's where the leukemia started, and it's important to sample that tissue so we understand how the marrow has been affected." She handed the procedure consent form to Betty. "The consent," she continued, "describes the procedure using a special needle to access the bone marrow. It specifies that we will take samples to be examined in the pathology lab. Some samples will be frozen for later use, a portion of the marrow will be sent to a central lab as part of the study protocol, where it will be mined for information about Richard's leukemia. A small portion will be stored indefinitely and may be available for a potential future study. All in all, about 2/3 of an ounce of marrow will be taken, the loss of that small amount should have little effect on Richie. I'll use a single-use disposable needle, and so the risk of infection is low, but not zero. There are risks of bleeding, very rarely needles can wind up in the wrong place and do damage because of that. All that is spelled out in the consent document. Do you have any questions?" she asked.

Betty was reading the consent as Sandra spoke. Betty signed the consent and handed it over to Richie.

"There is the part you must sign, Richie, the "assent" because you're not yet eighteen," Sandra explained. "It means you agree also. It doesn't have legal authority because you haven't reached the age of consent." Betty handed him the pen, and they waited.

"Yeah, I know, I'm not going to read the whole thing," Richie signed the assent and handed it back to Sandra.

"OK, I'm going to make sure everything's set in the procedure room, I'll see you in a few minutes," and Sandra walked out along with the rest of the team.

Rounds were finished and the team members dispersed to work on their respective assignments. Richie's nurse remained with him in his room. Drs. Gardner and Stanner made their way to the procedure room. There were things that needed to be set up to be ready for the exam.

The PICU intensivist was getting her equipment set.

The doctors quickly reviewed what would happen during the procedure. The sample trays were set. Selma was there to be sure that the correct study samples were obtained, and the hematopathology tech was ready to receive the samples to prepare slides for the analysis of his marrow. Drs. Stanner and Gardner scrubbed for the procedure and were ready for Richie just as he and his mom were being led into the procedure room.

The intensivist, Dr. Rachel Street, talked briefly with Betty and Richard. She had reviewed his medical record, and confirmed that there were no allergies, nor respiratory or cardiac conditions. She verified that neither Richard nor his mom, nor any first-degree relatives had ever had an adverse reaction to anesthesia. Betty and Richard signed the sedation consent and assent.

Betty and Madelyn stood together as they watched the medical aide and nurse help Richie transfer to the procedure table. Next his IV bag was moved from the IV pole on his wheelchair to the IV pole on the procedure table. He was connected to the monitors. Richie was then directed to lie on his left side, with his head to Sandra's left. His knees were drawn up and his back was toward her.

Everything in place, Dr. Street announced that she was starting to administer the propofol. "You'll feel a bit of burning as the medicine flows into your arm," she warned. Watching the monitors and Richard's breathing, she slowly advanced the plunger of a 10-cc syringe, forcing the sedative through the stopcock connected to Richie's IV tube. He felt the medicine burn as it flowed into his arm, but before he could say anything, he was asleep.

Madelyn turned to Betty, "why don't you give Richard a kiss, and then we'll walk out together."

Betty paused, she looked at Madelyn, looked at the staff, glanced at the monitor and then leaned over and gave her son a kiss. "Please take care of my boy," she said. She dabbed a tear with the tissue she held and walked out with Madelyn.

It was time for Sandra to start the procedure, she narrated as she proceeded. "I'm locating the site on his back at the right posterior iliac crest, deep to the dimple above the buttocks." Sandra located the superior aspect of the right hip, then slid her thumb downward toward the familiar spot. Using her thumb, she pushed around the site, until she was comfortable that she knew where the needle would go. She was grateful that Richard was a thin athlete, his habitus made it easy to find the best spot. "OK, I have it," she said. Now with her sterile gloves and mask on, Sandra reached for the betadine solution to prep the site where the needle would pierce. She swiped in circles, continuing as the clock's second hand made a complete revolution. The solution was then allowed to dry. It was as it dried that the betadine was most effective at eliminating the skin flora. She then placed a sterile fenestrated drape over his hip, with the hole lined up over the area she would sample from. She used an alcohol gauze to wipe off the dried betadine. She would use local anesthetic, infiltrating the skin over the bone, and then advancing deeper, pushing the analgesic lidocaine into the periosteum covering the bone. As she began, Richie stirred a bit. "He moved, Dr. Street, I think he needs a little more morphine." She waited.

"OK, I'm giving him 3 more milligrams of morphine. With that and the topical analgesic you just infiltrated, he should be OK. I can still give him a bit more if needed. Why don't you go on," Dr. Street suggested.

Sandra gave more of the lidocaine, and this time, he didn't move.

"He seems good now," she said. She placed the cutting end of the needle against the site she'd chosen and then advanced the needle perpendicularly to the pelvic bone. She leaned in with her weight, pushing on the handle as the sharp end of the stylet bit into the pelvic bone. She rotated the needle a few degrees clockwise, then counterclockwise, pushing and twisting as the needle advanced. Sandra stopped when she sensed an abrupt drop of resistance indicating that the business end of the needle was within the hollow marrow space. She removed the stylet and attached the empty syringe to the hub of the needle. When the syringe was firmly seated, she pulled up on the plunger. She watched as the marrow sample bubbled up into the syringe. As it filled the barrel, it looked like foamy, thick blood. Enough marrow was aspirated to fill three syringes, yielding all that was needed for the pathologist, for Selma, for special studies and the protocol requirements. Finally, having collected all the needed samples, Dr. Gardner pulled the needle out of Richie's hip, and using a sterile gauze applied pressure to the exposed site for a full minute. When she was sure there was no further oozing from the puncture wound, she placed a sterile pressure bandage over the area.

"Great!" said Dr. Stanner, "we should have everything we need. Thanks everyone. Thank you, Dr. Street, looks like we're done."

"OK," said Dr. Street, "the propofol will soon wear off and he'll wake up. His vitals have been rock-solid. That went well. Good job, Dr. Gardner. Let's leave him on his side, until he's completely awake. That's the safest position if he begins to vomit."

The pathology technician was packing everything securely to bring to the lab. Selma had her samples. Drs. Stanner and Gardner removed their disposable sterile garb and tossed them in the trash.

"Let's go find Ms. Samuelson and let her know everything went well."

13.

As Richie's sedation began, Madelyn escorted Betty into the parents' conference room. "How are you?" she began.

"I don't know, I'm scared, Richie is my world," Betty began. "I've been trying to put up a strong optimistic front, but inside, I'm jelly." With that admission, deep angst bubbled up and the long-suppressed tears flowed. Madelyn offered a box of Kleenex. "I don't know how any parent does this. I'm not sure I have the strength for this. I'm just barely holding on," said Betty.

Madelyn spoke softly to Betty, "what you're feeling is completely normal, there would be some deep denial or lack of understanding if you didn't feel that way. As I've been with you, just this short time, I sense that you have what it takes. You've been able to summon that strength when it was needed. Even if you're not sure inside, your ability to wear that mantle like a suit of armor will keep you going." Madelyn paused and then continued, "everyone needs help through this. We have resources in our division that can help you. There is a parent support group, which I'm in charge of, but which is really run by the parents. They'll be available to help when you're ready."

Madelyn paused and then asked, "Do you have any family that can help?"

Betty sighed, she took a deep breath and began, "My parents are dead, I lost my father 5 years ago, and my mother, it will be 3 years, next month. But even when they were alive, we barely talked. They recused themselves from our lives a long time ago. As soon as they learned that I was pregnant with Richie they disappeared. I wasn't married, and they couldn't abide that."

Madelyn continued, "What about the father, is he involved?"

"You want to know about his father? I'm not sure what you want to hear," said Betty.

"Whatever you want to tell me," Madelyn answered.

"His name is Dylan, and he's never seen Richie. We were together in college for a very brief time. It's a long story. I was very young, impressionable and naive. When I became pregnant with Richie, Dylan quickly disappeared and we've never talked again."

"That must have been hard" said Madelyn. "I will want to talk to you more about that, about your job and how I can help. You're going to need to take time off from work."

There were so many thoughts running through Betty's head. She couldn't seem to begin to sort out the crazy jumble cramming her brain, it hurt. She felt lost and powerless. She'd always managed to be the mom and help Richie when he needed it. But not now, this was different. Could she lose her boy? What would be left of her life without Richie? Speaking with a stranger without judgement, a professional, might be what she needed. It was hard to concentrate on what Madelyn was saying. Betty tried to focus.

"Work!" Betty exclaimed, "shit, I need to call my boss, and Richie's school."

There was a knock on the door. "That's probably the doctors," said Madelyn. "We'll talk again soon. Here's my card, it has my cell number, you can call anytime."

Madelyn and Betty stood up as Sandra opened the door and came in, "it's all done. Richard's fine, he's just waking up. I'll take you over to see him. We got all the marrow samples needed. There's a dressing on the right hip, just above his butt which should stay dry for 48 hours. If it gets wet or soiled his nurse can replace it with a new bandage. The area will be a little sore for a day or so, but it shouldn't bother him too much."

"OK, thanks Dr. Gardner," Betty said. "I'm ready."

Betty needed to compose herself a bit before seeing Richie, her talk with Madelyn had stirred up some old, long buried memories. She took a couple of deep breaths, shook her arms, called up her smiley face, and she was set. She was glad she hadn't put on any makeup, tears and mascara didn't mix well. Sandra walked with her over to the procedure room.

Dr. Street was finishing and packing up her equipment for the trip back to the PICU. "He did fine, Ms. Samuelson," said Dr. Street.

Betty went over to the table where Richie was beginning to stir. She kissed him on the cheek, and gave him a careful squeeze, "how do you feel?"

Richie was still hazy. He blinked a few times and let out a big yawn. "Are they going to do the marrow test now?"

Betty smiled, "I guess Dr. Street did her job, it's all done, Richie. They got everything they needed."

"Wow, really, I don't remember any of it," said Richie. As he started to move, he felt the bandage, and then added, "Oh, I feel it now, it's a little sore, but not bad. It kinda feels like when I fell last year jumping over one of the hurdles, well I guess it wasn't exactly *over* the hurdle."

"Please don't try to get up by yourself," said Dr. Street, "your nurse and one of the aides will help you."

Just as Dr. Street finished saying that, his nurse and the aide appeared. They supported him as he moved gingerly off the procedure table and into the wheelchair for the short ride back to his room.

"I don't think I need the wheelchair. I'm OK."

His nurse, Steve, said, "You must get in the wheelchair, that's the rule after sedation. In about 15 minutes, with my help, we can get you up and walking if you're ready. Remember, you still have a couple of items scheduled for the day, including placement of your central line catheter, which will also be under sedation. So, you still can't eat or drink anything until after that. The IV fluids will keep running, which should help until you're allowed to drink."

Betty watched as Steve supported Richie back into his hospital bed and actuated the control to raise the head of the bed. Talking with Madelyn had helped some, but she still felt lost. Only a couple of days ago everything was fine, her life was in order, she had their future mapped out. All of a sudden, without warning, that was all in danger. Her son was being pushed in a wheelchair, back to his bed, in a pediatric oncology unit. She began to feel angry, but had nowhere to direct it.

"Anything else you need right now?" Steve asked.

"No, I'm good," Richie responded.

"OK, I'll leave you now," Steve said, and he walked out of the room.

"Mom, how are you?" Richie asked.

"I was just going to ask you that," said Betty, she smiled, thinking about her son asking her how she was.

"I'm OK, my backside doesn't hurt too much. I'm comfortable enough, but I'm definitely hungry," Richie said. "Hey, I feel pretty good about everyone here in the hospital, don't you? Like I'm still scared and anxious, but not as much as I was when we first arrived. It seems like that was a long time ago, but it was only last night."

"I'm scared too, Richie, but I agree, we seem to be in a good place." She paused, and then added, "you know, Richie, while you were having the bone marrow test, I was meeting with the social worker, Madelyn. She asked me a few questions. She asked about your father."

"Yeah, Mom, I really don't have much interest in that, he's never been there for me. I don't need to know any more about him. You're my family."

"Maybe I could find him, I've never seriously looked for him. What do you think?" Betty asked.

"Gee Mom is that what you want?"

"This leukemia diagnosis, it's serious, you know of course, I just wondered if you felt, well, maybe you were missing something, and meeting him would help." Betty thought it was important to at least get it out in the open. It had been in the background for many years. There had never been any serious discussion about him. She wondered if Richie was protecting her by not broaching it. He likely knew that it wouldn't be a comfortable topic. Perhaps he really wanted to meet his father. Betty didn't want to be the reason that Richie didn't see him. She would try hard to find him if that's what Richie wanted. She could do it.

"OK, Mom, you know that you didn't answer my question."

Betty looked at her son again. "OK, Richie, no bullshit. I love you more than anything in the world and I would do anything for you, whatever it takes. For me, I don't care if I ever see that fucker again!"

Richie smiled at his mom, "Whoa Mom, now you're talking. I love it. I say, fuck him, let's leave him in the dark where he's been my whole life!"

Betty smiled, then she giggled, then laughed, a glorious belly laugh, that went on, and on. It was contagious and soon Richie was laughing too. They were peas in a pod, cut from the same cloth, and connected by their shared lives. It couldn't be explained, but it was real. The laughter was hard and loud, and cathartic. The sound carried through the unit, to the other rooms and over to the nurses' station.

Richie's nurse, hearing the commotion, came over and stuck his head in. "Hey, are you guys OK?" He looked at both of them and smiled, "I wasn't sure if you were laughing or crying."

Betty looked up at Steve, she put her hands over her mouth trying to squelch the laughter, but it was hard to do. As soon as she started to control it, the laughter erupted again. "I'm so sorry, Steve, we'll try to be quieter," Betty said, but even as she spoke, the laughter had to be muffled once more.

"Well, I'm glad it's laughter," said Steve, "we don't have too much of that, and frankly it's nice to hear. But maybe for the others, try to tamp it down a few decibels. Oh, and by the way, someone from Reproductive Medicine will be up shortly. They'll have some papers for you to sign and then they'll escort Richie down to their department. I'm going to hep-lock your IV. The tube will still be in your arm, but you won't be connected to the pump and IV bag. It'll be simple to hook you up later when it's needed." Steve disconnected him from the long IV tubing, and he flushed Richie's end of the tube with heparin, so his side wouldn't clot. Finally, he capped the end and coiled the tube, so it didn't hang loose. A small stretch sleeve netting covered the whole site. "You're all set."

Steve turned and left.

They were quiet for a while. Betty wondered about bringing up a teenage boy without a father. There were certainly challenges. It made her think about what a single father might say to an adolescent daughter. No doubt being a single parent wasn't easy. Anyway, they seemed to have managed without a man so far.

Betty remembered she had to call her boss and Richie's school, to explain their absences. She'd do that while Richard was down in Reproductive Medicine.

Soon, the food tray cart passed near their room. The lady behind the cart slowed as she came near, but she saw the NPO sign on the doorway, and instead of stopping she picked up the pace and moved on to the next room. Betty watched the food go by and glanced at Richie. She saw him track the cart as it passed. She felt the grumble in her stomach and imagined that it was happening in him too. OK, no food for them, this was something Betty could do to support her son. She was determined to be strong.

"Mom, I'm going to see if I can sleep a bit, that might help. At least when I'm asleep, I won't be thinking about food. Well, maybe I won't." He turned over, closed his eyes and was soon breathing soundly.

Betty looked at her son and was amazed that with everything going on Richie could just close his eyes and fall asleep. Whenever she closed her eyes, a million thoughts and worries flooded her brain. Rest was elusive. As she was trying to relax, one of the staff, pushing a wheelchair, knocked on their door.

"Excuse me, hi, I'm Shauna, from Reproductive Medicine, is this Richard Samuelson's room?"

"Yes, it is," said Betty. She stood up and went over to gently wake Richie. "Richie, it's the woman from Reproductive Medicine." Richie blinked a couple times, stretched his arms and sat up, seemingly wide awake at once.

"I believe you were expecting someone from our department?" asked Shauna.

"Yes, we were told you'd be here," said Betty.

"Then, I assume you know why I'm here. There is a consent to be signed, and Richard will need to sign the assent. Can I check his wrist band ID, please?" Shauna checked his wristband and used her scanner to verify that it matched the records. She asked Richard, "Can you please tell me your name and date of birth?" Richie did. "OK, good," said Shauna, "you should read the consent. It says that you will be providing a sperm sample, which will be processed, frozen and stored. Before the product is stored, a small sample will be tested to document the sperm count and assess its viability. We will be diligent in preserving and protecting the sample. But we do not guarantee that future access will yield a viable sample, nor do we guarantee that it will result in successful fertilization. There's a bit more to the consent, which you should read, but those are the important elements," said Shauna.

"Well, I guess there aren't many options," said Betty, "I'll read the entire consent later, but I'm sure that it's written in a way to minimize your liability. Richie, do you have any questions?"

"No, I'll sign it," he said. He signed, printed his name and dated it, then handed it back to his mom to do her part.

"OK," said Shauna, "I'll bring Richard down now." Looking at Richie, she asked, "can you please get in the wheelchair for me?" Turning to Betty, Shauna said, "he should be back in about 45 minutes."

Betty was about to ask if she could walk down with Richie, but then thought better of it. "See you later," was all she finally said, but she wondered. She had a dream of her golden years. She was at home. Richie and his wife would be visiting and three or four grandchildren would be in tow. She'd have sage advice for Richie. She would read stories to the kids, spoil them, watch them grow up. She had hopes. And now?

The Reproductive Medicine department was down on the second floor of the medical center. Once there, they were greeted by the clerk. He also asked Richie to identify himself, checked his wristband and looked over the consent.

"You're here to provide a sperm sample. There's a private room for that. I'll provide you with a container, and a cover, for the sample. There is a cot inside and a recliner chair for your convenience. Inside, there are some aides you may use if you need help," said the clerk. "Do you have any questions?"

Richie wasn't sure how this would all go, but he would figure it out. He said, "no."

The clerk said, "the sample would be best if it's been at least three days since the last ejaculation. When was the last time?"

Richie was thinking back. It seemed like forever, but he had come to the hospital less than 24 hours ago. He wasn't excited about having this conversation with a stranger. All Richie said was, "it's been more than three days."

The aide looked at him and checked off the appropriate box. "Here's the container, it has your ID label on it, when you're done, make sure to screw the cap on securely." He walked Richie over to the room and let him in. Without saying anything more he closed the door.

Once inside, Richie turned the privacy lock. He looked around. There was a rack with some girlie magazines, Playboy and Hustler, he noticed that the dates on the covers were several years old. "I guess they don't have a subscription," Richie thought. It wasn't the first time he had seen those, but he didn't usually need magazines, he could see all he wanted on the internet. He found the lotion and tried sitting in the recliner that had been covered with a clean paper sheet pulled from the roll at the top. He flipped through the Hustler magazine looking at the pictures, trying to get in the mood. He squirted a generous amount of lotion on his penis and started sliding his hand up and down along the shaft. Soon the magazine dropped to the floor. All he had in his head now was an image of Nancy, next to him, on the bench at the track. He imagined touching her breast, feeling her closeness. His hand became hers, touching him. Just as he was about to come, he remembered to bring the cup in place, and with a shudder, he released into the container. It was clinical and pleasurable at the same time. Soon after ejaculating, still breathing hard, he lay quietly for a few moments while the signals ebbed. All of a sudden he was tired and craved sleep. But he sat up. He made sure everything was tucked away. He put the magazine and bottle of lotion back where he had found them. Richie washed up at the sink in the room. Then he unlocked and opened the door. Richie handed the cup to the clerk.

The clerk checked that the cover was secure. "There'll be a sample analysis report in the EMR tomorrow. You'll be notified if we need another sample. An escort will bring you back to your room now, do you have any questions?"

Richie shook his head.

The escort was nearby with the wheelchair, and Richie was soon back in his room. Betty had tried but was unable to get any shut-eye.

"Anything you want to tell me, young man?" she asked.

"Ah, well there will be a report tomorrow," is all he said. And that seemed to put an end to any further discussion. With everything that happened, and still with no chance to eat, his body figured it might as well go back to sleep again. Richie laid down, closed his eyes and once again he was asleep.

It seemed that Richie could shut down whenever and wherever he liked. When Betty tried to sleep, her mind filled with what ifs and worst case scenarios. She tossed and turned, and though she was exhausted, falling asleep remained elusive.

Carol, from Child Life, came to see Richie and to find out what he liked, what video games, virtual reality sets or books. She wanted to find out more about him. She saw Richie asleep, and Betty wasn't. "Hey, how are you? I'm sure this has been hard," she said.

Betty didn't know how to explain what she felt, "this is the most difficult thing I've ever done. I'm so terrified I can't think straight. I've had to put my child's life in the care of doctors I've never met. I've got to trust them to do right. I've chosen not to eat, because Richie can't. Awful images appear unbidden, and I can't get them out of my head. So, how am I? I'm a hot mess."

Carol sat down. "Betty, I can't even imagine what you're going through," Carol paused. "I've been doing this for twenty years and I've seen many children like Richie diagnosed with leukemia. They usually do very well, and I expect that your son will too. It may sound cliché, but try not to look too far ahead, take each day as it comes. Ask questions and learn as much as you can about leukemia and Richie's treatments. Use reputable sources like the National Cancer Institute websites. Over time, you'll become part of the team, and this will get easier."

Betty listened. She couldn't imagine this getting any easier.

"I can be here for a little while, why don't you take a walk, get off the unit, it'll help clear your mind. You can go down to the lobby or the cafeteria, there's a gift shop to browse, there's also a chapel on the street level, it can be comforting, regardless of your faith. Take your time, if Richie wakes up, I'll let him know that you'll be back soon."

"I don't know," said Betty.

"You can't take care of your son, if you don't care of yourself," said Carol. She looked at Betty and nodded, "go on, just a short break. You'll be surprised at how much it can help. Let them know at the nurses' station, make sure you have a visitor sticker, and your phone."

Betty looked at Richie, sleeping comfortably, she looked back at Carol, "OK, I'll be back soon, thank you," and she left.

It was late afternoon, and the lobby was busy, visitors were lined up at the information desk finding out how to get where they needed to be. She walked past the line, and toward the cafeteria. Richie was getting IV fluids, she could certainly drink some water. She bought a bottle of spring water and took a nice long swallow. It was delicious. She walked along the corridors, stretching and loosening her tight muscles. It wasn't long before she came to the open chapel door. She had not planned to, but she stepped inside. Betty couldn't remember the last time she had been to a religious service. It wasn't a large room, there were five rows of polished wooden pews, the backlighting in the front and along the sides provided soft ambient color. The chapel was ecumenical, soft meditative music played in the background. Betty walked down the single center aisle. She was alone in the chapel. As she sat down in the second pew, a sense of comfort came over her. After a few quiet moments Betty felt the need to say something, though she doubted that anyone was listening. At least she would hear. Softly, barely louder than a whisper, she began.

"My son, Richie, is here in the hospital," she said. "I guess you know why he's here, probably you already know if he'll get better. I'm worried about him. He's all I think about. I have always known, but it is so clear to me now, that he's everything that's important to me. If I could switch places with him, I would do it in a heartbeat." Betty paused a moment, thinking, "Please help the doctors, nurses, and everyone else as they care for my son, and for all the other children up there. Whatever else happens, please, please don't let Richie suffer. I guess that's all. I can't ask for anything more than that." Betty felt calmer, a feeling of peace embraced her. She sat there for some moments, quiet and alone, with nothing more to say. She stood and looked upward, "thank you for listening," she said and left the chapel.

As Betty walked toward the elevator bank, her phone rang, it was the nurses' station. Betty held her breath and answered, she felt her stomach instantly knot up, "this is Betty Samuelson."

"Hi, everything's fine, your son's OK. I'm calling because the surgeon's up here and he wants to talk to you both about the catheter placement," his nurse Steve said.

The phone ringing instantly put Betty on edge again, it resurrected all her anxieties. She tried to calm herself, she took a few deep breaths, it helped, "I'll be there in two minutes, I'm at the street level elevators." Betty hung up and punched the 'UP' button.

As Betty walked out of the elevator onto the pediatric oncology floor, she passed the nurses' station, let them know she was back, and then turned to the right, headed for Richie's room. She saw a young doctor garbed in a white doctor's coat over green scrubs, a surgical cap on his head and a face mask dangling below his chin. He was waiting outside the room. Carol was with them, as she promised. Richie was awake. He appeared to be chatting with Carol, who was making sure that the doctor wasn't going to have a conversation with Richie until Betty was back.

"Thank you, Carol," said Betty. Then to the doctor, "I'm, Betty, Richie's mom."

"I'm Dr. Gilgood. Richard's next to come down to the OR for his central line catheter placement. I'm here to see your son, ask a few questions, explain what will happen and perform a quick exam," said the doctor.

Betty turned to Richie, "How are you dear?"

"I'm fine, ready to get this done so I can eat," said Richie.

"OK," said Betty, "what happens now?"

Dr. Gilgood continued, "I will listen to his heart and lungs, and ask about any allergies or medications. I see that after the transfusion, his hemoglobin was 9 gm/dL. That's a nice improvement, not normal yet but OK for the procedure. His platelet count is up to 65,000, which is also a good improvement, but I would prefer it to be a bit higher for the surgery. I'll ask his doctor to order another unit of platelets. He'll be cleared to have the surgery as long as the platelet transfusion has started when he comes to the OR. It doesn't have to be finished. His doctors have asked for a double lumen catheter to be placed in his subclavian vein. Richard looks big enough for that, but if there's a problem, I will put in a smaller single lumen tube. The procedure itself will take about 30 minutes, but preparation, and recovery will mean that he won't be back here for about 2 hours. I'll also be asking you and Richard to sign a consent form. Do you have any questions?"

Richie asked, "Will it hurt when I wake up? And what's that you said about the catheter, a double *lupen*?"

Dr. Gilgood replied, "It's a double *lumen* catheter, it means that there are two separate channels inside the tube, so two different solutions can run at the same time without mixing with each other, or one side can be used to draw a sample, while the other is being used for an infusion. It's likely to be a little sore at the site for a day or so, but after that it shouldn't hurt. When it's not being used, it can be curled up under a netting. If you're wearing a shirt, no one will know it's there. It's a temporary line, and it will be removed before you're discharged from the hospital."

"Richie does not have any allergies, he doesn't take medications and he's never had a problem with anesthesia. What else do you need to know?" asked Betty.

"Sounds like you've done this a few times already. Any bleeding or clotting problems with Richard or close relatives?" asked Dr. Gilgood.

"No," said Betty.

"OK, quick exam," Dr. Gilgood continued, "I'm going to close his door now and pull the curtains, if it's OK with Richard, Mom you can stay. I'm not going to be looking at any private parts."

Richie nodded.

Dr. Gilgood opened the top of Richie's gown, undraped the stethoscope from around his neck, and listened to Richie's heart and lungs. "OK, that's all I need. Let me show you where the catheter will go." Dr. Gilgood pointed to the area below his left clavicle, "it will be here, midclavicular, below the collar bone, about 4 or 5 inches of the catheter will remain outside of the skin. Once the central line is in place and functioning, the IV in his arm won't be needed. Usually, one of the nurses will take that out after he settles back up here."

"So, when it's done and I come back to the floor, I can eat? Right?"

"I think so," said Dr. Gilgood, "certainly from my point of view there would be no reason to keep you from eating." He looked at them both and when there were no more questions, he opened his binder holding the consent. Betty signed the consent, Richie signed the assent, and they were ready for the next step. Dr. Gilgood walked over to the nurses' station and briefly talked with his nurse. He then went to find the resident to make sure that another platelet unit would be ordered. One of the pediatric doctors on the floor would have to order the platelets; as the consulting surgeon, he was not allowed. He asked the resident to call the blood bank and make sure they knew he was going to the OR soon. That usually expedited the arrival of the platelets.

Betty and Richie looked at each other. It had been a very long day. It was hard to believe that it was only about 24 hours since he was admitted to the hospital, so much had already happened. "Well, what do you think you want to eat when you're back?" asked Betty, "maybe it shouldn't be too heavy right after the surgery."

"Gee Mom, I was going to say, two pork egg rolls, a plate of egg foo young and fried rice, but maybe you're right. Let's see, what can be lighter?" Richie wondered.

"How about a grilled chicken sandwich and a bag of chips, you can have a Dr Pepper if you want," suggested Mom.

"That sounds good, but I might be hungry again in a couple of hours."

"I'm sure I'll be able to find something for you if you're still hungry."

They were quiet for a while, each with their own thoughts.

Before long, Steve came by, with Richie's platelet bag. "When the blood bank hears surgery, they can move pretty quickly," said Steve as he checked the label on the bag and used his scanner on Richie's wristband. When everything checked out, he spiked the bag and watched as the platelets began their journey into Richard's vein. "Any questions?"

"When do you think they will be coming for Richie?" asked Betty.

"It should be very soon, the OR called up and said they're ready for him, so I expect to see patient transport any minute." No sooner had he finished speaking, than the patient elevator opened, and Steve watched a wheelchair come out, followed by the escort pushing it. She stopped at the nurses' desk and was directed to Richie's room.

"I'm here for Richard Samuelson," she said.

"That's me," said Richie.

Steve helped Richie get into the chair and then he transferred the platelet bag from the IV pole on the bed to the pole on the wheelchair, allowing the transfusion to continue. "We'll see you soon. There will be some food waiting for you," said Steve.

Betty followed Richie and the escort back to the patient elevator. Soon they were on their way to the pre-Op area. Once inside, the escort helped Richie get onto an OR gurney, carefully transferring the platelet bag again and the escort left.

Soon, another woman approached, "I'm Brianna, the Medical Assistant. I'll get you checked in." Brianna went through the standard questions, checked his medical wrist ID and completed a brief physical exam. Next the anesthesiologist was by and quickly completed her questions and had the consents signed.

Preparations continued like clockwork. The OR nurse came by. "OK, Richard, I'm going to wheel you into OR room #4. Mom, you can give Richard a kiss."

Betty looked around the pre-Op room. It was very busy, staff was hustling around, they all seemed to have jobs to do. What could go wrong inside there? She imagined all kinds of horrors in an OR. But, she tried to reassure herself. This was a good hospital, right? Richie's trusted pediatrician had recommended it, and everyone she'd met so far had seemed dedicated, and caring. So, she leaned over, gave Richie's hand a squeeze and kissed him on the forehead, "Break a leg, kiddo, I'll see you soon."

"We'll call you to let you know when you can come down to be with him in Recovery," the nurse said, as he pushed the gurney with Richie through the doors of OR #4.

Betty watched him disappear behind the swinging doors. She took a breath, crossed her fingers, and turned to leave, headed back to the unit to wait for the call from Recovery.

Back upstairs she found Steve at the nurses' station.

"I have a question," asked Betty, "Richie will be back from the OR in a bit, and as you know, he hasn't had anything to eat all day. You may also know that I joined him in fasting. We're in this together and we're both famished. I was thinking about ordering a couple of grilled chicken sandwiches so they're here when Richie gets back. What do you suggest?"

"Good timing." answered Steve, "several of the nurses are getting ready to place an order to the deli nearby, the food is good, and of course, they deliver. I can take your request, what do you want?"

"That's great. Two grilled chicken sandwiches on rye, mustard, mayo, pickles and lettuce. Two bags of chips. A Coke for me, and Richie likes root beer or Dr Pepper. Thanks again Steve, do you think $30 will cover it, with the tip?"

"That'll be fine, you should get change back," said Steve, "I'll bring the food over when it arrives."

"Thanks Steve, I'm going over to the room to lie down, maybe I can get in a quick power nap." She walked over and lay down on Richie's bed. Betty was exhausted. Her head hit the pillow, her eyes closed, and finally she was asleep.

14.

About an hour and a half later, Steve knocked on the door, "Betty, your delivery's here," he said with an impish grin. Steve was pushing a smiling Richie, seated in a wheelchair, back from Recovery and guarding a deli bag propped up on his lap.

"I've been smelling the food in this bag, and I can't wait any longer, it's time to eat." said Richie.

"Richie, how'd you get here? I thought that I was going to come down to Recovery to be with you when you woke up," said his mom.

"It's fine, I feel OK, just a bit sore near my left shoulder, but not bad at all. I woke up as they were wheeling me into Recovery. They were impressed, I guess, with how fast I woke up from the anesthesia." Richie was ready to eat. He'd been smelling the food wrapped up on his lap. His stomach was growling and his mouth was watering. After the long wait, the sandwiches would taste awesome. He could hardly wait.

Betty and Steve helped Richie stand up, careful not to put pressure on his left shoulder, and supported him as he gingerly stepped over to his bed. The head of the bed was elevated. Richie got in and Steve pushed the bedside tray table in front of Richie, positioning it so he had a surface to eat from.

"I'll leave you guys," said Steve, "my food is waiting for me back there. I'll check in later."

Betty thanked Steve again and told him not to worry about the change. She opened the bag and got the sandwiches, the chips and the drinks. Always with motherly advice, Betty said, "Richie, please eat slowly, give your stomach a chance to catch up with the food."

After not eating all day, the food tasted amazing. The chicken had grill marks. It was cooked well, but was still juicy. There were a lot of chewing and munching sounds, with drinking slurps interspersed, and despite the warnings, the food was dispatched quickly.

Soon, Sandra knocked on the door and looked in. "Looks like you've eaten, that's a good sign. How are you feeling Richard?"

"Much better after the food," said Richie. "My shoulder's just a little sore, and I've already forgotten about my butt."

Betty asked, "What's the plan for tomorrow?"

"We'll be accessing one channel of the new catheter so that you receive IV fluids during the night," said Sandra. "I've ordered only one blood test during the night, and it will be taken from the second lumen of his catheter, so Richard shouldn't be disturbed. Tomorrow, Dr. Stanner will talk to you about the test results and the planned treatment. As you may suspect, there will be more consents to sign. Any questions?"

Richard and Betty shook their heads, they had no questions. Richie was too exhausted to think about anything else. It was easier for him not to think about the disease, or about being in the hospital, about his school, or even about Nancy. He wanted only to shut off the blaring noise in his head.

"OK, I'll be leaving soon, and Dr. Belkin will be here this evening. Have an uneventful night, I'll see you in the morning," said Sandra and she left.

Steve came into the room after Sandra left. "Looks like the food is gone, was everything OK?"

"Fine,' said Betty, "we'll keep that deli in mind, good choice."

Richie asked if Steve could take the IV out of his arm. Steve managed that quickly and placed a band-aid over the site.

"Shift change is soon, and I'll be leaving," said Steve. "Dr. Gardner ordered intravenous fluids for the night, but I'll hold off for now and ask the night shift nurse to start it later. You have some visitors if that's OK."

Richie looked at his mom. She shrugged, "I don't know."

"I guess it's fine," said Richie, not knowing who they might be.

A minute later, Richie saw Nancy and an older gentleman walking towards them. He saw her looking around the unit. He imagined what she felt as she passed the rooms filled with sick children. But then, as her head swung back, their eyes met, and she smiled. She seemed to be dressed up. She wore a yellow blouse, open at the neck, with a gold pendant necklace, it was paired with a dark pleated skirt, falling to just above her knees and smart black shoes with kitten heels.

"Hi, Richie," said Nancy, and she introduced the man with her, "this is my dad."

Betty stood up as they approached. "It's Walter," said Nancy's father. "Nancy insisted we come out to see Richie, and I knew better than to argue."

Betty reached her hand out, "I'm Betty."

Walter shook her offered hand, "Yes, I know, Nancy told me. I'm so sorry to hear about Richie. I've heard a lot about him.

"Oh, Richie, how are you?" said Nancy, "I can't stop thinking about you. I've been imagining all the awful things they must be doing to you. When I stepped off the elevator, and looked around, all I saw were sick children, and I thought about how you were here, one of them." Nancy looked around, "I wanted to see you Richie, but I was also scared."

Richie wasn't sure what to say, "I was kind of scared too. But now that you're here, I feel much better." He couldn't stop looking at her.

Walter looked at Richie and Nancy, then he turned to Betty, "I think we can leave them alone for a little bit. Would that be OK with you Betty?"

Betty hesitated. Finally, she said, "OK," and Walter and Betty walked out, leaving the two moonstruck kids alone.

"Nancy, you certainly can make a kid with cancer feel good," Richie smiled.

Nancy came closer, she sat down on his bed and held his hand. She leaned over and kissed him, lingering just a moment on his lips.

"That was nice," said Richie.

"I feel it too. But, leukemia, I just don't even know what to say. What's it like?"

"I think that I've known for a while that something wrong. I could feel it in my bones, they ached. And I've been tired a lot." said Richie.

"But what will happen, Richie?"

"So far, they've just been testing, but I'm going to start treatment soon, you know, chemotherapy and they say it'll be difficult. But everyone here is nice, and the doctors are good, so I think it's going to be okay."

They sat quietly for a while, holding hands. Richie took comfort in her closeness. He could hardly believe that she was here with him. Somehow the girl he just met still cared for him. She had come to this place filled with children with cancer to be with him. Maybe she did feel the same connection that he did. All those dark thoughts crowding his head seemed to disappear when she was near.

"Richie, I already felt something special with you and now this. It's fucked up that this is happening to you."

"I know. It's really weird, like something alive is growing inside me. You know, something that doesn't belong. It's hard to describe. I worry about the treatment and how it will make me feel, but I also can't wait for it to start. Crazy, isn't it?"

"No Richie, it's not crazy." Nancy looked down, she seemed to be thinking. "I watched my mom get chemotherapy. It was hard to watch. I've been thinking about that a lot, now that you're in here."

"I'm so sorry, Nancy. I, uh, I didn't know." Richie wasn't sure what to say next.

Tears welled up in Nancy's eyes. She didn't try to stop them. She turned to Richie, and looked him in the eyes. "You'll be fine, Richie," she said between sobs. "I know it in my heart."

They were connected, for sure. Richie felt her pain. He reached out to hold her and they embraced. Her head resting on his shoulder. Richie and Nancy, together, a bond growing between them. Faces wet with tears, Nancy pulled back to gaze into Richie's eyes and then leaned forward to kiss him.

This kiss was different, Richie felt it. It wasn't just heat. Two souls were coming together. Richie knew right then that he would not lose her. They would be there for each other.

Their connection was strong. As their lips parted, still watching each other, they smiled, and then giggled at their changing relationship.

The sound of throat clearing along with the appearance of their parents in the doorway quickly brought them out of their own world. "It's good to see you both discussing Richard's health," said Walter.

Nancy stood up, she glanced down, and tried to dry her face. She smiled at no one in particular.

Nancy looked at Betty, "Thank you for letting me visit Richie, Ms. Samuelson," said Nancy. "I will pray for him to get better quickly. And I hope it will be OK if I can visit again soon."

"Well, I'm sure that Richie would like that, and it's OK with me too, as long as your father approves," said Betty.

"Richie, please text me when you can," Nancy said.

"Well young lady, we've got to get you back home," said Walter, "I think you have homework to do, and I suspect Richard will need his sleep. We should go." And to Betty he added, "I will also pray for Richard. It was very nice to meet you both, although I wish that it had been under different circumstances."

With that Nancy and Mr. Peters turned to leave the unit. Just before they passed out of view, Nancy turned and blew a kiss to Richie, and then they were gone.

Betty and Richie looked at each other for a minute.

"What?" said Richie, "I can smell the gears inside grinding."

Betty smiled, "Nancy seems very nice, and she's pretty. She made the trip to see you in the hospital and that probably wasn't easy for her, it took some courage. I also see that she genuinely cares about you, and clearly you like her too."

"And," Richie knew there was more.

Betty continued, "I don't want to see you hurt, you have a lot to go through now, and that needs to be your focus. Richie, I'm glad that she makes you happy, really, I am, but relationships can be difficult, especially early on and on top of everything else that's happening. So just be careful with your heart."

Richie had been feeling good just a few minutes ago. He stared at his mom. Why did she want to ruin that feeling? It made him angry. She had no business saying those things. He was nearly 18, had a god awful disease and what right did she have to interfere with the one good thing happening in his life. She couldn't know. "Mom," Richie replied, trying not to lash out at her, trying to calm himself. He needed his mom. "I know you've had your own experiences and I know you're trying to protect me, but Nancy is not like that. Besides, I don't know how to be careful with my heart."

"OK, Richie," she said, "I'm here for you, unconditionally." Betty hugged her son, there was nothing more to be said.

Richie tried to get that feeling back, he closed his eyes and thought of Nancy, and her kiss. It helped him feel better, the anger receded. Moms had to be moms, and he had to move on.

For a while, they were just quiet together.

Sometime later Paul stopped by. "How are you? It's been a long day, and you've been through a lot," he said.

"Yes, it sure has, and more than even you know," said Richie, "but I'm OK."

"I need to peek at the dressings over the procedure sites to make sure that they're not soiled or oozing. Does anything hurt?"

"They feel fine," answered Richie.

Paul examined the dressings, which appeared clean and dry. "You'll be starting IV fluids through your new catheter tonight. Dr. Stanner will be speaking with you tomorrow about the test results, the treatment protocols and the consents."

Betty answered, "Yes, we were told."

Paul continued, "I want to explain a bit about leukemia now, to prepare you for some of Dr. Stanner's talk. We've learned from studies that treatments sometimes failed because leukemia can relapse in parts of the body that we call sanctuary sites, places where leukemic cells can avoid effective treatment. Over many thousands of years, people have evolved a system of protection against inadvertent poisonings. Way back, when our ancestors ate something toxic, like a bad mushroom, it was an advantage to have those roadblocks. So, in a Darwinian way, those ancestors who inherited a mutation leading to the creation of a blood-brain barrier were more likely to survive and pass that protection on to their progeny. That barrier is comprised of a vascular system which restricts certain substances in the blood from reaching the brain. Under most circumstances that's useful. But in order to treat any cancer cells that could be hiding in your brain, we need to get around the blood brain barrier. Richie's treatments will include scheduled spinal taps. A needle is inserted into the lower spine, between two vertebrae to sample the fluid. A teaspoon or so of cerebrospinal fluid drips into a series of tubes which are then examined for disease. After collecting the fluid, we then use that needle already in place, to infuse intrathecal chemotherapy. The meds will circulate through the fluid that bathes the brain and spinal cord. That bypasses the blood-brain barrier and treats any leukemia that might be lurking there. So, tomorrow the treatment will begin with a spinal tap and intrathecal chemotherapy."

All those fears that he had started to control came roaring back. What did Paul say? Leukemia cells lurking in his brain. That couldn't be good. Chemo in his brain? What would that do to him? He had plans for the future, college and a high tech job. Chemo in his brain, that didn't seem to be good for his SAT scores. What kind of school would he be able to get into with a chemo brain, if he even survived? And there was the pain of another needle.

"It sounds painful. Will I be asleep for that?" asked Richie.

"You have a choice," answered Dr. Belkin, "I can arrange to have Dr. Street from the PICU come up and administer sedation. You would need to be NPO tonight, and not eat until after the spinal tap tomorrow. Or we can do this without sedation, often spinal taps are done that way. We're not puncturing bone, the needle goes through soft tissue, so it is not too bad. Instead of sedation, I can arrange for you to receive Versed, an anxiolytic which will calm you, though you'd still be awake. During the procedure, I'll also use a local anesthetic, which may burn for a few seconds, but then the area will be numb, and you shouldn't feel the spinal needle. Also during the procedure you'll need to bend into a tight ball, like you're doing a cannon ball splash into a pool. That'll be easiest if you're awake and can maneuver yourself."

"I'm not sure, what do you think, Dr. Belkin?" asked Richie.

"If you were less than 8 years old, I would suggest sedation, but I believe that you'll be OK without it," said Paul.

"Mom?" asked Richie.

"Can I be with him?" asked Betty.

"If you want, you can be in a chair, sitting in front of him. You'll wear a face mask with a shield, and a gown. From that position you won't be able to see the actual procedure, but you'll be able to talk to him, and hold his hand," replied Paul.

Betty looked at Richie, he nodded, and Betty said, "OK, we're good without the sedation."

"I think you'll be fine, Richie," said Paul. "I'm going to check on the other children, is there anything else I can do for you?"

"Thank you, Dr. Belkin," said Richie, "I hope you have a good night, and you don't have to come back out again tonight."

Paul smiled and left to see the other patients.

"I'm getting tired," said Richie, "How about you?"

"Yeah, but I'm not quite ready to go to sleep," said Betty. "Hey, let's see what's on TCM, maybe we can find something good. I can find some popcorn to make. Why don't you check the channels and I'll see if there's some snack to dig up." Betty walked over to the nurses' station to find out what was available.

Richie found the remote and the TCM channel, Ben Mankiewicz was talking about the movie coming up. Ben explained the general plot: Sidney Greenstreet played a Scotland Yard superintendent trying to solve a locked-room murder mystery, in the 1946 movie, "The Verdict."

The timing was good, just then Betty arrived with a steaming bowl of Paul Newman popcorn.

"What did you find?"

Richie said, "The Verdict, not the Paul Newman one, it's with Sidney Greenstreet. It's directed by Don Siegel, who also directed the original *Invasion of the Body Snatchers*. This should be good."

"That's cool, I don't think I've seen this one," let's go. Betty sat close enough to share the popcorn. The movie started with Greenstreet walking down a dark, foggy street, and they were hooked.

Transported to Sidney Greenstreet's world, Richie could forget that he was in the hospital, that he was sick. Movies were his sanctuary. He could hide and leave the worried world behind. While they watched the movie, his nurse connected Richie's new central line to a bag of IV fluids for the night.

An hour later the nurse came in to check. The movie was still playing, but Betty and Richie were fast asleep. She turned off the TV and the lights and picked up the mostly empty bowl of popcorn.

15.

Richie and Betty woke up as the medical team entered their room.

"Good morning," said Dr. Stanner, "How are you feeling today, Richard? Any headaches, nausea, or weakness? Anything at all that's bothering you?"

"No, I feel pretty good," said Richie, "I had a full day yesterday. I guess I was worn out."

"Dr. Belkin spoke with us last night, I'm sure you're aware. He gave us some idea of what would happen today," said Betty, "he told us you'd be talking to us about the treatment, and that hopefully we'll start that today. I was also wondering if you know about Richard's sperm banking report?"

Richie looked for a place to hide. "Really Mom," he thought but didn't say out loud.

"I should be able to look that up on Elsie, hold on a minute." Carrie hummed a bit while she scanned through screens on the rolling computer. "Here it is, one second. Yep, it looks good, the report shows adequate viable sperm numbers. So, the swimmers were moving, that's good. They've been frozen and stored and can be retrieved when needed."

"Thanks, Dr. Johnson," said Dr. Stanner, "after rounds I'll come back for a more detailed discussion, including Richard's testing results, information about the study treatments and answer all your questions. This is sometimes referred to as '*The Day*

One Talk.' Madelyn has reserved the patient conference room. Dr. Gardner and I will see you there in a little while."

Richie's nurse came over, "I'm going to draw a blood sample through your catheter, and then disconnect you from the IV pump. You'll be free to go to the conference room. There's a cart with breakfast sandwiches coming around, I suggest you get something to eat before the talk," she said, "you could be there a while."

"Thank you," said Betty. "Should I get something for you, Richie?"

"Thanks Mom," said Richard, "a breakfast sandwich and some milk with coffee flavoring would be great."

As they were finishing the egg and cheese biscuit, Madelyn let them know that Dr. Stanner and the others were ready. Richie and Betty got up and walked across the hallway to the conference room. Drs. Stanner and Gardner, and the pharmacist Stacy were already inside, waiting.

"Come on in," said Dr. Stanner, "make yourselves comfortable. I want to tell you a bit about myself, and some history of leukemia treatments. I think it's important for you to know how we got where we are today. Then I'll go over Richard's results and the plan. Finally, we'll talk about the details of the therapy, the consenting process, answer your questions and then we'll be ready to start treatment. Please stop me at any time if you don't understand something or have questions. OK?"

"We're ready, thanks Dr. Stanner," said Betty.

"Me too," said Richie.

"I finished my pediatric oncology fellowship nearly 30 years ago," Dr. Stanner began his talk, "it was here at Memorial Medical Center, just like Drs. Gardner and Belkin, so over the years I've taken care of hundreds of children with cancer. The outcomes for the vast majority have been good, but no one will be satisfied until we can cure every child. That means continued work and research. In the early 90's, when I started, cancer treatment consisted entirely of a combination of chemotherapy, radiation and surgery. There had been significant refinements along the way, but that triad of therapy was what had been available for more than 40 years. However, in the last two decades there has been a treatment revolution. We're now able to coax the body's immune system to attack cancers. There are also biologics that target cancer cells. Using these new technologies, we've been able to beat cancers in children and adults who we previously thought had no hope.

Betty asked, "I wonder why doctors talk about being in remission. I don't hear the word, *cure*, what's that about?"

"A good question," said Dr. Stanner. "The word *remission* may seem evasive. Remission means that through standard testing, we find no evidence of disease. We know that some leukemia cells can sort of hibernate and hide in the body during treatment. By staying quiet, those few cells may avoid the immediate toxicity of the chemotherapy. Years later, they may awaken, eventually leading to a relapse. So it becomes difficult to say when a child is cured. It's like combing through a haystack, trying to be sure there is no needle to be found. Likewise, it's very hard to determine if there are zero leukemia cells in someone. But we do know that if a child is still in remission five years after the treatment ends, the incidence of recurrence is extremely low, and we feel that is tantamount to a cure. Many families will celebrate that 5-year milestone."

"What did you find out about my leukemia, Dr. Stanner?" asked Richie.

"There are different types of leukemia, and if you had to have leukemia, the one to choose would be the precursor B cell Acute Lymphocytic Leukemia (ALL). And that is what you have. It turns out that the very youngest normal white blood cells and leukemia cells are somewhat confusingly both called blast cells. And although under a microscope they look the same, they are in fact very different. One matures into a normal functioning cell and the other is literally a dead end. There is molecular testing that we will use to tell the difference. It's normal to have up to 5% of the population of marrow blood cells identified as these baby cells. The appearance of more than 25 to 30% of the cells with those characteristics defines the diagnosis of leukemia. Your bone marrow sample showed that 80% of the white blood cells were blast cells. That confirms Richard's diagnosis."

"That sounds like a lot of leukemia," said Richie. Twists and turns churned inside Richie's head. He felt like he was riding an out of control roller coaster. Treatment hadn't even started, and he was nauseated. He wondered why all those shitty cells chose to wind up in his body, and what they were doing to him. Mostly he was scared that the doctors might not really be able to destroy all those fucking cells. Richie groaned.

"There are rules to assign a risk category for Richard's leukemia," answered Dr. Stanner, "but the percentage of leukemia cells in the bone marrow does not affect his risk, and while it's true that 80% is a lot of leukemia, it's not unusual.

The important criteria that we use to determine his risk category are the number of leukemia cells in a blood sample and his age. Later, genetic information about DNA mutations will refine his risk category. That important result will be available sometime later. But Richard must start his treatment now, we can't wait the week or so it will take for those results to be available.

As to age, the very highest risk is for infants less than one year old. Standard risk is for children from one to ten years old. So, although Richard's white blood count was less than 50,000, which is OK, his age at 17 years, unfortunately puts him into a high-risk category. This means we'll be tailoring his therapy according to the high-risk group."

"That doesn't sound so good." Richie drew his legs up, curled into a fetal position, and began to rock back and forth in his chair. A high-risk group, Richie's brain was screaming at him. That's all he heard. For the first time, he wondered what dying would feel like. How much would he suffer?

"Everyone does better when their treatment is tailored to the appropriate risk category. By using less therapy for the low risk, they improve with less side effects, and by using more therapy for the higher risk, they have better response rates. Most of the current data comes from studies done before the use of biologic agents and we expect that with the use of these new drugs we will see even better outcomes."

"What will his treatment be?" asked Betty.

"The new protocol most appropriate for Richard is available through the American Pediatric Cancer Organization, it adds Inotuzumab ozogamicin, which is only available to patients on study, to the previous standard high-risk protocol. Agents that end in 'mab' are monoclonal antibodies. These designer antibodies are created in a laboratory, and they target the unique proteins that dot the surface of cancer cells."

Betty said, "that seems amazing. Have you seen it work?"

Dr. Stanner replied, "we don't have the final report from this study, but there's interim data that shows a significant improvement. Every study is reviewed by a Data Safety Monitoring Board, independent of the study investigators. They evaluate outcomes from the treatment protocols in progress and have the power to stop it immediately if something concerning is discovered. This study began by randomizing children into two groups. One group received the antibody along with the previous high-risk therapy and the other group received only the standard high-risk chemotherapy. The DSMB found such a significant improvement in the antibody group that they stopped the randomization and now every high-risk child on study will receive the antibody along with the conventional high-risk chemotherapy."

"That's encouraging," said Betty.

Richie asked, "can this really work for me? It all sounds pretty awful."

Dr. Stanner responded, "Yes Richard, our data says that it often does work. Let me go on. The first treatment phase is called induction. The goal is to *induce* remission within the first 30 days of treatment. It's a very intensive cycle. We'll be prepared to respond to the inevitable complications.

We use some drugs to mitigate the expected side effects. Zofran will help with nausea, and there are other anti-emetics available if needed.

Most patients will experience nausea, hair loss, and bone marrow suppression. During the course of his therapy, Richard will require multiple transfusions of blood products."

"When do you think we'll start?" asked Richie. All he could think about was those leukemia cells slinking around in his body. It was them or him, and he wanted to fight.

"The treatment starts with the spinal tap," answered Dr. Stanner, "I expect that we can get that going in the next few hours. You spoke with Dr. Belkin last night and you're ready to proceed without sedation, is that right?"

"Yes," said Richie. He couldn't wait anymore. He stopped rocking, and closed his eyes. In his head he repeated his new mantra, "kill those fucking cells,' over and over. He pictured armies of chemotherapy agents battering all those sneaky cells. It was like a video game and he was ready to battle. "Dr. Belkin said I could get some Versed to relax me and you would use a numbing injection."

Sandra answered, "this morning before he left, Dr. Belkin, filled me in on the conversation you had, and I can make that all happen. I'll start with a numbing cream on the site."

"Well, I'm still nervous about this, but I'm ready," said Richie.

"OK," said Sandra, "while I get everything prepared, Selma will go over the signatures with you. Any questions before I leave?" Sandra waited and when there were none, she added, "if there's anything on the consent that you're not sure about, ask Selma to call me and I'll come back to address your concerns."

Richie looked at Betty, "I'm ready, let's slaughter those fucking cells."

With that, Sandra left and went to find Richie's nurse and the rest of the team. Steve was Richie's nurse again and Sandra found him at the nurses' station. "How are things, Steve?"

"I'm ready," Steve answered, "first up will be the spinal tap, right?"

"Yes, I hope to get that going soon, we'll be starting with the intrathecal Ara-C. Richard's decided to do this without sedation. His mom asked if she could be in the room during the procedure. She'll need a mask, a gown and a chair. I don't want to be managing a fainting parent. Any questions?" asked Sandra.

"That's fine, I think mom is pretty strong," said Steve, "but I agree with taking precautions. When are you expecting to do this?"

"In about an hour. I'll enter the orders and then call Stacy to make sure everything is prepared. I'm headed down with the team to see his marrow slide from yesterday. I'll be back after that to do the LP."

Sandra went into the fellow's room to work on the orders. She then called Dr. Stanner to ask him to review them before they were finalized.

Once back up on the unit after reviewing the marrow slides with the team, Sandra found Steve to check on progress. She then spoke with Stacy to be sure the chemotherapy, starting with the intrathecal Ara-C, was ready. The Ara-C would arrive on the floor in a sterile syringe, which was labeled, bagged and then sent in a padded capsule through the hospital's pneumatic tube system. The label would have Richie's name and medical number and warn: "For Intrathecal Use," as part of the safety steps to protect patients.

Sandra then called Selma, "are the consents signed?"

"Yes," said Selma, "I have Mom's consent, and Richard's assent and Dr. Stanner signed as the Principal Investigator. The APCO center has everything it needs, so Richard is enrolled on the study and has a protocol assignment number. The study drug will be available shortly. Stacy can make sure everything is set."

Sandra then called Dr. Stanner, "Just checking with you," she said, "I'm ready for Richie's LP. He's officially enrolled. I expect that you've reviewed the chemo orders. Anything else?"

"Great job, Sandra," said Dr. Stanner, "yes, it all looks good from here. I know you can do the LP. I'll only be there as backup. I'll be up in about 20 minutes, does that sound OK with you?"

"Fine, Dr. Stanner, see you then," Sandra hung up.

She walked over to Richie's room, "we'll be doing the LP in the next 30 minutes or so, do you have any questions?"

"You'll be giving me some stuff, so it won't hurt?" asked Richie.

Sandra thought back to her time in the hospital with mono. She was a few years younger than Richie is now. There were a few days back then when they thought she had leukemia. Of course, it turned out that she didn't, but she still remembered that fright. It must be ten times worse for Richie. The possibility of dying would be very real to someone nearly 18 years old. Doubts, uncertainty and fear would be filling his mind. Still, no matter what was going on inside, Sandra saw a young man on the outside doing what needed to be done. She had watched families debate the need for chemotherapy. Forgoing chemotherapy would be a disaster, Richie would be dead in a month without treatment.

"Yes, first you'll get IV Zofran, for nausea," said Sandra. "You'll get the Versed once you're in the procedure room, which will relax you, but you won't be asleep. You'll be able to respond to my directions and maneuver into the best position for the spinal tap. I'll apply the topical numbing cream now. That'll help when I inject the lidocaine at the site to complete the analgesic effect. OK?"

"Sounds good," said Richie.

"And I can be there with Richard, right?" asked Betty.

"Yes," said Sandra.

"Let's get you in the right position and we'll start by putting the LMX-4 numbing cream on your back. It should take about 30 minutes to achieve full effect. First, I'll lower the head of your bed so that it's flat, then you'll need to turn onto your left side, facing away from me."

Richie did as Sandra asked, "like this?"

"Perfect," said Sandra, "we talked about getting into a position like you're going to do a cannon ball jump, sometimes I describe it as making your back curve like a Halloween cat. Before you do that, please pull your shirt up above your waist and tug your scrub pants down just below the top of your hips."

"How's this?" asked Richie.

"Good," said Sandra, "just for a few seconds, practice, wrapping your arms around your knees and drawing them up to your chest." Richie did that. "OK, you can relax, you don't need to be in that tight ball now, but later during the spinal, you'll need to do that. I'll put on exam gloves and then you will feel my fingers hunt for right the spot." She put on the blue nitrile gloves from a box in Richard's room, then she felt the top of his right hip bone and slid her fingers down along an imaginary vertical line connecting the tops of his hip bones. She found the midline spot where his spine sat. Gently probing further, she found the space just below that imaginary line and between two lower lumbar vertebrae. She opened the LMX-4 kit, which contained a small tube of the topical anesthetic and an occlusive dressing. She spread the cream into a circle about the size of a half dollar, and then covered it with the clear occlusive dressing from the kit. The cream would sit there on his back and begin to numb the area.

"That's done, you can stretch out now," said Sandra, "later you'll have to find that position again. Try to avoid pushing on the dressing for a bit, we don't want the cream to ooze out. I'm going to talk to your nurse and get everything else ready. Any questions?"

Richie and Betty both shook their heads, they were more than ready to get started.

Sandra went to find Steve. "We're going to start soon, I've put the LMX-4 on Richard's back. Has the Ara-C arrived?"

"Yes, we got that about 5 minutes ago," said Steve.

"OK, good," Sandra replied, "Dr. Stanner should be up shortly, and we can then move Richie into the procedure room. I'll need an adult LP kit."

"That's all set up for you, Dr. Gardner, the monitor's ready so he can be hooked up as soon as he's there," said Steve. "What size gloves do you want?"

"I'll need the small latex-free gloves." Dr. Gardner double checked the syringe containing the Ara-C, confirming the 70 mg dose for Richie. She made sure that it was the only chemotherapy in the room during the procedure. The saline drip was ready in one arm of the 'Y' connection, the anti-emetic Zofran was infusing through the other, as they met in the same catheter lumen. The Versed was available and ready to be given just before the LP started.

When Dr. Stanner arrived on the unit as Sandra's back-up, they were ready to go.

Sandra rechecked the most recent lab results. His WBC count was 48,000, not much of a change, and his hemoglobin was better at 10 gm/dL, his platelet count was over 90,000. It was safe to do the spinal tap.

"It's all good," said Sandra, "we can bring him into the procedure room."

Everything set, Richie lay on the procedure gurney, on his left side. Sandra thought he seemed anxious but ready. She knew he wanted to get this over and done. Betty sat in front of him, holding his hand and began talking. She asked him to picture a fog covering the horizon on a dark stormy sea. In a calm, quiet voice, she continued, "now you see a light breaking through the fog, a brilliant red globe pokes up over the horizon, cutting through the fog. The skies light up and the ocean becomes quiet, a flat blue mirror reflects the rising sun, and seagulls dance lazily across the sky." Richie seemed lost in the image, his breathing slowed, a serene look transformed his face. A set of leads pasted on his chest, a sphygmomanometer around his arm and a pulse oximeter probe on a finger, all sent telemetry to the monitor.

Sandra asked Richie to get into the position he had practiced. The occlusive dressing was removed, and the LMX-4 cream wiped off. Sandra put on a sterile gown, a face mask with shield and donned a pair of sterile gloves. The LP kit was opened. Sandra swiped the betadine, serially using 3 soaked sponges, to clean the area for the puncture. The sample collection tubes were lined up in their tray, ready to receive the fluid from the needle hub. She covered the area with a sterile fenestrated drape allowing the working site to be accessed.

Steve tipped the open bag holding the syringe of Ara-C letting the chemo gently drop onto Sandra's sterile field.

"OK, Steve, everything looks set, and he's in good position,' said Sandra, "please start the Versed."

Soon, Richie told Betty that he could feel the drug. "You should definitely try this Mom," he said with a giggle. Betty just smiled and held his hand.

Sandra wiped off the dried betadine and began to infiltrate lidocaine into the site. "How are you, Richie?" she asked.

"Feeling pretty good," said Richie.

Betty smiled, softly speaking encouraging words, continuing the imagery to distract him.

Sandra picked up the 20-gauge spinal needle. Richie couldn't see the needle behind him, and Sandra kept it low enough so that Betty couldn't either. Spinal needles were scary long if you weren't used to seeing them.

"Here we go," she said. She slowly advanced the needle. From time to time, she would withdraw the central stylet to see if any CSF flowed. Finally, Sandra felt a subtle pop indicating decreased resistance. She knew she was in the right place. Now when she removed the stylet, crystal clear fluid dripped from the spinal needle's hub. As she collected the fluid, it reminded her of trips to watch the maple sap harvest in Vermont. She collected the spinal fluid in three serial tubes, each one numbered and labeled. Each sample would be sent for a different test. The fluid looked clear, like water. In addition to white blood cells, the fluid also contained glucose and proteins. She had a silly thought that if she gathered gallons of it and boiled it down, the result might be like that Vermont maple syrup. She smiled to herself, only a doctor might think of something that strange.

Once the fluid was collected, she briefly replaced the stylet, hanging halfway in the sleeve. Sandra then picked up the syringe containing the Ara-C and checked it once more. She removed the stylet again and then fit the nub of the syringe into the hub of the spinal needle still in place. Slowly she advanced the plunger, so that the Ara-C was pushed through the LP needle and into the subarachnoid space just below his spinal cord. It would then circulate throughout his CSF, killing any leukemia cells that might already be there. Once the Ara-C instillation was complete, Sandra smoothly withdrew the needle and syringe with one hand and covered the site with a sterile gauze using the other. The gauze was replaced with a band-aid and the procedure was complete.

"OK, it's all done Richard, you can stretch your legs out, and turn on your back."

"That was OK," said Richie, "I may have felt a little bit, but that medicine made it pretty cool."

"The fluid looks very clear, and that's good," said Sandra. "In the lab a drop of the fluid will be spread on a microscope slide and examined to see if there are any leukemia cells. We will also test for glucose and protein. Steve will move the table into a Trendelenburg tilt, head slightly lower than your feet, so that the medicine, which is denser than spinal fluid, will flow from the puncture site near your hips, down toward your head. We want the medicine to circulate throughout the central nervous system. After about ten minutes, Steve will straighten you out, though you should remain flat for another 20 minutes. We'll plan to start the rest of the day's chemotherapy in about an hour."

"Thank you, Dr. Gardner," said Betty, "that seemed to go well."

"Once you're sitting up again, you can eat if you're hungry, but try not to eat too much too quickly, pace yourself," said Sandra.

"Good work Dr. Gardner," said Dr. Stanner. "After you get these CSF tubes on their way and take a few moments to get settled, we'll meet in the fellow's room."

"OK, I'll see you soon," said Sandra.

Sandra then spoke with Steve, "have you cleared time for the chemo infusions? That'll start soon, the dexamethasone infusion and then the vincristine should each run over no more than 10 minutes. After that he'll receive the antibody, to run over an hour. We'll need frequent blood testing. Are you covering any other patients this morning?"

"It's all set," said Steve, the vincristine and the first dex dose are already up here. And I don't have any other patients this morning, I'll only have Richie as long as I'm needed."

"That's excellent, I'd like to be called when you're ready to infuse the vincristine, just to make a final check. I also want to be close by when the antibody starts. Though it's been humanized, it's still a mouse-based antibody, and he could react. We should have the crash cart on standby," said Sandra.

"OK, I got it," said Steve, "we had another patient about six weeks ago who got the antibody, she did OK, but I'm prepared. I think that Richie has been in Trendelenburg long enough, I'll raise him back to flat. He still needs 20 more minutes on his back, but he can finish that in his room."

"I'll be in the fellow's room, with Dr. Stanner, don't hesitate to call me if you need anything or have any concerns," said Sandra.

16.

Richie was in his room, laying on his back, the heart monitor, quietly pinging away, the 20 extra minutes were nearly done. He texted Nancy. "Finished spinal med, lying here, waiting. I was very nervous, seemed 4ever 2 get started. But now happy it's done. Not so bad. Can almost hear those bad cells screaming as the chemo hunts 'em down. It's like one of my video games. Kersplash. Pretty soon his phone was dinging. Richie smiled as he read the texts and dashed off responses. He was in his world now.

Steve came in the room, "how're you feeling?"

"Walk in the park." Richie answered.

Steve smiled, "I can raise the head of the bed now. You can get up in a few minutes."

"OK, maybe after the treatments are done for the day, I could get something to eat."

"Yep," said Steve, "the rest of today's therapy should start soon," and he left to check the meds.

Betty asked, "are you really feeling OK? No symptoms?"

"Yeah, I'm good Mom, how are you?" It was a real question, he wasn't looking for an auto response. Richie worried about how his mom was with all this.

"It's hard to believe that we came in on Wednesday evening, and it's only Friday morning, so much has happened. I've been anxious," said his mom, "but seeing how you've handled all of this, makes it easier for me. I've also seen how much you've grown up. Honestly, I'm kind of amazed."

"Mom, I want to talk to you about a couple of things."

"OK, I'm all ears."

"First, you are the best mom ever, and being here for me, has made all the difference in the world, I have no idea how I would have managed this on my own."

Betty smiled, "Thank you for saying that, but it kind of sounds like the good part of a critique sandwich, what else?"

"Can't put anything over on you, can I? There's more, but I meant what I said."

"OK, I'm ready to swallow the rest of the sandwich, what gives?"

"So, one thing's about you, and the other's about Nancy."

"Go, on."

"OK, so you've been here, with me, for almost two days, continuously, giving me support, even joining me when I couldn't eat. You've been trying to sleep in that chair, and that can't be very comfortable. There's still more therapy today, and I know you'll be here for that. But tomorrow should be a quiet day, nothing too dramatic should be happening, and if I feel OK in the morning, it would be all right for you to go home, you know, overnight and you could come back on Sunday. There's stuff you need, and getting a good night's sleep at home, that would be important. And it would make me feel better to know that you have a little time to yourself, recharge the batteries, so to speak."

"Richie, I think you're telling me you need some space."

"Ah, yeah, you've been great. But this is my disease, and I feel everybody watching me, including you. I'm like under a microscope and it's a bit suffocating. So, I do think I need some time by myself to process everything."

Betty turned away, but Richie saw the tear before she wiped it away.

"OK, Richie, I get it." Betty took a deep breath, "there's a lot going on here. I feel it too and I can probably use some of that space too. I do love you Richie. What's the other thing, about Nancy, you wanted to talk about?"

"Well, you remember she came to visit me last night with her dad," said Richie, "and you left us alone for a little while."

Mom was looking at Richard, she appeared anxious. Richard could tell she was worried about where this conversation was going.

"OK, Mom, I don't like where your head's at right now, please, she is not pregnant, OK!"

"OK, Richie, that's good. So what's this all about?"

"Well, I worry about her. We've connected, and it's amazing how quickly that's happened. She said something about watching her mother get chemotherapy and I know that her mom is gone. So I'm thinking about what she's going through watching me, and what dark memories that must bring up. It must hurt."

Betty watched her son. "It must be awful for you, Richie. I'm not sure what to tell you about Nancy. Your leukemia is affecting lots of people. I think that you both must be going through some difficult times."

"Mom, I don't want her to hurt because of me."

Betty looked at her son. She seemed to be digesting everything Richie just said. For now at least, she didn't say anything in response.

Just then, Steve came in and announced that the other medications would be starting soon. "Dr. Gardner wanted to be here, so I'll call her. First, I'll hang the dexamethasone, that can start without her, but she wants to be here for the vincristine, and the antibody. You should be finished with today's chemo in about 2 hours. Well, there will be a second dexamethasone infusion tonight, but that shouldn't be a big deal." After checking the label, and scanning Richie's wristband, Steve started the dexamethasone "that should be done in about 10 minutes," he said, "I'll be back." Steve walked out to call Sandra and let her know the other meds were ready.

Just then Richie got a new ping on his phone. He read Nancy's words to himself. "Maybe I shouldn't have told you about my mother, but it felt right at the time. You're going to be fine, Richie. It didn't work for her, but it'll work for you. My heart is with you."

It was the perfect text, at the perfect time. He read it over and over. Maybe he was in love.

Soon Sandra appeared, "how're you feeling, Richie? Anything bothering you, nausea, headache, chills?"

"Well, I guess I'm a bit hungry, I only had one egg sandwich, like forever ago," answered Richie.

"Hunger is a good sign." Sandra smiled.

"I also wanted to let you know that one weekend a month, us first-year fellows have time off, and that's tonight. A couple of the senior fellows will be covering. Monday, Dr. Belkin will be back as the daytime fellow, and I will be covering the nights. We switch night and day coverage each week. But I'll still be here until this evening."

"Thank you, for everything you've done," said Betty, "and I hope you get a chance to rest up and maybe have some fun this weekend. It's important. Speaking of recharging, you know, Richie wondered if I might go home overnight tomorrow, and return Sunday. I'm not sure if he was concerned about me or trying to get some space for himself. Anyway, I wonder what you think?"

"Being here can be overwhelming, I do think it's good to get out," said Sandra. "If things look stable tomorrow morning, it should be a safe time to leave. On Monday, Richard will get another new chemotherapeutic agent, called pegylated asparaginase, another element in his therapy cocktail. I don't expect any significant problems, but I think that you'd want to be here for that. Does that make sense?"

Betty didn't answer. Richie watched his mom. He thought she was still hurt from his request. But his mom was strong and well, he needed the space.

Sandra refocused on Richard's chemo and monitoring his reactions. She explained, "we're expecting to have to manage something called tumor lysis syndrome. The cells are like tiny packages, and as his leukemia is attacked, the packages break open and their contents are dumped into his blood stream. We could see dangerous increases in his normal blood salts, particularly potassium and uric acid. There are ways to address those changes and we are set to intervene as needed."

"How long do we have to be worried about that?" asked Betty.

"It could have started already, we'll check labs after the antibody infusion is finished. We'll be watching carefully over the next 48 hours."

"By the way," said Sandra, "the antibody infusion is about half over, how are you feeling, Richard?"

Richie glanced at the monitor, wondering what Sandra was looking for, "I feel fine."

17.

Betty was also watching Sandra as she studied the EKG on the monitor. The tracing repeated over and over. Betty couldn't tell anything from the screen, it looked like a lot of squiggles to her. But she didn't like the look on Sandra's face. Sandra lifted the stethoscope from around her neck and listened to Richie's heart. She took out her phone and called Steve, "can you come back here, I want you to send the labs I ordered right now. Also, bring the crash cart over. Thanks."

Betty's expectations about the side effects of therapy had, until now, been theoretical, like reading the warnings on a Tylenol package insert. But Sandra's request for the crash cart abruptly brought her to reality. The color drained from her face. She felt her heart banging in her chest. She sat down to make sure that she didn't pass out and wind up on the floor.

Sandra spoke, "I see changes in Richard's EKG." She pointed to a segment of the EKG that looked like a little pointy spike. "This is the 'T' wave, when it gets bigger and pointier, it means that his potassium blood level is climbing. We're prepared to manage that. In a way it's good, it means his cells are breaking up in response to the treatment. But if the potassium levels become too high, it can lead to dangerous heart arrhythmias, or even cardiac arrest. I'm going to check his chemistries now. I'll also increase his fluids and give Lasix which will make him pee out some of that excess potassium. I may soon be requesting an insulin and glucose solution. The insulin will signal the normal cells to suck up some of the potassium in his bloodstream. That'll help lower his blood level."

As his nurse arrived, Sandra asked, "Steve, please draw the labs I ordered, maybe you can hand them off to someone to make sure they're sent off, stat. Then I want you to give 10 mLs of 10% calcium gluconate, over 3 minutes, it should be on the crash cart. That'll help stabilize his cardiac muscles."

Betty was in complete panic mode. She heard Sandra on the phone asking for medications, something about glucose and insulin, followed by more requests. The rapidly unfolding events seemed like alarm bells blaring. The crash cart, the orders being barked out to Steve and over the phone, the look on nurses' faces, none of that looked good. Betty couldn't tell how much trouble her son was in. Was he dying right now in front of her? She had watched medical dramas on TV. *Code Blue* would be announced and doctors would appear out of the woodwork. Chest compressions would begin, all clear shouts, electric shocks, patients bouncing on the gurney, a flat line on the monitor, doctors shaking their heads and then a sheet covering the patient. All those images flashed through Betty's brain.

"Steve as soon as you're done with the calcium gluconate, let's give 40 mg of IV Lasix, and please turn up his normal saline IV rate to twice maintenance, that should be about 160 mL/hr. I'm going to get on the horn to the lab to be sure we get those lab results back ASAP."

Sandra was back on the phone, asking for lab results. Betty heard her say, "I need those now."

Betty watched as Sandra looked up at the monitor again. She shook her head briefly and muttered something that Betty didn't understand. Weren't those pointy mountain waves Sandra showed her earlier, still there, were they bigger? Betty couldn't tell, she imagined they were worse. Her heart was in her throat, her mouth was dry, all she could think was "please be OK."

"How do you feel Richie?" Sandra asked. Again, she pulled off her stethoscope and listened to his heart. Just then the monitor alarmed. Sandra reached up to silence it. It would alarm again if nothing changed in the next 5 minutes.

"I can feel my heart racing." Richie said.

"Any palpitations?" asked Sandra.

"I dunno know, what's that?"

"Steve, have you given the calcium gluconate and the Lasix yet?"

"Yes, both are onboard," Steve replied.

"Palpitations are a feeling that the heart is beating too fast, or irregularly or skipping beats," Sandra answered Richie's question while reaching for her phone. But before she could dial, she heard the nurses' station's phone ring.

The nurse came over quickly, took a breath and reported, "I have the following panic values: potassium is elevated at 7.2 mEq/L, his uric acid is high at 12 mg/dL, phosphate is elevated at 5.5 mg/dL and his calcium is too low at 6 mg/dL."

"Not surprising. None of those are good. Please bring over the full print copy." She speed-dialed Stacy who answered on the first ring, "OK, I need the sugar-insulin bag right now. I'll also need the Rasburicase, but get the insulin first, OK?"

"Dr. Gardner, you asked about palpitations," said Richie, he had his hand resting against his chest, "mostly my heart is beating fast and hard. It's very fast, Dr. Gardner. It could be skipping beats, it's hard to tell. I feel really weird, like something bad's going to happen. It's very scary."

Betty couldn't think. She couldn't sit still. She paced around the small room, finding corners to lean on. Betty scanned the monitor, watched Sandra and fixed on Richie. She was in full panic mode.

"It's because the potassium is too high. We're going to fix that. Let me know if you feel any other changes," said Sandra. "Your blood pressure is good, and so is your perfusion, so you're

OK, for now. The abnormal lab values are from tumor lysis. The meds I'm giving you now will help, they just need some time to work. Remember, the results we just got are from the blood that was drawn before any treatment," said Sandra. The monitor alarm began again, and she reached up once more to silence it.

"How worried should we be?" asked Betty. She could barely get the words out and she wasn't sure she was ready to hear the answer.

"Everyone's working on it, Betty. I have two more meds to use, and then we'll check labs again," said Sandra.

One of the aides came over with a bag of fluids, "this just came over for Richard," she said.

Sandra checked the label on the bag, "OK, Steve, this is the glucose-insulin solution. Please run this over 30 minutes."

"Got it, 30 minutes," said Steve. All the nurses were now on full alert, focused on the acute events in Richie's room. There was no need to call a code, not yet. But it had certainly crossed their minds.

Again, she called Stacy, "As soon as you can, please send up the Rasburicase."

Richie announced that he had to pee. Sandra smiled, "that's good, it means the Lasix is working." Steve brought plastic urinals for Richie who hid under the sheets and quickly filled the vessels.

"Richie's filled two urinals," Steve reported. "I've got all his fluids charted, everything going in and coming out."

"What's the balance?" asked Sandra.

"He's positive 500 mLs," answered Steve.

"Good, we have room to get more off, I may repeat the Lasix in a few."

A few minutes later an aide came over carrying the bag with the Rasburicase.

"Steve, how much time is left on the glucose-insulin bag? And how much urine have you collected?"

"He filled four urinals now, about 4 liters, and we have 15 minutes left on the glucose-insulin."

"Good, as soon as that's finished, flush the line with saline and hang the Rasburicase, also to run over 30 minutes." Sandra had to reach up to silence the alarm again. Each alarm deepened Betty's fear. She watched the EKG tracing as it danced across the monitor. She was now able to pick out those nasty T waves from the rest of the squiggles. Was anything else changing? She couldn't tell. Her stomach was in a knot, it hurt. She imagined the worst, a low, deep guttural groan emerged as she tried to hold on.

"What are you feeling Richie?" asked Sandra.

Betty also wanted to know. She didn't like hearing the alarms blaring. Betty was frantic, but she had no way of helping. It wasn't a good feeling.

Richie answered, "about the same, my heart is racing, pounding. I still feel jittery, like I drank too much coffee."

Sandra explained, "the Lasix helps Richard pee out some of the potassium, the glucose-insulin will force some of the potassium into his cells and that hides it from his heart and kidneys. His heart sees less of it because more potassium's been tucked away. We need more time. Richard will get the Rasburicase next, a synthetic form of uric oxidase. It's what makes bird poop white. The Rasburicase enzyme will chew up the uric acid in his blood and that will protect his kidneys."

Richie had to pee again.

Steve brought more urinals, working under the hospital sheets, Richie promptly filled two more.

"Excellent," said Steve. "There's about 5 minutes left on the glucose-insulin infusion, as soon as that bag's finished, I'll flush the line with saline, then spike the Rasburicase bag, and hang that."

"Thanks," Sandra responded, "keep the saline running in the other lumen. Send another set of chemistries right now."

Steve pulled off another set of labs, and then started the Rasburicase. He handed the tubes to the aide to be run *stat*.

Betty now saw the beginning of a smile on Sandra's face as she looked up at the monitor. "The T waves may be just a bit softer, the QRS waves not so broad and his heart rate has begun to slow. The rhythm is more regular. I haven't had to shut the alarm off in a little while, that's all good."

Betty liked the news, but she remained on guard, she wasn't ready to relax.

The fluids continued to run, as Steve started the Rasburicase. Richie filled more urinals. Sandra kept her eyes peeled on the telemetry.

Betty watched Richie. Did he seem less anxious? She was finally able to come out of the corner and over to him, to sit by his side and hold his hand. "I'm here for you Richie. You've got this."

It wasn't long before the latest results were back. His potassium was down from 7.2 to 6.9, his uric acid dropped from 12 to 10, his calcium improved a bit from 6 to 6.5 and his phosphorous was down from 5.5 to 5. Everything was moving in the right direction, his glucose level was acceptable at 90, but they were still not where they needed to be.

Sandra seemed to be considering the latest information, she turned to Richie and Betty. "These results are better. The meds are doing their job. We're not out of the woods, but we've managed the worst of it. We need to continue to be vigilant. The tumor lysis, albeit at a lower intensity, will continue for days."

Sandra looked up at the monitor again. She continued with orders, "when the Rasburicase is finished, flush that lumen, stop everything for 5 minutes, and repeat all the labs. Make sure there's a CBC too, I want to know how his white blood cell count has changed, it was 49,000 this morning, before the therapy started. Once you've drawn all those labs, restart his D2.5W, normal saline at 160 mLs/hr. You can stop his allopurinol, the

Rasburicase will be filling that role. Continue the Lasix, every 6 hours for the next 24. Also please make sure Richie steps on a scale every 6 hours, I want to know how his weight is changing with all those fluids coming and going. Steve, only when he's awake, OK."

Betty waited for Richie. What Sandra was saying sounded good, but she was anxious to hear how Richie was feeling.

"Dr. Gardner, I'm feeling a little better, not so jittery and less pounding in my chest." Richie managed a slight smile.

Steve saw the difference too, "good job with this." Steve smiled and gave a thumbs up to Sandra.

"Thanks, Steve, we've managed this together, but we're not done, there's more to come. I'm going to the fellow's room. I want to update Dr. Stanner. All the meds, doses and times should be documented, so I'll see them in the EMR, along with the most recent lab results. I'll be back in a few. I have my phone, call anytime." She turned to go.

"Dr. Gardner," it was Betty, as she stood up. She was pale as a ghost, her face was sprinkled with tiny beads of sweat. "I'm glad you didn't have me hooked up to the monitor just now, I think it would have been alarming like crazy." Betty came a bit closer to Sandra. She wondered what went through Sandra's head as she performed her medical magic. Betty was a mess, but Richie's doctor seemed cool as a cucumber. Was she really like that inside? Betty didn't know, but she was grateful. Something was beginning to change in Betty's head. These were no longer strangers caring for her child. A connection was growing that would transform their relationship. "Um, would it be OK if I gave you a hug?"

Sandra reached out, and Betty came to her, wrapping her arms around Sandra. She whispered in her ear, "thank you." After a few moments Betty let go, she smiled at Richie's doctor, and watched her as she left for the fellow's room.

Betty sat down next to Richie. She was drained. She looked at her son, who seemed comfortable, and at least for the moment didn't appear to be in danger. Betty watched the monitor, the heart tracing looked better to her. She was learning. As best as she could tell, the pattern seemed normal, anyway there were no roaring alarms blasting away. Thoughts raced through Betty's head, reliving the last hour, how quickly things had changed, how danger seemed to arise without warning. She wondered how close she had been to losing her son. She looked at him again, at rest, peaceful for now. She felt that mother's love, as it washed over her, it was wonderful and disturbing, all at the same time.

Betty had been through so much with Richie, and yet he was just a teen, a young man who deserved to have much more life ahead. She realized that all those experiences that should be his, might not ever happen. Love with a woman, children of his own, building a life, watching his children grow up and start their own lives, all that should be ahead of him, and the chance that it might never be, brought some quiet tears. As those thoughts ran through her head, she watched Richie, tranquil for now.

Richie looked at her, "Mom, what's going on?" he asked.

"That was kind of scary."

"Yeah, I was worried for a while," said Richie, "but Dr. Gardner was awesome, don't you think? I feel OK now."

"Richie," said his mom.

"Yeah."

"Remember what we talked about before?" His mom continued, "as to me going home tomorrow, I don't know. We'll see."

18.

It was the end of the school day, the end of the school week, like no other that Nancy ever had. So much had happened, the active shooter's drill, the moments on the field behind the school, the kiss, Richie's diagnosis, seeing him in the hospital. Images swirled in her head. It was hard to sort out. A frisson of déjà vu passed through her. She couldn't help what she felt.

Just then she got a text from Richie, and she shot one right back. "I've been thinking of you," she said, "call when you can." She sent smiling heart emojis.

Nancy was in the shot gun seat with her dad driving home.

Walter watched his daughter, busy on her phone. He was pretty sure it was about Richie, but he worried about intruding on her privacy. Instead he asked, "how did your library committee meeting go today?"

"It was pretty good. I'm so glad I signed up for that when I started here. And I really like the librarian, Ms. Shute. You know she's into world history too and we've been talking about adding to the library collection, particularly books about Asia."

Walter glanced at Nancy and sighed. "I hope that all those stories I've told you about my service during the Afghanistan War were not too graphic." He seemed to gaze off into the distance, transported to somewhere far away. "I still have nightmares. Sometimes, out of nowhere, I feel like I'm hunkered down in those frigid mountain ranges, taking cover while an unseen enemy is shooting at us. It was horrible."

"It's OK, Dad. That time is part of who you are. The history of that part of the world's been very complicated. It helps me to learn as much about it as I can."

"I worry that some of the troubles you've had in schools are because of my stories."

Nancy was surprised. "Gee, Dad, I didn't know you worried about that. It's fine. All of what you had to do is part of why I'm interested in history. And that's going to be my major in college." She smiled at Walter, "and then, of course, law school."

"I'm so proud of you, honey."

Nancy was quiet, thinking about all that's happened. Her phone rang. Nancy had programmed a unique ring for Richie. "Hi, Richie," she answered, "is everything OK?"

"I just love hearing your voice," Richie answered, "and I can't wait until the rest of you is here. I feel good right now, but it's been a wild ride, like it was crazy here for a couple of hours, like a horror movie. Dr. Gardner was awesome, and like the whole team was in action, working on me. I felt like Frankenstein's monster, strapped to the table with lightning crashing and exploding around me. The only things missing were electrode bolts sticking out of my neck and Dr. Gardner, wearing eye goggles and screaming at the heavens. Anyway, I'm alive. It was scary for a while, but it's cool now. Mom was pretty freaked, but Dr. Gardner was a cucumber."

"Oh, Richie, you've got me all worried again," said Nancy.

"It's OK, I'm fine, maybe I souped up the imagery a bit," said Richie, "but I'm really OK. They know what they're doing here. Nancy?" said Richie.

"What?"

"It's nice to hear that you're worried about me."

"Yes, well, I do worry about you, and I don't think you need to make the danger seem any greater than it already is, thank you very much. I'm riding with my dad, we're on the way back home."

"That must be nice, the school week's over for you."

"It's OK. Are you really all right? I worry when I don't hear anything."

"I'm good, really, and it's just the steroid tonight and through the weekend. The next new chemo won't be until Monday," said Richie, "they got me peeing like a racehorse, it helps get the potassium out. There's a slew of urinals that I keep filling up."

"TMI, Richie."

"Sorry. Here comes Dr. Gardner, I gotta go."

"OK, I'm thinking of you, call me later, and I'll see you tomorrow." Nancy rang off but she couldn't stop worrying about Richie. Every time she thought about him in the hospital it reminded her of her mother's harrowing experiences and her treatments. She closed her eyes and cried.

Betty was sitting next to Richie, reading her book about mid-century modern art. Several clients at the gallery were interested in that period, and the background information helped her close sales. She tried not to listen too closely to his conversation. Richie was clearly smitten with Nancy, a "first love," whatever that meant at seventeen. So much going on. She saw Sandra approaching and closed her book. Betty looked up at the monitor, as far as she could tell it seemed OK. She noticed Sandra carrying a paper and stood as she approached.

Sandra didn't waste any time with formalities, "I have the newest lab results. How do you feel Richie?"

"Pretty good, my heart seems regular, and I've been peeing, cause I know that's what you want."

Sandra smiled. "It does sound like you're better, and the labs back you up. First, the white blood cell count is already down from 49,000 to 25,000, that's great, so the leukemia is responding nicely to the treatments. I knew it would be better, because of how things were unfolding with the tumor lysis, but I wasn't sure how much better. It's quite a nice response."

"What about the other labs," asked Betty, she was quickly learning what was important.

"Right," said Sandra, "his potassium is down from 6.9 to 6.0, his uric acid is down from 10 to 8, and that should continue to get better with the Rasburicase onboard, his calcium improved a bit from 6.5 to 7.5 and his phosphorous is down from 5 to 4.5, so all the labs are improving. I'm quite happy with these results.

Richard will receive the dexamethasone tonight and twice daily for the rest of the induction month. I'll keep the fluids and the Lasix going for the next 24 hours and then those might be adjusted. We'll continue to check his labs every 4 hours through the night, and as things stabilize, we can increase the interval between checks. Richard can eat whatever he wants, well no bananas, too much potassium, and he can walk around the unit. He'll have his IV pole as an escort wherever he goes, at least for a while. Remember to save all the urinals. Your nurse needs to record everything. You're still getting the anti-nausea medicine, Zofran, around the clock, though depending on how you feel we may be able to cut that back. Any questions?"

"Do you think we'll be going through another event like we did this afternoon?" asked Betty.

"Not anytime soon, not this weekend. But it could happen again, especially after next week's antibody infusion, on day 8. We'll be prepared," answered Sandra.

That wasn't the answer Betty was hoping to hear. The thought of going through another crisis like that made her feel sick.

Sandra looked at them and waited a moment to see if there were any more questions. "I have a few more hours today, and then I'll be signing out to the senior fellows covering the weekend. Dr. Solomon, and Dr. Friedman will be splitting the coverage, I'm not sure how they're divvying it up, but one of them will always be available. They will, of course, have backup from Dr. Stanner. Dr. Belkin and I will be back on Monday, but next week, as I said, he'll be covering the day and I'll be here at night."

"Thank you, Dr. Gardner, I'm sure we'll see you before you go, but I hope that you have a wonderful weekend, and you have our deepest appreciation," said Betty.

"Ditto for me," said Richie.

Sandra smiled and turned to walk back to the fellow's room.

Betty looked at Richie again, she hadn't spent this much time with him since he was a toddler. She watched the news most days and heard about awful things happening to other people, and of course she understood that bad things could happen to anyone, but now this crisis was not happening to anyone, it was happening to them. Cliché as it may be, it hit home, reminding her of what was truly important. When Betty looked at Richie, she felt something inside, not something new, but that old feeling that began way back in her college days, when he was growing inside. That feeling had grown and developed, as he did, blossoming with his birth. Those first weeks of his life, she held her breath each morning as she checked his crib to be sure he was still breathing. Betty breastfed him, cuddled him and talked to him constantly. She read those first books to him, pointing to the pictures as he followed along. She heard those first words and watched him take his first steps. Back then, there was nothing more important in her life. More recently she'd been distracted by the worries of daily life, work, budgets, and so much other stuff. Other stuff, whatever that was, she couldn't even remember now. These events, however awful, had pushed all that other stuff into a distant background, tucked away, where it should have always been. Life was precious, fragile, and yet also tenacious, and it was more important than anything else. This would be a new beginning for her, priorities reoriented, a new/old way of seeing things. It was sad that it required a crisis to wake her up, but there it was, she was determined not to lose her compass again.

Betty also thought about her job, it provided for their lives. She knew she needed to talk to her boss again. She would find Madelyn this afternoon. Suddenly she heard her son calling, it brought her back from her reveries.

"Mom, yoohoo, Mom, ... where are you?... Earth to Mom, come in Mom!" Richie had been trying to get her attention.

Betty turned and smiled at Richie, "I guess I was pretty far away," said Betty.

"What were you thinking about?" asked Richie.

"Oh, you... us, everything, life, I dunno," Betty answered.

"I guess you *were* pretty far away."

"Well, maybe not so far," said Betty, and she reached over to touch her son. "Were you trying to say something?"

"Well, I am getting hungry, so I guess that's good."

"Oh, OK, that does sound like you're better," said Betty, "I need to talk to Madelyn. I'll go over to the nurses' station and see what I can find out about her and food. Maybe they're going to order out again. Any requests?"

"The chicken sandwich was good, I could go with that again, but I'm fine with whatever you pick, Mom, just, you know me and Michelangelo, no anchovies, please."

"OK," said Betty, "still a Ninja Turtle, huh." Betty walked over to the nurses' station.

Meanwhile, Richie began texting Nancy again. Still in the car with her father, Nancy's phone lit up. "My doctor was here, she's awesome. I just had some good blood test results. She's happy, Mom's happy, everybody's happy,"

"Thanks for the update, sounds good," texted Nancy. "I'll C U tomorrow."

"What time?"

"Not sure, talk more 2 nite, OK?" Nancy pushed send and followed with more smiling emojis.

Nancy's dad was still driving, but he couldn't help noticing all the texting. He decided to venture a question. "You really care about him, don't you?"

"Yeah, Dad, it's real. He's nice and sweet, and kind of cute. I feel something when he's around, you know."

"Maybe we should have a talk?"

"Oh, Dad," Nancy giggled, "it's not necessary, I know all that stuff. I had the talk with Aunt Ruth, quite a while ago."

"Oh, I see," said Walter, "that's good. But there's more than just ah... the mechanics, I'm here for you if you want. You may not believe this, but I had those feelings too."

Nancy looked at her dad, "what was it like, with Mom, when you met her? Do you remember?" They had talked about this before, but Nancy was in a different place now, and ready to hear the story anew.

Walter glanced at her, quickly returning his eyes to the road, "like it was yesterday, I remember everything about the first time I saw your mom. It was at a school party. I saw her across the room, her eyes twinkled, and the rest of the world vanished. I wasn't sure if she saw me, or what I should do next."

Nancy listened. She couldn't remember the last time that they talked to each other like this. Nancy wanted to hear more. "Dad, I kind of feel like that with Richie."

Walter glanced at his daughter again. "I think Richie is nice, but just be careful, honey."

Careful? What the fuck does that even mean? Her dad was not seeing her. She wasn't a little girl anymore. Had he been careful when he first met Mom, or when she was sick? Nancy was upset and frustrated with her dad, again. She thought about Richie and what he was going through, it brought a strong feeling of déjà vu. Once again, she loved someone in trouble. A frisson of dread shot through her. She was way passed being careful.

19.

Betty was at the nurses' station, chatting up the evening charge nurse. She was a bundle of nerves and it helped to have someone to talk to even if the nurse only listened.

"Thank you for listening, Nurse Somners, I actually came over to see if I could get in touch with Madelyn," said Betty.

"I'll have her paged, she may still be around. Anything else I can do for you?"

"Yes, last night the staff was ordering out for dinner, I was wondering if you guys might be doing that again tonight. Richie and I are getting pretty hungry."

"We're just getting ready to order some pizza, from nearby, I can take a request."

"That would be great, maybe we could get a large cheese, pepperoni and mushroom pie, a Coke for me and a Dr Pepper for Richie. I've got some money in the room. I'll be right back."

Meanwhile, Sandra was walking towards Richie's room and saw Betty. "How are you, Ms. Samuelson? I know we focus on the patient, but the parents are really patients too."

"Betty, please," she answered, "I was just talking to Nurse Somners, she's a good listener. I hope I can talk with Madelyn later. They said they would page her.

The whole thing is crazy, I doubt that anyone could really be prepared for this, but I'm managing and that's mostly because Richie seems to be doing well and because everyone here seems to know what they're doing. I can't ever thank you enough, Dr. Gardner."

"Thanks for the kind words. We have another set of labs cooking right now," said Sandra, "I expect they'll show continued improvement. We'll go over those results before I leave. Ms., I mean Betty, I don't usually do this," Sandra reached out with her business card, "but here's my cell phone number, you can call me if you need to."

That was so unexpected, Betty was not sure what to say, all she managed was, "thank you Dr. Gardner, I will do my best to respect your time off."

"Just tuck it away somewhere, I'm probably not supposed to do that. Let's go see how Richie is."

Richie was busy texting Nancy when his mom and Sandra came over.

As they were walking over, Richie's nurse handed Sandra the most recent lab report. Sandra looked over the report, she smiled, "these results look very good. Potassium is down to 5.5, uric acid is 4, and that's in the normal range, his calcium has improved to 8.0 and phosphorous is now 4, these are all better, and very nearly normal. His white blood cell count is down to 20,000, so the chemo is continuing to do its job. Richard's hemoglobin has fallen to 7 gm/dL, normal for him would be at least 12. That won't improve on its own, so he'll need an RBC transfusion. His platelets are OK at 50,000. By the way, Betty, I also looked up the results of his spinal tap. The glucose and protein levels were normal, and there were no red blood cells or blast cells in the CSF, so that's all very good news."

Betty smiled. She'd been wound tight as a drum. Hearing the new numbers brought some relief. The difference was palpable, the furrow in her brow relaxed, the tension in her shoulders gave way, the knot in her stomach eased. Even the pitch in her voice dropped a bit, "that's wonderful. Thank you Dr. Gardner, for everything."

"Dr. Gardner, I've been peeing like crazy," said Richie, "do you still need to give me so much fluid? I think that medicine is making my kidneys work overtime."

"I'm going to order the red blood cell transfusion for you," answered Sandra, "and I'll have the IV fluids turned down while that's going. If the next set of lab tests also looks good, the order will specify that the nurse can turn down the IV rate and increase the interval between Lasix doses. That should make it more comfortable for you," said Sandra.

Richie reached up to high five his doctor, and she responded. Betty watched, she smiled at the display. Betty was astounded at the human capacity to adapt. Just a couple of days ago, they were faced with a potentially lethal diagnosis, and now, anyone watching them would have no idea that that had been so. Betty watched Sandra as she left to find Richie's nurse and then over to her computer to place the orders in the EMR. Betty turned to her son, and raised her hand for a high five, but she hesitated. "Fuck that!" she said, and gave Richie a big bear-hug squeeze, "I'm happy, Richie. It's all good news." They held each other for some time. It was an emotional roller coaster, and this part of the ride was good.

"Hey Mom," said Richie, "I think this is the first time since all this started, that you seem OK."

Betty looked at Richie, seeing him again. It seemed she was doing that more than any time since he'd been in the crib. "Well, I'm not sure if I'm OK, but this moment feels good. Hey, there should be food coming, I ordered a pizza for us. And I asked to see if I could get Madelyn to talk with me."

"I'm hungry, pizza sounds excellent," said Richie. Out of nowhere it seemed, he asked, "are you worried about your job?"

Betty was about to answer. She had not considered that Richie was thinking about her. But just then the food delivery guy appeared. He carried several large pizza box sized insulated containers. That created a buzz. He unzipped the bags and pulled out at least a half dozen pizzas, unloading them onto the counter. There were also several sub sandwiches, and lots of drinks. Apparently, the crew was hungry because most of it disappeared into the back very quickly.

"We'll talk about that, Richie," said Betty, "but I'll go get our pizza first, we should eat it while it's hot."

The pizza was indeed hot, and tasty. With each luscious bite, a trailing string of melted mozzarella had to be managed. "Hmm, good," said Richie as they chowed down. He made three slices disappear quickly. Madelyn showed up while they were enjoying their pizza.

"That looks good," said Madelyn, "their regular pizza place, I see."

"Yeah, it's good," said Betty, "you want some? We have plenty."

Madelyn said, "No you enjoy, you can save the leftovers. You might be hungry later."

"Thanks for coming by," said Betty, "I was hoping to talk to you."

"I can come by later, when you're done eating," said Madelyn.

"No, it's fine, I sated the hunger beast, let's do it now." Betty looked over at Richie, who nodded.

"OK," said Madelyn, "we can go to the parents' conference room to chat."

Betty stood up, "that works," she said and followed Madelyn.

Pretty soon Betty was using the Kleenex box again, she could keep it together in front of Richie, but here, with Madelyn, behind closed doors, the tears flowed. "Sorry, I'm sorry," said Betty between sobs and tears.

"There's no need to say that," said Madelyn, "it's OK to cry. People are always asking, '*how are you doing*?' but I'm not going to ask you that, first, because most people really don't know, and second, because words are often inadequate to express those feelings. I see you functioning on the outside, but I know that inside, it's probably not going quite as well. There are no right or wrong feelings. Betty, I've done this for a while and I know that there are two patients named Samuelson on the unit. Your son already has lots of medical people caring for him. It's part of my job to help the other Samuelson."

"Yeah, I do need the help," said Betty.

"I asked you before about family support, and you said that there's no family," said Madelyn.

"There really is no one."

"What about friends, co-workers?"

"Richie has some friends," said Betty, "they hang out, play video games and seem to have a good time together, but I don't really know their parents. Between my work and Richie's school, and just managing the house, I really haven't had much time for friends. Maybe that sounds kind of sad, I guess, but we've been OK, Richie and me."

"I want to talk about your work in a minute," said Madelyn, "but before I do, I want you to know that you're not alone. We have a support group, parents of children with cancer. They know what you're going through, they've all been there, and they can be an excellent resource. I can connect you. In addition to emotional help, they may also be able provide some financial support. Money comes from local groups, but there are also national groups with deep pockets. Mostly they work quietly, but they have some clout," said Madelyn, "I'll introduce you, when you're ready."

Betty tried to listen but her mind was elsewhere. She wasn't ready to meet a new set of strangers. It was enough to focus on Richie's treatments and what she would say to her boss at the gallery.

What about your work, Betty? You've been here a few days. I imagine you've discussed your absence with your boss. Tell me about your work, the more I know, the more I can help."

"I have degrees in art and business. I help manage an art gallery," said Betty, "it's a small business, but we have some high-end clients. I've been on the phone several times with my boss. So far, she's been supportive and understanding, but I don't know how long that will last."

"How long have you worked there?" asked Madelyn.

"It's been seven years, and recently, Shelley, my boss, seemed to have hinted about a promotion. She likes my work. But then all this happened."

"There are laws that are designed to protect you when there's a catastrophic illness in an immediate family member," said Madelyn, "but I hope that we don't need to use those. In my experience, people can be very understanding. I can help with Shelley if you want. I can provide her with details about the time that you'll likely need based on Richard's diagnosis. OK?"

"That might help, I'll let you know."

"Do you think that you can do some of your work remotely?"

"I probably can do some online, especially the bookkeeping. Of course, with the pandemic and all, I've had a lot of experience with that already."

"Good, you should explore those options with Shelley," said Madelyn. "Have you talked to Richard about when it would be OK, for you to leave the hospital for a bit?"

Betty smiled, "my Richie can still surprise me, he's growing up so fast," said Betty, "he's already brought that up. And that's one of the reasons I was looking to talk to you."

"I've been impressed with what I've seen of your son," said Madelyn, "I think that says a lot about you."

Betty smiled, "there is no other Richie."

"When Richie brought that up, he was thinking about you, and himself," said Madelyn. "You both need some space, and only you can provide that. Tomorrow is Saturday, why don't you start with just a single day away? Do you think you can do that?"

"In theory, it sounds like a good idea," said Betty, "but I'm not sure."

"What's making you hesitate? Is it about you or Richard?"

"I guess he seems OK, for now, and he's in a hospital with oncology experts. So, he's in the safest place anyone could imagine. But it's me. If something should go wrong, and I wasn't here, I don't know if I could ever forgive myself. Maybe that's silly."

"Betty, of course that's not silly. But returning to normalcy, starts with small steps," said Madelyn, "doing things that are normal, even if they don't feel normal, just doing them starts the process. Waking up in your own bed, getting dressed, putting on makeup, doing the usual chores, showing up for work, even if it's just a few hours, that's the way back. And you can do it."

"OK, I think I'll feel guilty about leaving, but I guess I'll have to do it some time. So, if Richie seems all right tomorrow, I'll go home. Clean up, put on some fresh clothes, and head out into my other world." Betty was psyching herself up. "I can probably go to work for a few hours tomorrow afternoon, Shelley would like that."

"Good, you have my cell number, it's OK to call me on the weekend, if you need to talk." Madelyn stood up.

As they walked out together, Betty turned toward Madelyn and said, "thank you, it helps to talk."

Betty stopped in the bathroom before going back to Richie's room, she washed her face, trying to erase any evidence of her meeting with Madelyn. She looked in the mirror. She appeared worn, "you can do this," she told herself. A big breath, a shake of the arms, and Betty stepped out.

Back in Richie's room she saw that the RBC transfusion was about halfway through. Richie was busy playing a video game. He had his headset on. He was working the controller, pushing buttons, moving the joystick, bobbing and weaving side to side, telling the machine to behave, trying to beat the game, whatever that one was. He was so involved he didn't notice that she was back.

"Hi, Richie, I'm back, how's the game?"

"Gee, Mom, I didn't hear you," said Richie, "it's good. This one's new for me. There are lots of tricks to learn."

"Can you pause it for a minute?"

"Sure, what's up?" Richie paused the game. "How was your talk with Madelyn?"

"It was good, Richie. We talked a little about you, but mostly about me. She asked me about work and when I thought it might be OK to leave the hospital for an overnight, and of course I told her that you had already mentioned that. Madelyn thought it would be good for both of us."

"What did you say?"

"I've been thinking about it, and if you are all right in the morning, I'll go home, as long as I still have your permission. I'll call Shelley this evening and see if I can come in for a few hours tomorrow afternoon. Anyway, I'll be back early Sunday morning."

"That's good Mom, I'll be fine. There's a couple of things I need from home, including my laptop and some school stuff."

"I'll feel a little guilty leaving you."

"It's cool Mom, don't feel bad, there's really no chemo til Monday, just the decadron, and I'm OK, I can keep busy. And I think I may have a visitor," Richie smiled.

"I see, maybe I shouldn't feel guilty. Is Nancy coming?"

"She said she would try to come."

Betty noticed that Sandra was approaching. "I guess your day is almost up Dr. Gardner," said Betty.

"Yes," Sandra replied, "very soon. I see that Richard's red cell transfusion is almost done. How are you Richie?"

"I feel great," said Richie, "do you have another test result?"

"Yes, everything's continuing to improve, so I'll tell the nurse to lower your IV rate and decrease the Lasix. Overnight, we'll just check labs every 6 hours, instead of every 4. It's all good."

"Thanks for everything, Dr. Gardner," said Betty, "everyone here's been wonderful, and I hope you and Dr. Belkin have a good weekend off, you certainly deserve it."

"Thank you, I'll see you Monday evening. Have a safe and medically boring weekend." Sandra turned to leave, Richie and Betty, could see her heavy backpack with all of her medical stuff slung over her right shoulder. They waved, but Sandra had already turned and disappeared into one of the elevators.

It had been a very long day, with perhaps too much excitement. Betty would try to leave those events to memory and just veg for the evening. She still felt conflicted about leaving in the morning. Her heart said one thing and her brain had a different idea. Logically, leaving was the right thing to do and she was bound and determined to walk out as long as he was safe.

20.

Richie and Betty had a surprisingly quiet night. On the night shift, the required blood samples were taken from his central catheter and Richie slept undisturbed. He woke up once to pee, he reached for the urinal at his bedside, used it and fell quickly back to sleep. He'd adapted to the hospital routine remarkably well.

Betty stirred hearing a smaller skeleton team of doctors as they gathered outside their room for weekend morning rounds. She reached over alerting Richie to their imminent entry.

"Good morning," said Dr. Stanner, "I think you know everyone here except Dr. Solomon." Dr. Sarah Solomon, one of the upper year fellows, raised her hand. Dr. Stanner continued, "Dr. Solomon will be covering today and tomorrow during the day. At night it will be Dr. Friedman. The regular team will be back on Monday."

"How are you feeling today?" asked Dr. Solomon.

"I feel good, I slept pretty well," answered Richie, "how were my labs last night?"

Dr. Carrie Johnson, at the C.O.W. said, "they're all improving. A few are in the normal range." She read each chemistry value, though the team had already reviewed them outside the room.

Betty listened to each of the lab results, ticking them off in her head. She'd always been a fast learner and the numbers were beginning to mean something to her. Even without the doctors saying, she could tell that the results were good. She felt more confident about her decision to go home for the day.

Dr. Stanner said, "we'll be taking another sample soon, and depending on those results, we may be able to make some changes that will make the next few days more comfortable. We'll check the complete blood count and the usual chemistries with the next blood draw. There's a new blood test for today, in preparation for the PEG-asparaginase on Monday. Since that medication can affect the way your blood clots, we're going to check your coagulation system. That'll tell us if you need vitamin K, to shore up the clotting factors. Unfortunately, this test can be unreliable if it's taken from the catheter, so someone will be taking a blood sample using a peripheral needle stick."

Richie said, "no problem. So, if my tests are better, can I be unleashed from the pole for a while today?"

"We'll see, it's possible," said Dr. Stanner, "you'd have to keep drinking though."

"I will lug a tank of water around on my back if that means I can be unhooked," said Richie.

Carrie performed a cursory exam, listening to his heart and lungs, and declared that everything was fine.

"Dr. Solomon will be here for the day, and I'm available if she has any problems," said Dr. Stanner, "do you have any questions?"

"If this next set of blood tests are OK, I may go home for the day and come back tomorrow morning," said Betty, "do you think that would be all right?"

"Richard's stable, now, and I don't anticipate any big changes," said Dr. Stanner. "He may need a red cell or platelet transfusion, depending on today's results, but I don't expect there to be any significant problems. His nurse can call you if anything comes up.

"Thank you," said Betty, "I haven't decided for sure. I'll wait for the next lab report."

Dr. Solomon said, "I'll be here all day checking in on Richard frequently. I'll let you know if anything comes up, but we'll likely have a quiet day." With that, the team filed out.

It was about an hour later, when Richie and Betty were nearly finished with their breakfast, that Dr. Solomon came by with the next blood test results.

"Everything looks good," Dr. Solomon said. "His white count is down to 5,000, which is great, his platelet count is only 30,000, he might need a platelet transfusion tomorrow, we'll see, but nothing today. The chemistry labs are in the normal range. The coagulation studies are still pending. Depending on those results he might need vitamin K. He can come off the IV fluids for a while as long as he keeps drinking. We'll check his labs later to see if they remain stable. Medically speaking it should be a boring day." Dr. Solomon seemed happy.

"What about the Lasix?" asked Richie, he didn't want to be carrying the urinal around.

"I think we can hold off on that for now, we'll see with the later lab results," said Dr. Solomon. "Ms. Samuelson, if you are still interested, I think your plan for the day should be fine."

"Thank you, Dr. Solomon," said Betty, "I'm going to talk to Richie, but I think I'll be going. I'll have my cell phone, so please call me if anything comes up."

"Will do," said Dr. Solomon, "we'll take good care of Richard," and she turned toward the nurses' station.

Betty looked at Richie. "I'm fine," said Richie, "please don't feel guilty, it's OK, nothing will happen overnight. I'm in a pretty good place anyway, you know, it's a hospital."

Betty sighed. She knew Richie was right. But the devil was whispering in her left ear. "If you go home, something will happen to him, and you'll blame yourself." She hated that guy. She knew the right thing to do. She knew leaving would make Richie happy, and her boss Shelley happy. She had things to do.

"OK, you're right. I can bring some things back for you. I know you want your laptop, maybe some of your textbooks?

"Yes, that'd be good, I probably need my math and French books, you can call me before you come back tomorrow."

"I'll call you tonight anyway," said Betty. She stepped over and sat on the bed next to him. Betty put her arms around him and squeezed, "I love you Richie, you are my world."

"I love you too, Mom."

21.

Richie's nurse came over, "Dr. Solomon said I could unhook you for a while. I'll flush both lumens of your catheter, and cap them off so you can be free. Sound good?"

"Yes ma'am," said Richie.

"Please don't call me that, it makes me feel old, just call me Annie, OK."

"OK, Annie OK," pleased with himself, he smiled at the joke.

Richie was alone. His mom was usually hands off, letting him figure things out, sink or swim. But she was definitely a helicopter mom since his diagnosis. He felt the gusts from her whirling rotors. Today was just an intermission, a bit of freedom from his mom and from anything too heavy in the hospital. Richie was determined to enjoy the break. He walked around the unit, exploring it for the first time since his admission. He found the Child Life room, it was packed with books, board games and puzzles. There were also several video games, which could be hooked to the TV in his room. Walking further along he came across the small snack area with all kinds of eats. Further on down the unit he found the medical supply room with boxes of stethoscopes, blood pressure cuffs, thermometers, and pulse oximeters. Other shelves were filled with medical tape, bandages and sterile nitrile gloves lined up next to stacks of IV fluid bags and cartons of tubing. Poles and pumps stood crowded in the corner. As he moved on, continuing his tour, he came to the procedure room where he had his LP and bone marrow exam. Now, without sedation, he was able to see it clearly. It triggered hazy memories. He'd been knocked out for the bone marrow exam, and then he was awake, but drugged, for the spinal. There'd been a swarm of gowned people behind masks. He remembered the smells of antiseptic and his mom sitting in front of him. Images played in his head. He was the center of attention, but not in a good way. He decided it was better not to dwell on that too much. He moved on. It didn't take long to complete the small circuit around the unit.

As he came up to the nurses' station again, Richie's nurse came by and said, "don't forget to keep drinking fluids, you need to pee more."

"OK, Annie," said Richie, "will do."

"Here comes Dr. Solomon," said Annie.

Richie turned around to see his doctor walking over.

"Everything OK over here?" she asked.

"I'm good."

"Your coagulation lab tests came back and one of the tests called a PT, was a bit prolonged," said Dr. Solomon, "so I've ordered a dose of Vitamin K for you. Your nurse will access your catheter and you'll get it through the IV line."

"You mentioned that test before," said Richie, "what is that?"

"Well," said Dr. Solomon, "your body has a coagulation system, to control bleeding. There are two parts. One part is made up of the platelets, and the other arm consists of a series of proteins that work sequentially to produce a clot to stop bleeding when there's an injury. The platelets are tiny cell fragments, normally slick like Teflon, but they become sticky when you're injured. If their numbers get too low, you're at risk of bleeding. To prevent that you receive platelet transfusions, like you've already had a number of times. The other arm of the system, made up of a series of proteins, helps the platelets form a plug to fill a laceration and stop bleeding. That part is called the coagulation cascade, because one protein activates the next. Think of dominoes lined up. As one is pushed over, it pushes the next, and the one after that, and that continues until the last domino falls. That's when the clot forms. We know how long it should take for all those dominoes to fall, and if it takes too long, well then one of those dominoes, or in this case one of the proteins, is missing, or not produced correctly. So, the vitamin K will help fix that."

"I see," said Richie, "I'm on the school track team, it sounds like a relay race, handing off the baton from runner to runner, until someone crosses the finish line."

Dr. Solomon smiled, "that's a good way to think about it," she said. "What we found is common and nothing to worry about. It's easy to fix by giving you the needed vitamin. OK?"

Richie gave the thumbs up. He sat down on his bed, took out his pad and colored pencils and began to draw a new comic strip. It featured a lost space traveler trying to navigate around nasty green alien creatures and giant black toppling dominoes. Maybe he could turn it into a video game. He was soon completely absorbed in his work.

22.

Richie was sitting in his room, busy with his comic strip when he was abruptly torn away from the aliens. He looked up to find that he had visitor.

"Hi, Richie," said Nancy, "I see you're drawing another comic strip. What's it about?"

"I've been thinking about you," said Richie, "yeah, it's something I had an idea about."

"It looks scary," said Nancy. "How're you feeling?"

"Well," Richie smiled, "my lips feel kind of lonely."

"We can't have that," said Nancy, and leaned over, pressing her lips against his.

"Hmm, that was nice," said Richie. "Sit down next to me." She sat down on the bed, as close as she could.

"You smell good," said Richie. He thought of a summer breeze and newly blossomed purple lilacs. He leaned toward her, with his nose to her neck, breathing in her perfume, and then kissing her softly right there.

"Richie," she giggled, "I keep thinking about you. That feels good, but I also worry."

"I'm OK, Nancy," said Richie, "but it's kind of nice to know you worry."

"I do. What's happening to you has me terrified," Nancy sighed. "Dad dropped me off at the lobby. He's got some business in town. He'll come by to get me in about an hour, so we have some time together. Where's your mom?"

"Mom went home this morning, she'll be back tomorrow," said Richie, "I told her she should go. She needs a recharge. Anyway, not much is happening here during the weekend, at least treatment wise. I'm going to get a new chemo drug on Monday, but Mom will be here by then."

"You look good, Richie, maybe a little thin on top," said Nancy, "is the medicine really bad?"

"It's not so bad, they put a tube in my chest, so the medicine goes through there," said Richie, "sometimes I can taste it after it goes in."

"That's kind of weird," said Nancy, "it goes in the tube, into your body and then you taste it in your mouth."

"Yeah, I guess it's all connected," said Richie.

"Does it hurt where the tube is?"

"Nah, maybe for a little while when it first went in, but not anymore."

"Can I see?"

Richie pulled his top up, showing Nancy where the tube came out from under his collarbone, he wore a chest sleeve netting that kept the end of the tube from dangling.

"Can I touch it?"

Richie nodded. Nancy reached up, and put her hand on the tube, tracing along it, and touching his chest where it emerged. She felt the tube and his chest, a merger of human and plastic. "Does it hurt, when I touch you?"

"Your fingers feel nice," said Richie, "I like it, wherever you touch me."

"Well, Richard J. Samuelson, you are sounding normal." she smiled. "It's good to see you like this. At home I have all kinds of shitty, dark thoughts about you. It freaks me out. Aren't you worried?"

"I'm sorry about that, Nancy. I get freaked too, thinking about those cells traveling through my body. But I don't want you to feel bad. The doctors are telling me that the medicine is working. The white cell count is way down, and that's good news."

"I guess so, but I wish this never happened to you. You know, it brings back bad memories. When my mom was so sick, I watched her. I didn't really understand it back then. But now I do. I couldn't stand it if you..., well you know."

"Nancy, that's not going to happen." Richie tried to reassure Nancy, but he was also trying to convince himself.

"I know."

They held onto each other. Richie didn't want to let go. He felt safe with her in his arms. He was sure nothing bad could happen as long as they were together.

23.

Betty was at the gallery trying to focus on her work, but it wasn't easy. She kept thinking about Richie alone in the hospital. It didn't help that news traveled in a small town. It was nice to think they cared, but every time she heard, "*I'm so sorry. We are praying for Richie*," it ratcheted up her angst. She thought that if she heard that one more time she would scream. Betty wished that her son didn't need anyone's prayers.

Her boss Shelley came over, she looked concerned. "Why don't you take a break. Maybe go in the back and call Richie. Take as much time as you need."

Betty was grateful that she had an understanding boss. She went into the back room and pushed Richie's speed dial button.

Nancy had already left and Richie was back working his drawings when his phone rang. "Hi Mom."

"Hello, Richie, how are you?" she asked.

"I feel fine, really, like normal. I did find a few more clumps of hair on the pillow. And I guess they gave me some Vitamin K, through my tube, but I feel OK, I've got an idea for a new video game. Where are you?"

"I'm at work, but I've been thinking about you, Richie," said Betty, "I feel like I should be there."

"Mom, I'm fine, really, I miss you too, but I've been busy, and I'll see you tomorrow morning, right? You don't have to worry about me. How's work?"

"It's good, Richie, it's a little hard to concentrate. I keep thinking about you. Shelley has been incredibly understanding. She's going to let me do more work remotely, I'll probably have to come into the Gallery a few hours during the week, but she said that'll depend on how you are."

"I wish you didn't worry about me. It's been a quiet day.

"That's nice, so you're really all right?"

"Yes," said Richie. "Nancy came to visit."

A new girlfriend on top of everything else, Betty worried that Richie would get hurt in his budding relationship. "I see. That's nice, Richie, a lot of girls probably would have just moved on after what happened, it means something that she hasn't."

"She's not like any girl I've ever known, Mom. Course, I haven't known many. Nancy makes me feel special." Richie took a breath, "you know, we can talk about anything. I'm comfortable when I'm with her."

"I'm glad," said Betty, "and of course you are special."

"Are you almost done at work?"

"Yes, I'll be going home soon, probably stop for groceries on the way. I'm looking forward to taking a nice bath, and getting a good night's sleep."

"Maybe a glass of wine, huh, Mom?" said Richie, he smiled.

"Yes, I do think you know me, maybe too well."

"OK, yeah, anyway I guess we'll talk again before you go to sleep."

"Absolutely, talk to you soon. I'm glad you're feeling OK. You know, I can still come back tonight if you want."

"I know you could, Mom, but I'm really OK, and it makes me feel better that you get some time for yourself."

"All right Richie, somewhere along the way, I seemed to have found a way to raise a good guy. I'm so proud of you. I gotta go before I start crying. Talk to you soon, bye."

"Bye," said Richie, and they ended the call.

That night Betty was alone in their house. She couldn't remember the last time that happened. Everywhere she looked, she was reminded of her missing son. His jacket hanging from the hook in the entryway, the fridge stocked with enough food to feed an army, all his clothes scattered around the TV room, they all poked at her heart. She sat down at the kitchen table, laid her head down on her crossed arms and cried.

24.

Richie must have fallen asleep working on his drawings. The next thing he knew was that his mom was there, running her fingers through his hair, "good morning, Richie," said Betty, "sleepy head, it's almost 10."

"I guess, I was pretty tired, huh," said Richie, trying to rouse himself.

"I see some strands of hair coming off on my hand, so that's going as expected," said Betty, "maybe I should find a buzz shaver and do it all? We'll get you looking like Telly Savalas."

Richie smiled, a fan of the old TV shows that were now streaming online, "I'd need a Tootsie Roll lollipop."

"I guess you would." Betty leaned forward and kissed the top of his head, "are you OK?"

"I'm good, and I really did miss you. I'm glad you're back." Richie enjoyed the space he had yesterday, but he was very much relieved to have his mom back. He didn't need to put on a brave face with her, he could just be Richie. And right now he needed his mom to be there for him. She was his rock. "Whenever we've been up against it, it's been you and me, Mom. We're the A-team, right? I'd be lost without you."

They sat together, drawing strength from each other. It was a quiet moment that they both needed.

"I brought you what you asked for from the bagel store." She opened the bag and took out the two bagel sandwiches and the drinks, hot chocolate for Richie and café au lait for her.

"Mom, can you turn around for a minute, I really have to pee."

"Sure," said Betty, she stepped out of the room, until she heard the 'all finished' clearance from her son.

"Look," said Betty, "I also found something I thought you might like in the Black Light store, near the gallery."

Richie pulled off one of the metal ends of the cardboard tube and found the rolled-up poster inside. He extracted the gift and unrolled the paper.

"It's a movie poster for the Creature from the Black Lagoon," Betty said. "I know you don't have that one. I thought you might like it while you're here. Later it could go in your room at home, next to Count Dracula."

"Wow, that's really cool, Mom," said Richie. "It's from 1954, with Julie Adams and Richard Carlson. The creature on the poster is carrying Julie. Like Godzilla, you could see it was a guy in a costume." Richie was full of information. He loved telling what he knew. "The actor, Ricou Browning, was the diver for the underwater monster scenes. It was shot in 3-D. Everyone wore those colored glasses, with the red and green lenses. When they hunted the creature in the water, they used harpoon guns that shot deadly spears. With the 3-D the spears seemed to come right at the audience, everyone ducked and screamed, I guess. Hey, you know what else? There were two actors playing the creature. Ricou was kind of small, so they used Ben Chapman, a bigger guy when the monster was chasing Julie around on the boat deck.

Thanks, Mom, this is great. I'll hang it up later," said Richie. He was hungry and dove into the bagel with the works. "Mmm, this is good, and the hot cocoa goes perfectly." He was still chewing, but between bites, he managed, "so your day was OK?"

"I did miss you, Richie, but I guess I needed to spend some time at the gallery. Shelley's been sweet and she asked about you."

Betty was drinking her coffee and eating a much simpler plain bagel with cream cheese when she saw Dr. Solomon approach.

"Good morning, Dr. Solomon," said Betty, "I brought a bag of bagels and two tubs of cream cheese, chives and regular, it's over at the nurses' station. Some of the bagels are still warm."

"Thank you very much," said Dr. Solomon, "I'll check those out in a bit. How are you both?"

"We're OK," said Betty, she looked at Richie, "aren't we? I just got here a few minutes ago."

"They told me you'd gone home yesterday," said Dr. Solomon, "is everything all right at home?"

"It's fine, Dr. Solomon, thanks for asking. Richie told me you wanted to talk to us. How is he?"

"Richard has been responding very well to the treatments," said Dr. Solomon. "His chemistries have been good. His blood counts are dropping as expected. Richard's platelet count this morning is less than 20,000 so he'll need a transfusion. His hemoglobin is OK at 9 gm/dL, which is low, but not low enough to need an RBC transfusion. His WBC, white blood cell count, is very low, as expected. It's now less than 1,000, which is part of the reason he needs to stay in the hospital. Although we can transfuse platelets and red blood cells, it doesn't work so well for white blood cells. Those cells live for only about seven hours, so a transfusion of white blood cells won't last long enough to provide much benefit. It will be a while longer before his marrow is healthy enough to produce those cells.

At some point we may need to use antivirals for Richard. There can be fungal infections as well, which require their own type of drug. Now that his WBC count is so low, we need to be even more vigilant for signs of infection. I told Richard yesterday that it's important to let us know if he feels hot, or chilled or if he notices anything different. We should screen all his visitors, to bar anyone with any signs of illness. All visitors should wear masks."

"Should I be wearing a mask?" asked Betty.

Dr. Solomon answered, "if you've been outside for the day, it may be worth wearing one for at least the first 24 hours that you're back, until you can be sure you haven't picked up any new bugs."

Richie immediately wondered about visits with Nancy and how careful he needed to be. Wearing a mask would definitely put a damper on those saliva swaps. He'd have to figure out a way around that.

"Richie said you were going to talk about his chemo tomorrow," said Betty.

"Yes, he's going to receive a drug called PEG-asparaginase, it's one of several important medications in the ALL treatment cocktail. The medication has two parts, first the active moiety, the enzyme L-asparaginase, and secondly, the enzyme is pegylated, which means it is covered with a cloaking substance, a modified form of polyethylene glycol, the stuff in *MiraLAX*. That keeps the enzyme hidden from the body's immune system. That allows the drug to last longer and to be less likely to trigger an allergic reaction, two good things. The second part, the enzyme l'asparginase, breaks down one of protein's essential amino acids, asparagine. Since normal human cells make asparagine, and leukemia cells can't, it selectively inhibits protein synthesis in the leukemia cells and so it only, well mostly only, destroys the bad cells. But one of the significant side effects is that it can increase the risk of blood clots. That's why we checked his coagulation system and gave him a dose of vitamin K yesterday. He'll need a second dose today."

"Thanks for that information," said Betty.

"Do you have any other questions?"

Betty and Richie shook their heads.

"OK, I'll check in on you guys later."

"Thanks, Dr. Solomon," said Betty as she watched her walk away. Betty turned toward Richie, "did you get all that, Richie?"

"Well, some of it," said Richie, "I understood the low white cell count stuff."

"I got that too, and I also heard that all visitors should wear a mask," said Betty. "I'll go get one right now, be right back."

Betty was back in a few moments, "it seems the bagels I brought are disappearing quickly. Richie, I also brought some of the things you asked for. I have your textbooks, your laptop, and some clothes."

Richie rummaged through the new stuff. He thought about all the schoolwork he'd already missed, and the effort it was going to require to make it up. "Ugh," he sighed. Everything had been piling up and all of a sudden it seemed overwhelming. The new drugs, worrying about his low white count and wearing a mask to prevent infections. And final exams coming up at the end of his junior year. His thought about French class was summed up in one word, "merde."

Sitting there, tired even before he started, he watched as Annie delivered his yellow bag of platelets.

"Is that my chicken soup?"

The nurse hung the bag of platelets on the IV pole and connected its tubing to Richie's central line. "That'll take about an hour," she said. "You know, now that you mention it, it does look kind of like chicken broth. I guess it's good for what ails you," she chuckled.

Richie and his mom settled in for what they hoped would be an uneventful Sunday afternoon. Richie's platelet transfusion was almost done, and his nurse would follow that with his second vitamin K dose. His line would then be flushed, and he could be disconnected from the IV pole for a while. He was still behind on his schoolwork and knew that he needed to get back to work. In his head he heard his mom saying, *'it's not gonna get done by itself, Richie.'*

He opened his laptop, connected to the hospital Wi-Fi, using the password he was given: Well1234. It wasn't very inventive, but it was the guest Wi-Fi and he thought security was probably not a high priority, likely there was little information to hack on the guest Wi-Fi. He had his Horace Mann HS website lined up among his screen icons and clicked on that.

The junior year teachers were listed. He clicked a teacher's hyperlink and found everything he needed for that class. Per his usual strategy, he chose to start with French. He wore his headphones with the attached microphone to practice his skills.

Betty left the room and set up her laptop in the day area. She had her own personal hotspot so she could log in to her worksite securely, www.PikchureThis.com. There was a public access icon on the website to explore the Gallery, but there was also a private tab to click, bringing her to a password protected login for employees. Betty clocked in and started catching up on the bookkeeping.

Richie worked on his French, practicing pronunciation. "La plume de ma tante est sur la table," the program would decide if he said it correctly. It was bad enough that he had to be graded by his teacher, now the bot was assessing his work too. Just as he was getting started, his phone rang, a welcome distraction. It was Nancy's call ring, "Frére Jacques, dormez vous?" he answered immediately, "Hi, Nancy, watcha doin?"

"Just sitting at home, thinking about you and wondering what you're up to."

"I feel like I'm in school again, I was practicing French. I don't think the bot likes my accent."

"Fuck the bot, Richie, who's the human here?" she giggled.

"You're right, what's the world coming to?" said Richie, you know, I've only missed three days of school and it seems like there's a shit load of work to do just to catch up and even more will be added tomorrow."

"Don't worry about it, Richie," said Nancy, "you're taking high school classes and battling leukemia at the same time, you're doing way more than any of us. The teachers know. Maybe I could come over after school this week and we could work on some stuff together. Would you like that?"

"Well, I definitely would like to work on some stuff with you."

"Richie, you bad boy," she giggled, "it's still you inside, I like that. But I imagine all kinds of awful things happening to you."

Richie was trying to focus on the positive. It was all so stressful. Right now, he just wanted to talk about anything else. "Really Nancy, you don't have to always worry about everything that might go wrong," said Richie. "I'd rather not even talk about that."

"I'm sorry, Richie. I didn't mean to get you upset."

Richie realized that he'd been sharp with Nancy and he immediately regretted what he said. "It's just hard to keep thinking about all the bad things. I shouldn't have snapped at you."

"It's OK, Richie. I can't even imagine what you're going through. Maybe we can talk about it more tomorrow. I'll just say goodbye til then."

Richie heard her start to cry just before she hung up. He started to call her back, but then thought maybe he better not.

It was an hour later and Betty had done what she could for the Gallery, she packed up her stuff and came back to their room, "I got a lot of work done," said Betty, "did you get a chance to go through some of your school assignments?"

"I started the French, but, you know, it seems so foreign." He started to mention the phone call with Nancy, but he wasn't really in the mood to talk about it.

"Yeah, well I guess it does," said Betty.

"What should we do?" asked Betty, "want to find a movie to watch? I saw a collection of DVDs in the Child Life room."

"Sounds good," said Richie, "I'll walk over with you, and we can pick one out."

Richie was looking forward to sitting down and just vegging with a movie. His mind was a jumble, his head hurt, there seemed to be trouble from every direction. It was hard to think straight. It seemed that everything was going wrong. His blood counts were tanking, he had to wear a mask, he worried about his mom, he had a ton of school work and final exams, and he was probably an asshole during his last conversation with Nancy.

25.

Betty and Richie must have been very tired, once again they couldn't finish the movie. No more than fifteen minutes into the film, they were both asleep, and the next thing they knew the full medical team was coming into their room for rounds. It was the same team as last week, except Paul was leading the rounds, not Sandra.

"Good morning, how're you feeling?" asked Paul.

"We're fine," said Richie, he wondered how many times someone had asked him how he was feeling. It was a lot.

"Good to see you this morning, Dr. Belkin," said Betty, "I hope you enjoyed your weekend break and I expect it'll be nicer for you on the day shift."

"Thank you for asking, I did enjoy the weekend," Dr. Belkin smiled.

"Richard will be getting the intravenous pegylated asparaginase. He'll get Zofran first, but that chemo is not very emetogenic, so he likely won't have much nausea."

"So, that's the last new medicine for me?" asked Richie.

"Well, on Friday," answered Paul, "you'll have another LP, and the intrathecal medicine will be methotrexate, instead of the cytarabine. You'll continue to get the dexamethasone twice every day. But, other than the methotrexate in the LP on Friday and the PEG-asparaginase today, you'll have seen all the induction chemotherapy drugs at least once."

"How are the lab results?" asked Betty.

Carrie was there with Elsie, and she said, "I have them right here. The chemistry results are all fine," she said, "the CBC, shows the hemoglobin is 9 gm/dL, reflecting last night's transfusions. The platelet count is only 17,000 and the WBC count is zero."

"Zero? That doesn't sound good at all. Can it really be zero?" asked Richie.

"Yes," said Paul, "with the strong chemotherapy you're receiving, zero is pretty much par for the course. It will be like that for a while. You'll have to very careful, but there are germs everywhere. They live throughout your body, and no matter what you do, the likelihood is high that one of those bugs will cause an infection," said Paul. "I'll order a single donor unit of platelets for you after rounds. The chemo and Zofran are already ordered," he looked at Stacy, who nodded in confirmation.

Dr. Stanner added, "Richie, we want to start antibiotics as soon as possible after a fever develops, so it's important to let us know if you feel anything different."

Paul added, "the nurses are ready for this. There's a *Golden Hour,* and survival improves dramatically if the antibiotics are started within the first hour after the appearance of symptoms. Here in the hospital, of course, antibiotics will be started quickly, usually within 10 minutes or so. The problem is if you're home when the fever starts or you go to a typical ER, where you might sit for a while before anyone gets to see you. We'll talk more about that before Richie's discharge."

Richie struggled to think positively. But his doctor was talking about *survival.* There were so many ways he could die. His leukemia could kill him, he could die of infection, or bleeding or maybe his kidneys could fail, or his heart might stop. Dark thoughts crowded his head. It might have been macabre, but he wondered which would be the best way to die.

"Do you have any questions?" asked Paul.

"I don't think so, Dr. Belkin," said Betty, "you're all very good at explaining stuff, and that's much appreciated."

As the rest of the medical team left the room, Madelyn stayed behind.

"When you get a chance," said Madelyn, "I hope that we can talk for a few minutes, I'd like to hear about your weekend."

"Sure, I think we can do that here in the room, I've nothing to hide from Richie."

"OK," said Madelyn and went to get a chair so she could sit with them. Once back she started, "Betty, you went home on Saturday, how did that go?"

"I was a little anxious about leaving Richie, but he encouraged me, and it was fine. I think we both got a needed break from each other. I got a lot done."

"Did you talk to your boss?" asked Madelyn.

"Shelley, she's my boss at the Gallery, has been very generous with me. I was there for a few hours Saturday afternoon, and we talked. She told me that she understands that my number one job is to help Richie and that I should take all the time I need. We discussed how I can do more of my job remotely and only come into the gallery when I'm comfortable. I think I'll be using some of my vacation time, but we didn't really talk about money. I presume that you have a better understanding of how much time Richie would be here, and when it would be important for me to be close by."

"It sounds like your employer is being very nice," Madelyn responded. "Of course, some of that's required by law. It seems that you didn't discuss some of the details, which is understandable on your first day venturing back. Eventually, you may want to have a written agreement about how you will be managing your time at work. It'll be up to you how you want to proceed. If you choose, I can talk to her about that. I've done that many times. Sometimes it's easier for an objective, outsider with no skin in the game to speak on your behalf. If you're interested, just let me know."

Richie tried not to listen too closely, this was between his mom and Madelyn. But he couldn't help thinking that all these problems were his fault. If he hadn't got leukemia, if he didn't need to be in the hospital none of this would be happening.

"Thank you, Madelyn," said Betty, "let me think about it. If I ask you to do that, I'd want to give her a head's up. It's better if she's expecting your call and understands why I might be asking for your help."

"Of course," said Madelyn, "I know we talked about support when we last spoke, it doesn't appear that you have any family or friends that you could turn to. Have you had a chance to think about contacting Richie's father?"

"After we talked, I spoke with Richie," said Betty, "and I asked him what he thought about that. Richie has never seen him, or been in contact with his father. After a bit of discussion, we agreed that neither of us had any interest in reaching out to him."

"I guess we're done with the father," said Madelyn. "Richie's already seen most of the chemotherapy agents for this induction cycle at least once, and he'll be getting those drugs several times more. You should be prepared for the complications of Richie's treatment. They can be severe. Sometimes a child will need to be transferred to the intensive care unit, to manage blood pres-sure or breathing problems. Do you remember the doctor who helped with the sedation for the bone marrow test? That was Dr. Street, she would be your doctor in the ICU. So, I know you've heard this before, but it can't be emphasized too much: let the doctors or nurses know if you don't feel right, OK?"

"Yes, I know," said Richie. He was tired of hearing, *'let me know'* or *'how are you feeling?'* Did they think he was demented, after all, how many times did they think he needed to be asked that same question?

"Is there anything you want to say or ask?" When Madelyn only saw heads shaking, she said, "OK, we'll talk again soon." She got up to leave as Paul was coming over.

"I've ordered the platelet transfusion," said Paul, "that should take about an hour. After that he'll get Zofran for nausea before receiving the PEG-asparaginase."

"I hope he'll be OK," said Betty, "with his white count so low, we're hearing ominous warnings. What do you think?"

"If he becomes febrile, we'll cover him with very powerful antibiotics, we'll do our best to keep him safe," said Paul, "I wish I could say more."

"I understand," said Betty.

Paul started, "Remember to..."

But before he could get the words out, Richie finished the sentence for him, "tell you if I feel bad. I will Dr. Belkin." He was tired of all the reminders about what could go wrong.

"OK, nuff said," Paul knew when to quit, he smiled and walked away.

"What are you thinking?" said Richie, "you looked, I don't know, far away."

"Huh? Just everything, being here, you and Nancy. So many things. It's overwhelming.

You know, Richie, I think I'd like to speak with Mr. Peters," said Betty, "the next time you talk to or text Nancy, can you please get his number for me."

"Sure, Mom, I'll check with Nancy now."

Soon, Richie had the number, and held his phone up so his mom could see.

"I got it."

Betty walked out of Richie's room, to a corner of the unit and dialed the number. Walter answered on the second ring. "Hi, it's Walter." Nancy had obviously let her dad know she'd be calling.

"Hello," said Betty, "how are you and Nancy?"

"We're fine, more importantly how is Richard? We both worry about him, and Nancy talks about Richard constantly."

"Richie's the same. He's always talking about Nancy, they really seem to care about each other, don't they?"

"They certainly do," said Walter. "And this all happened so quickly. Richie seems to be a very nice boy, and I'm praying for him to get well. But I'm also concerned about how this might affect my daughter. It seems to be more than just a casual high school romance."

"That's the reason I wanted to speak with you," said Betty. "Richie is excited about her. She's made him happy, even with all that's going. It's incredible, really. I see how he is with her. And I know that she's more than a friend, but she is also a friend. It's all new for me, Richie with a girlfriend. But it all could change in literally a heartbeat, and now I worry about Richie and also your daughter. So, I'll be supportive, even if I can't help being worried. I was hoping to know what you think about all of this."

"It is complicated for me too, Betty," said Walter, "I think that you should know a bit about what Nancy's been through. My wife, Martha, Nancy's mother, died about five years ago. She had a brain tumor, a glioblastoma multiforme. And as you certainly can appreciate, for me, and for Nancy that was devastating. We've moved several times since then, and while we usually tell people it's because of my work, it's really about Nancy and how difficult it's been for her. It had been hard for her to focus on school with the specter of her mother's death looming over everything. Walking through the hallways, she would feel the other students looking at her and she imagined them thinking, there's that poor girl, Nancy, her mother died. She's been to multiple therapists, but she's never been able to connect with them. But it's changed here at Horace Mann, and mainly since meeting Richard, she's been a different girl. She seems alive again, excited, smiling, and happy. And I don't know how to protect her from what might happen."

"I'm so sorry to hear about your wife, Walter." Betty thought back to some of what Richie had told her about Nancy. She was beginning to understand that the attraction between her son and Walter's daughter had very deep roots. Somehow fate had brought these two souls together. "I can imagine that losing a mother at that age would be awful for a young girl. It must have been very difficult for both of you, even with help. I don't think Richie knows how difficult it's been for Nancy. I'm pretty sure he would've said something to me. Walter, it seems that neither of us is alone in having special children who need us. Thank you for trusting me with this information. I understand much more now. I think we're very much on the same page. I won't mention any of this to Richard, I'll leave that up to Nancy, when and if she decides to tell him."

Betty was off the phone and returning.

"Gee, Mom, you and Mr. Peters, seemed to talk for a while."

"We were talking about you guys of course," said Betty, "and I wanted Mr. Peters to know how much I care about Nancy. He's a good father."

"It seemed that you were being kind of secretive." Richie was pretty sure that his mom was not happy with his new girlfriend. Dads, who knows what they think? He didn't. Richie began to suspect that they were plotting to break them up.

"Just parent stuff, I expect that one day you'll understand," said Betty.

The chemotherapy was an assault on every part of Richie's body. He was tired all the time. He needed lots of sleep, but it got interrupted often. Feeling like he couldn't stay awake any longer, he lay down and closed his eyes.

Richie had been sleeping for only a few hours when something woke him up. He was disoriented as he picked his head up and looked around. He couldn't figure out what woke him. It felt like late afternoon. His mom wasn't in the room. Richie tried to clear his head. He checked the time. Nancy would be done with classes, so he called her. "Hey, how was school?"

"It was OK, Richie. I've been doing stuff on the library committee. Ms. Shute and I are looking at getting some new books. But I miss you. How do you feel?"

"I feel OK, it's kind of weird, everyone keeps asking me how I am, and I just feel like regular me. I'm beginning to wonder if it's OK that I don't feel bad. But I do feel bad in a certain way, and that way would be totally fixed if you were here."

"I feel like that too, Richie."

"Nancy, I can't help thinking about you, it's like all the time and I'm sorry about what I said last time. I didn't mean anything, I guess I was just tired. You know when I think of you it's like you're here, with me, and it's comfortable."

"It's OK, Richie, I know. When I think about you, and that's a lot, it also feels comfortable, like I've known you forever. I could be doing just anything, and you appear in my head. It's like we're connected."

"You're in my head right now, Nancy. Sometimes I get mad at this disease, cause it's keeping us apart."

Nancy used her ultra-sultry voice, "Richie, I wish you were better, and we could just sneak off together and be alone, just you and me."

Richie knew that he needed to stop picturing Nancy in all sorts of delectable ways. He hoped that there'd be time later to revisit that fantasy. "I know, I want that too. It will happen. I promise that the first chance I get, I will come to be with you."

"I'll be waiting for you, Richie. I gotta go now." Nancy kissed the phone and disconnected.

Across town at her home on leafy Bennit Street, Nancy sighed. Things were complicated. She was scared that something would happen, and Richie wouldn't be able to keep his promise. She didn't know what to do or think.

She left her room and came down the steps to find her dad. He was down in the living room, in his big comfy chair, reading the paper. Nancy watched him for a while, wondering what he was thinking. She walked over and sat down next to him.

"I guess you were talking with Richie's mom," said Nancy. "Ms. Samuelson is kind of pretty, don't you think? She seems nice, and smart too. You've been on the phone with her a couple of times that I know of. You seem a bit secretive about your talks with her."

Walter smiled, "Yes, she is kind of pretty and smart, and a good mother, too. But it's not like that."

"Dad, do you think Richie's mom likes me?"

"Oh, yes, she likes you a lot and she's very happy for you and Richard to be together."

"Dad," suddenly Nancy started to well up with tears, "do you think Richie is going to be OK? I worry about him a lot, and I get scared sometimes." Nancy sobbed, her voice broke down. It was all too much, like watching her mother in treatment. She remembered her mom coming home from the clinic, weak and sick looking. Nancy watched her waste away, unable to eat, eventually unable to walk or sit up. And her pain, that image of her wouldn't go away. Nancy shook her head, and wiped the tears. She looked at her dad, searching for answers. It was hard to get the words out. "I don't know what I would do if, you know, something bad happened to him. I just couldn't do that, again."

"Come here, baby," her dad held his arms out.

Nancy came to him, wrapped her arms around his neck and curled up in his lap, like she hadn't done in so many years, the tears flowed in earnest. She tried to describe how she felt, but the words wouldn't come.

"It's OK, Nancy, you don't have to say anything." Walter held her, rocking his daughter, gently stroking her head, and rubbing her back, trying to ease her pain. "I know this must be hard. It's OK to cry, let it all out. I'm right here. I'll always be here."

Any notion of restraint was gone, she let it all out, blubbering like a little child, the tears rolling down her face. Walter's shirt became wet where she lay her head, "Oh, Daddy," she wailed, "I'm so scared, what's going to happen?"

"Of course, we don't know, Nancy. Life can be scary sometimes, especially when we're worried about someone precious to us.

You know, we never told you this, but both your mom and I knew, from the first day of her diagnosis, that her brain tumor was incurable. She underwent surgery, radiation, and chemotherapy, all trying to delay the inevitable, so she could be with us, as long as she could. Mom endured a lot to have a few more months with you. Toward the end, when she was very sick, she told me that she wasn't afraid to die, but she was sad that she would not get to see you grow up, not to be at your wedding, she would never see her grandchildren. Mom cried about her loss of your future. You were her world, Nancy."

"Oh, Daddy, I didn't know." She was stunned to learn this, so many years later. Nancy had always wondered why her mom kept going back to the clinic. Even then she understood that it wasn't helping, she wasn't getting better. And now, at 17, she finally was able to see. "Oh, Mommy," was all she could say.

"You were not quite 13 years old, and your mother and I discussed this. We both agreed that there was no need for you to know that she had a terminal disease. We wanted you to have time with her, without feeling that shadow hanging over you."

"All this time, you never said."

"Well time passes, and I guess at some point I would have told you, but it seemed like the right time now. We don't know for sure what will happen, but leukemia in a young person is curable. Richard's disease is very different from what your mother had, and there's every reason to have hope."

Nancy used her sleeve to dry her eyes, "oh Daddy," she looked down, "and look, I've gotten your shirt all wet." She tried to dry it with the tail of her shirt. "There, that's a little better. It must have been very hard for you, taking care of Mommy, keeping her comfortable, and protecting me, and all the while you must have been hurting too. You've always been my protector and shield, haven't you?"

"You're my love, Nancy, and that's what daddies do."

"Yes, I love you too, but not all daddies are so good. I feel better now, I'm glad you told me about Mom. But Daddy..."

"What is it?"

"I understand what you did, and I think it was okay when I was like 13. And I know I'm not all grown up at 17, well nearly 18, and I still have lots to learn, but you should know that if bad stuff happens, I won't break. I need you to promise that you won't hide stuff from me anymore, OK? We're family and we share the good and the bad."

Walter smiled, she was right, in many ways Nancy was very nearly an adult woman, though indeed, she still had a ways to go, "I promise."

26.

Back at the hospital, Betty put her phone in her pocket and walked back to their room. She looked at Richie, and then reached up to squeeze the IV bag and read the label. She was learning. "Your PEG-asparaginase is nearly finished."

"Gee Mom, please don't ask how I feel, I promise to let you know if I don't feel OK."

Betty could tell how hard this was for Richie. He was being assaulted all day long. There were drugs, fluids, blood, pokes, constant interrogation. He was under a microscope every moment. He was at a hard age to be going through this. A younger child would not have so much insight into what was happening. An older person should have the maturity to handle the onslaught and he would have some perspective on what he'd already accomplished in life. But not Richie, he had neither innocence nor experience. If she could switch places, she would.

"Alright, Richie," she smiled, "can I ask if you're hungry?"

"Yes, you can, and I am. What do you have in mind?"

"Let's ask your nurse if you can walk down to the cafeteria, maybe we can find something scrumptious."

"Good luck with the scrumptious hunt, Mom, but I'm all in for trying."

"Here comes your nurse," said Betty as Annie approached. "It looks like his chemo is just about finished, do you think we could walk down to the cafeteria when he's done."

"Yup, he's just finishing, I'll flush his line and draw the lab samples that Dr. Belkin ordered. I can hep-lock him and disconnect Richard from his IV pole. You can go down to the cafeteria and look around, but Richard has to wear an N95 mask and a gown when he's off the unit. He'll have to come back up here to eat."

"Thanks, Annie," said Richie. When Annie was done, and Richie was freed up, he put on the N95 mask and gown. Together mom and he walked to the elevator bank. They got out on the lobby level where the cafeteria was located.

"Hey, Mom, can we just walk around a little before we go to the café?"

"Sure, let's do that."

As they walked through the lobby they passed the chapel, and the gift shop. Although it was an effort to keep up, Richie, at least initially, seemed to savor the sense of freedom. But he was very weak and the effort quickly became a struggle. "I'm tired, maybe we need to get over to the cafeteria and pick something up."

Betty saw how much trouble Richie was having, her mind flashed back to the tumor lysis crisis and how scary that was. Now he was struggling after walking just a short distance. Maybe this hadn't been a good idea. The lobby, even in a hospital, was not the best place to need medical care. She was worried. "OK, sure," said Betty.

They backtracked a bit and were soon in the cafeteria. They chose a couple of dinners to-go and made their way back to the unit. By the time they were upstairs, Richie was exhausted. He needed to sit down.

"This is really taking a toll on you, Richie. Let's go slow."

Betty opened the bag and handed him his dinner and set hers down in her lap. She had a cheeseburger and fries. Richie had ordered the grilled chicken sandwich. Betty watched Richie slowly unpack his sandwich. He looked at it and turned it over a couple of times before taking the first bite. It was work just to chew a bit of the sandwich. He was soon breathing hard. "I really don't feel so good, Mom. I don't think that I can eat any more. Maybe you could put this away for later. I need to lie down."

"Go ahead, I'll take care of your sandwich." Betty went over to tuck Richie in. She placed her hand on his forehead, "you don't feel warm, try to get some rest." She kissed him on top of his head. She was worried. He was paler than usual, not well looking at all. Betty wondered if the walk downstairs was a bad idea. She wrapped up his sandwich and carried it with her as she walked over to the nurses' station. She told Steve that Richie didn't seem well. Steve asked a few questions and said he would come by to check on him. Betty saved his sandwich in the unit fridge, before walking back to their room. She found him already asleep and breathing heavily. She touched his forehead again, it wasn't hot, but still, she didn't like the way he looked. Betty sat down and waited.

A few minutes later, Steve came by, and he too watched Richie for a minute or so. "His breathing seems labored, he's breathing fast, and he looks paler than usual. I'm going to get his vitals." Steve checked his temperature with the temp gun. It was 97.4°, just a bit low. Using the sphygmomanometer, his blood pressure was normal, pulse and respiratory rate were elevated at 96, and 32. The pulse oximeter showed his O_2 saturation was low at only 93%. "I'm going to call Dr. Belkin with these results, he should be right over."

Steve stepped out of the room and punched in the speed-dial for the fellow. In a few seconds, he was talking with Paul. Steve described what he saw, the vital signs and his impression. He listened for a short time, and then poked his head back into Richie's room. "Dr. Belkin will be over in a minute."

Paul soon appeared. He took a quick glance at Richie. Immediately, Betty saw the look of concern on Paul's face. "How long has he been like this?"

"Well, maybe a half hour ago, we went for a short walk to the cafeteria. He was wearing his N95 mask and covered with a gown. We didn't stay long because Richie was feeling tired. We bought some to-go food and came right back. He took one bite of his sandwich and said that he was too tired to eat. I felt his forehead, he wasn't hot. He laid down and was asleep almost as soon as his head hit the pillow. That was like ten minutes ago."

"I see," said Paul, "first, he's not sick because you went for a walk. Since his white count has been zero for several days now, this was bound to happen. We're walking Petri dishes covered with bacteria, and without our immune system, infections are virtually inevitable. The delicate balance has tipped in favor of the germs."

Paul woke Richie and asked him to sit up. Paul examined his eyes with his penlight. He pulled the stethoscope from around his shoulders and listened to his chest in front and in back. He took Richie's hand and raised his arm so that it was level with his heart. He checked his pulse at the wrist. Betty watched as he briefly pressed down on Richie's index fingernail. He asked Steve to recheck his pulse oximetry.

Richie looked around and he blinked a few times. It seemed hard for him to stay awake. "I'm going back to sleep," is all he said. He lay down and turned to his side. He was asleep in seconds.

Paul continued, "his lungs sound OK, I don't hear any rhonchi or crackles. However, that can be absent because those sounds would be the result of his immune system fighting a lung infection. Since his WBC count is zero, his immune system is not functioning well, and he can still have a lung infection without the typical findings. His heart is pounding, and his pulse is bounding. His pupils are responsive, but he's very pale, and when I briefly push down on his finger, it blanches, but then it takes a few seconds for the pink color to return. That should happen in less than 2 seconds. These may be early signs of a brewing infection. I'm ordering a portable chest x-ray. Steve will get a full set of labs from one of Richie's central line lumens, including a CBC, chemistry profile, blood culture and a repeat type and cross. He'll likely need several units of packed red blood cells, we'll know soon. I also want a blood culture from the second lumen. A bacterial infection could begin in only one lumen of his catheter, so we need to culture both sides to be sure we don't miss anything. I'm not ready to start antibiotics yet, unless I find something on the x-ray, or he spikes a fever. But he needs fluid volume because his perfusion, that is, his blood circulation, is poor. I need to know what his hemoglobin level is before I decide whether to give him volume using crystalloid or red blood cells. For now, he'll get maintenance normal saline. Steve, make sure all the tests are sent stat, OK?

Ms. Samuelson, this was expected, we're going to take care of Richard," said Paul, "but I want you to be prepared for the possibility that he may need to be transferred to the pediatric ICU, it depends on how he responds to our treatments. Do you have any questions?"

"I don't really know what to ask," said Betty. It was hard for her to get the words out. She was cold and clammy, beads of sweat formed across her brow. The color had drained from her face. "I'm afraid to ask the most important question."

"I know this is scary, but we're prepared for this," said Paul. "The decision to transfer him to the PICU would be made if he either needs blood pressure support that we can't manage on the unit, or he requires respiratory support that can't be done here. It's a bit of a cliché, but we have to take this one step at a time."

"Respiratory support?" asked Betty, "does that mean you'd be putting a tube down his throat and connecting him to a breathing machine?"

"A ventilator," said Paul, "not necessarily, sometimes all that is needed is high flow ventilatory support which can be done with a nasal cannula, just a pair of short tubes in his nostrils. That could be just temporary, and that may be all he needs. We'll try simple first, before we think about intubation. We wouldn't need to transfer him if that's all he needs. But we don't know yet. You'll know as soon as I do.

Steve, please set up some blow by oxygen, and make sure he's on the monitor, I want telemetry, OK?"

Paul explained to Betty, "we'll try the scoop mask first, it sits below his chin, and provides a little extra oxygen, easing his respiratory effort." Paul watched a moment longer, looking at Richie and then Betty. With no further questions, he turned and walked back toward the fellow's room.

While Steve went to work obtaining the blood samples that Paul had asked for, Betty sat down and held Richie's hand. It felt cool. She tried to warm his hand by gently rubbing it with hers. She brought his hand up and pressed her lips to the back of his hand. "I'm here for you Richie. I need you to be strong," she sobbed. "We will lick this fucking monster." She lay her head down, resting on Richie's arm and began to pray.

27.

Paul came back to Richie's room, watching and checking the monitor. "His hemoglobin is very low at 5.5 gm/dL, that certainly can explain a lot of what's happening, he can't very well carry much oxygen when it's that low," said Paul. "His platelet count is 25,000, so that can wait, but he needs red blood cells."

Betty already knew Richie needed a transfusion. Her son was pale as a ghost, and icy cold. She could feel his heart pounding and hear his heavy breathing.

Paul continued, "we must do that slowly. If he's transfused too quickly, the extra blood volume will become too much for his heart that's already taxed by his anemia. That load could cause fluid to back up into his lungs, putting him in congestive heart failure. If the lungs become wet they can't absorb the oxygen he needs. But there's no choice, with a hemoglobin of 5.5, remember it should normally be at least 12 gm/dL, he needs more blood. His kidneys should be able to remove the extra fluid and avoid volume overload if we transfuse slowly and give enough time between blood units for his body to equilibrate. We may have to help get extra fluid off with Lasix."

"I understand, Dr. Belkin, please do what you have to do. Make my Richie better." She was exhausted and could hardly think. She knew her son was in trouble. All she could do was put her trust in the doctors caring for him.

"Steve, I'll order 3 units of irradiated, leukoreduced, packed RBC's. Each unit should be given over 4 hours, with 4 hours rest between the units. Let me know if he's not peeing enough, OK? Let's be sure he's using the urinals, and saving them. If we're careful, his oxygen saturation will improve. Let me know if it drops. I'll be in the fellow's room for a bit, call me if anything changes."

Many hours had gone by. Several units of blood had been slowly transfused while Betty and Richie slept together in the hospital bed. Not much had seemed different, which was good. As evening fell, shifts were changing. Betty stirred when she noticed that Sandra had entered the room.

"Hello, Ms. Samuelson, I heard from Dr. Belkin that Richard was having trouble today. How does he seem to you?"

"This is the worst I've seen Richie since his diagnosis, though he seems a little better since the oxygen and the transfusions. He's completely wiped out. I'm worried."

"Yes, of course, but we'll take good care of him.

Dr. Belkin went over Richard's day with me, including his recent change. We saw his chest X-ray, which has no suggestion of pneumonia. As of now, with no fever and stable blood pressure, there is no reason to move him off the unit. The plan is to continue the red cell transfusions through the night and carefully monitor his vital signs. Dr. Belkin is getting ready to leave for the night, and I'll be here. Do you have any questions?"

"I have lots of questions," said Betty, "but I suspect that no one really has the answers to what I want to know. I guess, Dr. Gardner, you and I will be here all night long and we'll be watching."

"Yes, I won't be far," said Sandra.

"I hope Richard feels better," said Paul and he turned to leave.

Betty watched the blood cells drip. As the transfusion proceeded, she watched for any changes. She watched the monitor. She studied his EKG tracing as it danced across the screen, repeating over and over again and remaining unchanged. His oxygen saturation had improved to 96% with the scoop mask. Betty figured it would be a while before the transfusions made much difference. His hemoglobin was awfully low. She wondered how that happened. Well, he wasn't making new cells, and the transfused cells didn't last as long as the homemade kind. She tried to stay alert, but the steady beep of the monitor, the unchanging rhythms, his deep steady breathing, were soporific. As she watched Betty became hypnotized by the repetitive beat, her eyelids became heavy, and closed several times. For a while she was able to shake herself awake, but that became harder to do. She was soon asleep.

28.

It was not a restful sleep. She moaned and fidgeted, twisting, and repositioning herself in the chair. She had horrific dreams, monsters lurking about, danger closing in on her, she tried to escape. She had to navigate long dark twisty corridors. The many doors and windows along the way were locked. Whatever was chasing her was getting closer. She was assaulted by unsettling banging noises. Only a few at first, but then more insistent, more frequent, steadily closer and louder. Betty struggled to surface from the dream. It felt like Richie's bed was moving, banging, and bumping into things as it rocked side to side like a ship caught in a wicked storm, the waves pounding, lightning crackling, explosions of deafening thunder clapped around her. It was dark and disturbing, she tried to cover her ears, she tried to flee.

And then, all at once, she was fully awake, she rubbed her eyes. As she looked toward Richie, they were alone, in his room, not in the ocean, but Richie's bed was indeed shaking. She tried to focus, what was happening? Richie was shaking violently, so strongly it shook his bed. Her first thought was that he was having a seizure, and she ran to the nurses' station to get help.

Betty was in full panic mode. For a moment all she could do was point toward the room. She had to take a couple of deep breaths before she could spit the words out. "Richie's having a seizure, his bed is banging and shaking. Please come, quickly!" She ran back to the room and saw it still going on. Betty wanted to help but she didn't know how.

One of the night nurses yelled out to call Sandra, and she followed Betty into Richard's room. The nurse saw Richie shaking violently, he was moaning, his eyes were open, and his lips were quivering, his hands tightly gripped the bed sheets, she heard him groan. With chattering teeth, he was repeating, again and again, "I'm so cold."

"He's conscious. He's not having a seizure, those are rigors, violent shivering probably from an infection," his nurse said. She shouted to bring the crash cart over.

Very soon, Betty saw Sandra emerge from the fellow's room and walk over quickly. She made a quick assessment, looking at Richie and the monitor.

The nurse, Camille, said, "Dr. Gardner, this just started a couple of minutes ago, it looks like rigors to me."

"I agree," said Sandra, "please stop the infusion, take the blood cell pack down, bag it to be sent to the lab for culture and analysis. Don't flush the line, please, we don't want to push anything more through it, not just yet. Let's get his vitals again. Call pharmacy to get 2 grams of Ceftazidime up here immediately. I want you to draw a full set of labs, CBC, chemistries, a haptoglobin level and a blood culture from one lumen of his catheter, and just a blood culture from the other lumen. Send a urinalysis when he pees. We'll find out if he's reacting to the transfusion. Tell me his vitals, please.

Both night nurses were helping now, and they called for a back up to come over from the nearby adult unit. "Dr. Gardner, should we call a code?"

The word, code, brought all kinds of nasty images flashing in Betty's head. All those medical TV shows had graphic depictions of what would happen. It usually didn't end well. She held her breath and watched.

"Not yet, talk to me, what have you got?"

"His temperature is 39.4° C, pulse is 120, respiratory 36 and his BP is 90/60.

"OK, he's pretty hot. I don't like any of those numbers. After the antibiotic Ceftazidime is in, we're going to give him IV acetaminophen and 10 mg of Demerol to ease those shakes. Until we get the shivering under control we can't give him anything per mouth. He's breathing too fast. He could aspirate if we tried anything oral." Sandra listened carefully to his heart and lungs, she checked his pupillary responses, and felt his hands and feet. They were ice cold. Pressing his fingernails, the cap refill was delayed. "Let's get some blankets," Sandra ordered.

"Richard," said Sandra, "you're OK, right now, I'm getting some medications up here to help you. I've stopped the transfusion. It's possible that we'll wind up moving you to the PICU, remember Dr. Street? But not yet, your vitals are not so bad, you're not going anywhere, at least for now. We're going to watch you like hawks."

Just then, Camille came with the IV bag, "the ceftaz is here," she checked the label, "Richard Samuelson, Ceftazidime 2 grams."

"Please infuse the antibiotic, over 10 minutes," said Sandra. I'm going over to the workstation to enter the orders: all the labs, the 'ceftaz' and 650 mg of IV acetaminophen followed by the Demerol. I'll also order vancomycin, to follow the acetaminophen into the same side of the catheter.

Vancomycin will provide better staph coverage, including MRSA, just in case. I want you to alternate lumens with the antibiotic infusions, so the next dose should go into the other lumen, let's call them A and B. Please repeat all the vital signs after the antibiotic and the acetaminophen are in. Any questions?" When Sandra didn't hear any questions, she looked directly at mom and added, "Betty, he's OK for now. I'm going to the work station to put in the orders he needs. I won't be far and I'm coming right back." There was a pause while Sandra waited for some acknowledgement. Betty's face was a blank, pasty green. Sandra leaned forward, face to face with Betty, and placed her hand on Betty's shoulder. Sandra needed to get to work on the orders. "Betty, look at me and nod if you understand." Another pause, a blank stare back. And so Sandra began to nod, which was finally followed by Betty's answering nod.

With that response, Sandra exited the room to do what was needed.

Betty was more numb than anything, she didn't know how worried she ought to be. She watched Sandra manage the last crisis when Richie had tumor lysis and that worked out OK. She certainly seemed to know what she was doing. And Betty could tell that the nurses were comfortable following Sandra's orders. Betty would have noticed some hesitancy or furtive glances if the nurses thought she wasn't handling the situation correctly. Sandra was young, but she had an air of authority about her as she worked, her orders were issued rapidly, clearly and crisply. She seemed methodical and confident as she assessed and responded to the crisis. Betty decided that there was nothing more she could do, except be there for Richie, be his mom, reassure him, talk to him quietly and lovingly, hold his hand, gently brush the little hair he had left off his forehead, and say some silent prayers. She watched as the antibiotic finished and the IV Tylenol and Demerol infused. The shaking subsided, and his oxygen saturation improved. He seemed to be breathing easier. As her hand gently swept across his brow, he seemed cooler, not like the red-hot firecracker he had been moments before. She thought he was a bit better already, but was that just the mamma wanna see, or was that real?

Betty watched Camille as she rechecked Richie and repeated his vital signs. She dared to ask, "what do you think?" she asked, "how's he doing, Camille?"

"He's better, the big thing was stopping the infusion," said Camille. "His rigors have stopped, his temperature is down to 38° C, which is a lot better, his BP is now 105/68, so that's good.

His oxygen saturation is stable. All in all, I'd say things are moving in the right direction."

"It looks like that to me, too," said Betty, "but I'm certainly biased. It seems Dr. Gardner knows what she's doing."

"Oh, yes, she's excellent," said Camille, "I'd let her take care of my kids any day. Though, of course, I hope they would never need a doctor like her." Camille looked at Betty, "sorry, maybe that came out wrong. I shouldn't..."

"It's OK, I understand. Thank you, Camille, for everything," said Betty, and she allowed her absolute vigilance to ease a tad, the tension dialed down a smidgeon. She still watched carefully. Betty became aware of how tense she had been, her muscles were sore, her neck was tight, her head ached, and her mouth was dry. She reached for the bottle of spring water by her chair and took a few sips, slaking her thirst and chasing away the desert dry mouth. Betty felt that she needed to talk to someone, but she didn't know who that might be. Usually, it would have been Richie. She thought of Madelyn, of Shelley at work, even Walter came to mind. But she didn't typically turn to anyone for help. She had gotten used to managing her own problems. In the past it had seemed a weakness to reach out. She prided herself on not needing anyone. It was just her and Richie against the world. But the armor she'd been wearing had developed chinks. It was tarnished, and she felt vulnerable. Would she now have to rely on others? Well, maybe that wasn't so bad. She struggled with her new reality. But it was hard to let the curtain down, she was tempted, but she was not quite ready to reach out, not yet.

"Mom?" said Richie, "what's going on?" He started to sit up. "What time is it? I think I had a bad dream, but I can't remember it. I have to pee, and I'm thirsty."

Betty smiled, a big ear to ear grin, and got out of her chair. She sat down next to him, a few tears of relief fell. She leaned over and gave him a big bear hug and a kiss on his cheek.

"Welcome back, buddy," said Betty, "here let me get your urinal, please don't get out of bed, I'll hold the covers up to give you some privacy, and then I'll tell you what's been going on." She found the urinal, handed it to Richie and held the sheet up.

From behind the curtain, she heard that he was done, and out came his hand offering the full container. She put it aside, knowing the nurses were keeping track. "Are you decent, can I lower the sheet?"

"Yes, it's fine. It looks dark, what time is it?"

"It's about 3:30 in the morning, and truth be told, you've scared the shit out of me for the last few hours. And I guess we have Dr. Gardner to thank, again, for helping you through this particular rough patch. And when I say rough patch, that's quite a toned-down version of how I would have described it just a little while ago."

"I don't really remember much. I know we got back with some to-go stuff from the cafeteria, and I remember being tired, and that's it. Wait, I remember being cold, like very cold, and shaking, like I was trapped in a freezer. That's the last thing I remember."

"Well, Richie, you put me through some shit. I'm not trying to blame you, but I was pretty scared. I'm just now feeling a bit better, but I'm not ready to go through it all again by reviewing it with you, not now anyway. Someday, hopefully we can laugh about it. I just want to let your nurse know that you're alive and kicking, I'll be right back."

Betty got up and walked over to find Camille. Betty wore a great big smile. She could barely talk without starting to cry, "Thank you so much," she said, "when you get a chance, come on by and see, he's alive again. I could kiss you."

Camille asked the secretary to call Dr. Gardner and then she walked back with Betty. Camille was almost as happy as Betty when she saw Richie sitting up and indeed, very much alive.

The fellow's room door opened and out came Sandra, she walked at doctor's pace over to Richie's room. She had a pleased, satisfied look as she saw Richie, sitting up in bed, engaged in an animated conversation with his mom and Camille.

Betty looked up and saw Sandra watching them. "Well, Dr. Gardner, I would say that you get a triple A plus rating in my Facebook. In my humble opinion, I think that you've saved Dr. Street some work tonight," said Betty, "don't you think?" Betty stood up, "And I hope you don't mind if I give you another big hug, Doctor."

At first, Sandra seemed stiff in Betty's arms, but that soon gave way, softening as she accepted the embrace. Betty figured that Sandra probably wasn't accustomed to receiving physical thank yous from her patients." As Betty held Sandra, she whispered in her ear, "you are my hero, thank you so much."

"Richard does look much better, but we're not out of the woods, yet. For tonight, we'll continue the antibiotics, alternating lumens by dose. Starting tomorrow, we will alternate lumens every 24 hours. There'll be no more blood transfusions tonight, but will start again on the day shift. I'm very happy to see Richard looking well again and as long as it seems to be a bit quiet, I'll go back to my room and see if I can get a little shut-eye. Call me immediately if anything changes." She turned and started walking back to the room.

Richie and Betty, sang out in unison, "Good night, Dr. Gardner."

"OK, guys," said Camille, "let's try to get some rest. I'll turn off your lights, and partially close the curtains." She walked back to the nurses' station.

"OK, Richie," said Betty, "we have orders. Let's try to get some sleep." Betty settled in her chair. For now anyway, she was feeling better, and she soon fell into a quiet, dreamless sleep.

To Betty, it seemed she had just closed her eyes, when morning arrived, and she saw Paul poke his head in.

"Good morning, Dr. Gardner reviewed the events of the night with me before she left." He watched Richie sleeping and breathing comfortably, he glanced up at the monitor, assessing the display.

"From what she told me, it sounds like things were a bit hairy for a while. His blood testing from earlier this morning showed the expected low hemoglobin and platelet counts, his chemistries were mostly normal but his low haptoglobin seemed to indicate that he had a reaction to that red cell unit. It happens sometimes. It was very good that Dr. Gardner stopped the transfusion when she did.

But Richard looks good now, what do you think, Ms. Samuelson?"

"Call me Betty, please. I'm very happy right now. Your colleague is an excellent physician." Betty hastened to add, "not that you aren't, but she has rescued Richie from at least two harrowing close shaves."

"No worries, Betty. You'll get no argument from me. I totally agree that Dr. Gardner is excellent."

"So, for today," he continued, "in terms of his ALL treatment, there's only the twice daily dexamethasone. We'll continue the antibiotics until his white count begins to recover, or he's completed a course of antibiotics for a positive blood culture."

"That works for me," said Richie.

Betty looked over at her son. She hadn't noticed that he'd awaken and so she was surprised to hear his voice. "Well good morning Richie. Glad to see you joining us."

Paul continued, "Richard will receive several blood transfusions today, both RBC's and platelets. I hope we get in as many of the planned transfusions as we can during the day so we can avoid giving any blood during the night shift. Any questions?"

When Paul saw they had none, he turned and walked on to check the next patient.

"Mom, I'm getting hungry, I'm starting to wonder about breakfast."

Betty was about to answer when her phone rang. She looked at the screen and saw the number was local, but she didn't recognize it. Normally she wouldn't have, but she decided to answer. "Hello," she waited to see if it was a bot calling.

"Hi, Ms. Samuelson, it's Nancy. Dad gave me your number, I was worried about Richie, and a little afraid to call him. I hope you don't mind. Is he OK?"

"You're so sweet Nancy, and it's fine that you called me, Richie had a hard night but he's much better this morning. You can call him, he's awake and I'm sure he'd love to talk with you. I'll add your number as a contact for next time."

"I get very anxious thinking about Richie in the hospital. Ms. Samuelson, you've been very kind. I just can't imagine how worried you must be. And you're staying there with him day and night. I think you're a great mother."

It was nice of Nancy to say that. Betty thought about this young girl, who seemed to have grown very close to her son. She was sticking by him, despite his serious diagnosis and despite all the memories that relationship had raised. A young girl without a mother. Betty wondered how Nancy saw her.

"Thank you," Betty answered, "I'm not sure I'm a great mother, the best I can do is care and be here, and hopefully that's enough. Anyway, Nancy, I'll let you go, I'm sure you'd rather be talking with Richie. It's OK, to call me anytime, if you're worried or you just want to talk."

"Thanks, Ms. Samuelson, I'll call Richie. I like to hear his voice. Bye."

When Betty heard Richie's phone ring, she grabbed her purse and left the room.

Richie waited a beat until his mom left before answering. His spirits lifted whenever he heard her ringtone. He could talk with her for hours. It really was amazing how quickly they had grown close. Her voice was sweet and comforting and all his worries seemed to melt away as soon as she said hello. "Hi, Nancy," he said into the phone.

"Hi, Richie, I was just talking to your mom, she said you were pretty sick last night. I was worried, again."

"Yeah, I guess so, I really don't remember much of it. But they said I had a fever and chills, and I was shivering so hard that the bed shook. It was kind of like the *Exorcist,* when Regan is possessed, and her bed does all sorts of tricks."

"You're funny Richie, you know lots of strange things, and you do sound like your regular self."

"I feel OK, and even better when I'm talking with you. When can you come over?"

"I'm not sure, I have to talk to my dad to see when he's coming that way. I guess I've been afraid to come see you because you've been so sick. I get pretty scared sometimes just thinking about what's happening to you."

He loved talking with Nancy and how she made him feel, but her angst bothered him. Maybe he was feeling sorry for himself, "I guess this isn't what you imagined, back when we first kissed. Now you're worrying about a boy with leukemia. Some guy who may not make it passed the next few months. You should just be happy now, excited about the end of the year, mixing with the whole class, looking forward to summer. I hadn't thought about how hard this must be for you. Maybe you'd have been better off, if we never wound up next to each other in French class."

There was a moment of silence. "Fuck you, Richard. That's what you think, really, so little of me. That's the most hurtful thing I've ever heard. You have no fucking clue! I guess you don't really know anything, do you?" Nancy was sobbing,

"You're just an asshole with leukemia!" and she slammed the phone down.

"Nancy... Nancy?" There was no answer. Richie was stunned. What just happened? He wasn't sure how he had gotten there, but it was obvious that he was in a shit load of trouble. That's certainly not what he expected, that wasn't his intention. He cared about her, and he had been trying to be...? What? What was he trying to be, chivalrous? He tried to think, but nothing made sense. He called her back, and the phone just rang and rang. She wasn't going to answer, he waited for the voicemail prompt, and all he could think to say was, "I'm sorry Nancy, please call me back."

He sat, trying to understand how he had gotten into such a deep hole. For sure he had said the wrong thing, or he didn't say it right. He wished he could go back and do it over, whatever it was, he wanted to fix what he had broken. He hoped he could.

As he was thinking about his fight with Nancy, his mom came back from the cafeteria. She was carrying a cardboard tray with wrapped sandwiches and two steamy, hot drinks. Betty started, "I've got some..." but she saw that Richie looked troubled, "what happened, are you OK?"

Richie looked up at her, "Ah, Mom, I fucked up, Nancy hates me now."

"Oh, I see. Well, I'm sure she doesn't hate you."

"Oh, yes, she does," said Richie, "I think I really pissed her off, we had a fight. Just suddenly, we were talking nice and all, and then I said some stuff, and she went ballistic. She said all kinds of shit, and then hung up. I tried to call her back, but she won't answer."

Betty put the tray down and sat down next to Richie. She put her arms around him and held him. "It's your first fight. Honey, both of you are under a lot of stress, and I'm sure things were said that were not meant. Sometimes in the heat of the moment, in a relationship, when someone feels hurt, they will fight back, using their words as weapons. Whatever happened, if she didn't care, she wouldn't have gotten so angry. Tell me everything. I need to know the exact words you each used, as best as you can remember."

Richie took a deep breath, and sat a moment, trying to recall the conversation. He tried to go through the sequence with his mom, telling it as accurately as he could. How abruptly the call changed, and how very angry Nancy had become. Just talking about it with his mom seemed to ease his tension.

Betty listened carefully to his recounting. "I do think you're in trouble with Nancy. But the good news is that you really didn't intend it and I think you guys can work it out. But you have some work to do. It seems that you were feeling sorry for yourself, and you fucked up. And the first thing you need is to understand what you did wrong. Do you think you can do that?"

"I'm not sure, I was trying to understand her situation, but somehow, I got it wrong. I thought I was going to make it easier for her."

"OK, that's good, you were trying to understand her worries about you. And *you* wanted to make it easier for her. But knowing other people isn't easy, and even after years together, one doesn't ever really know someone. Maybe you used your own feelings and projected them onto her, I don't know. Listen, you've only known Nancy for a short time, and you have no idea what she's been through. You presumed to know her and what she wanted, and you offered her a way out that she didn't ask for. That she didn't want. You decided that you knew what would be best for her. And, honestly, your offer implied that she was a shallow person, who would be better off leaving you because it was the easier path. It made her feel that you didn't think very highly of her. All of us need respect, and you didn't show her any.

I'm pretty sure that's not what you meant to do, you probably thought you were being gallant or something noble. But there you were, in fact, trying to make yourself look better at her expense. It's called unintended assholeness."

"Shit, Mom, she was right, I was an asshole, wasn't I?"

"Richie, you're not an asshole, but you sure were acting like one. Call her back, she probably won't answer, but she'll listen to your message. Be honest with her, and sincere, admit how you were wrong, and... well, it's your message. It may take a little time, but I think it will work out, cause you both care about each other."

"Thanks Mom," he gave her a big hug. He was even able to smile, now with some hope of repairing the damage.

"I'm going to leave you with your sandwich and the phone." Betty stood up, taking her food and giving him some privacy.

Richie picked up the phone and called Nancy again, it rang and rang until it went to voicemail. "Nancy, I'm so sorry, I said some stupid things. I feel really awful about what I said. It's our first fight, I guess I'm hoping that it's not also our last one. Maybe you're listening."

Richie pictured Nancy sitting in her bedroom. She would be really pissed at him, maybe she'd been crying. He hoped that she was listening. "You know, you said you were worried about me, and it bothered me to know you were worrying, I didn't want to think about you, being unhappy. But I was wrong, people who care about each other worry. I worry about you. I'm worrying about you a lot right now. I was wrong to say that you would be better off if we never met. That was really stupid. I don't even know why I said that. To care about someone means you worry about them, and I really want you to keep worrying about me. I know that I'm better when we're together. Nancy, I can't even imagine what it would be like if I'd never met you. I think about us all the time, I think how lucky I am that we found each other. I think about the times we've been together and talked. And held each other. I think you're beautiful, funny, and smart. I wish I could erase those things I said, I really hope that you can forgive me. You know, you are my first girlfriend and I guess I've got a lot to learn. You were right to call me an asshole. I can do better."

Nancy picked up the phone, "So you think you can do better?"

"Hi Nancy," he took a deep breath. "Yes, I'm sure I can be an asshole less often."

"Hmm. I hated it when you said that I'd be better off without you. You just don't know. You have no idea what it's been like for me. You presumed to make a choice for me, and that was disrespectful. It's been years since I've been as happy as I am with you. I think about us almost all the time. And I do worry, Richie, I can't help that because I care. And somehow you thought I would be better off if we never met. That hurt."

"I am truly sorry Nancy, you're right. I don't know what I was thinking, I should never have said that. I didn't really mean it. I certainly wouldn't have been better off if we never met. You've stuck with me through all this, and that tells me a lot about who you are, and how you feel. And I just wish we weren't fighting anymore, and I wish you didn't hate me."

"Richie, I don't hate you. I guess it's been hard for you. I can't imagine what it's like in that stupid hospital, day after day and all that stuff they're giving you. I wish that I could make that all go away, and we could be together."

"That sounds nice, Nancy. Does that mean we're OK? I hope it does."

"You've wiggled your way out of it this time, buster. But you better watch your ass, cause, I can be your worst nightmare!"

They both giggled.

Richie and Nancy talked for a while longer, laughing and remembering shared moments, they were happy again. "Oh, my god, Richie, look what time it is, I've got to get ready for school," she kissed the phone, with a loud smack and said, "electronic kiss now, a real one later, bye," and she disconnected.

Richie, laid back on his bed, happy and relieved. He thought about Nancy getting ready for school, he pictured her hurrying, picking out something to wear, getting her backpack, careening down the stairs to meet her dad. Well, he'd never been to her house, but he imagined she had stairs to careen down, maybe they were curved, with a newel post at the bottom. He thought about what her room might look like. Would it be all pink and full of stuffed animals, with posters on the walls of female artists? Or, maybe not, maybe less fluffy and more toned down, quiet and reflective. There were probably pictures of her family on shelves, or on her desk. Pictures of her mom? He thought about how her mom must have suffered with her disease and about all of her dreams that would never be fulfilled. What had they talked about when she was healthy? What did they talk about when she was sick? Nancy had been a child with a sick parent. He had a parent with a sick child. What was it about their lives that drew them together? He realized that there was so much he didn't know about Nancy. Should he ask? No, probably he should wait until she was ready. Conversations to be had later, he hoped. Was he in love? How would he know? He thought maybe he was. What if he said that to her? It felt like danger. His mind filled with questions.

And then he remembered the sandwich his mom left, and yes, he was hungry now, very hungry.

He eagerly unwrapped the bacon, egg and cheese on a toasted English muffin. It was no longer hot, but he didn't care, it turned out he was famished, and it tasted wonderful.

While he was busy with his meal, his mom came around, cautiously poking her head in the room to see if it was safe. She watched him inhaling the sandwich, and smiled, "it seems you're hungry, and not moping around in grief, two promising signs."

He was bent over the sandwich, and he picked his head up as she came in. "Thanks Mom, you're the best. I called Nancy and just started talking, telling her how I felt, you know, and she didn't answer at first, I was on her voicemail, but she was listening. Finally, she did pick up, and she was really mad at me, she told me how hurt she felt. We talked for a while. I was really scared that she might never want to see me again. But, Mom, you helped me understand how all those stupid things I said hurt her. Anyway, we talked more, and I told her how sorry I was, probably a hundred times, and how I didn't want to lose her. Finally, I guess, she still really does like me, I'm not sure why, she's so great. Anyway, by the time we finished talking we were all better again."

"I'm glad for you. Try to hold onto her, Richie, she's a very special young lady. You're in a relationship under difficult circumstances, and it would be easy for her to just move on, but she hasn't. Don't hurt her again, it may not be so easy to fix next time."

"I won't Mom. I want to do something special for her. Will you help?"

"Sure, Richie, maybe, the next time she's here you can give her something, a gift."

"That's a great idea, Mom. I wonder what she would like. Hmm, I don't know. Hey girls like jewelry, I guess, but I can't afford too much."

"Well, she might like a nice little charm bracelet," Betty suggested, "with dangling trinkets. A heart or a key, that will have some meaning. It would be nice if you added a personal note, something about how you feel."

"I have some money. Can you help me pick out something that she'd like."

"Sure, Richie, I can help you with that. I'll give you some ideas, but you have to make the final choice."

"I want everything to be perfect for her, Mom."

"Maybe perfect is too much to expect, and likely not what she's looking for. Let's not spend too much time worrying about it. Speaking about worrying, Richie, how are your school assignments coming along? We do want you to be promoted."

"Oh, oh, you're right. Richie had been in the stratosphere, thinking about how he survived a crisis and still had his girl. But the thought of school quickly brought him crashing down to Earth. "I'm going to need some courage for that, especially the French. I should get to work."

"And I need to work on my Gallery job. Maybe we both can have a few hours of quiet time."

They buckled down to business. While he worked, the blood transfusions and his antibiotics continued. So far, the blood cultures remained 'pending, no growth to date.' There were no new fevers or rigors. Things had settled back to routine, at least for now.

Paul came by to check on Richie. He examined him briefly, listening to his heart and lungs, checking his cap refill, carefully scanning the monitor and its telemetry. "You seem better. How do you feel Richard?"

"I'm good, except for this French, but I don't think you can help with that."

"I took Spanish in high school, so you're right, I don't think I could be much help. But I'm happy with your physical exam and vitals right now. I'm hoping that the blood cultures remain negative, so far, those are all pending and negative. The next big event will be Friday's chemo, a repeat of the first treatment day. For your last LP we didn't use sedation, only the Versed. Do you want to do it the same way?"

"Yeah, that's fine, and I won't need to be NPO, right?"

"That's right. You can still change your mind, and let me know, up until the day before. The plan is still for you to get at least two units of packed RBCs and one single donor platelet transfusion, during the daytime."

"Dr. Belkin," said Betty, "how can we keep Richie safe, with his white cell count so low?"

"Make sure that all his visitors are wearing masks. That'll help," said Paul. "But many infections in people on therapy come from their normal flora, the germs that live on our skin, in our mouths and in our gut. There's no way to protect against that. Being careful is the best he can do."

"We'll try to make sure that everyone who comes to see Richie is wearing a mask," said Betty. "Maybe I'll put a sign up and have a box of masks, right here. When will you be checking Richie's blood again?"

"It'll be done 4 hours after his next red cell unit finishes. Please remember to save all his pee, we're still tracking his output."

Except for the multiple transfusions, it turned out, as Paul expected, to be a quiet morning. Betty and Richie were able to get a lot of work done. After lunch, Carol came by to check in.

"I heard that Richard had a tough time during the night, he looks pretty comfortable now," said Carol. "Do you feel as good as you look?"

"I'm doing OK, Carol," said Richie, "but I have a couple of questions."

"What do you want to know?"

"As you can see, my head is looking kind of funky, with some random, straggly hairs. So, I was wondering if you have any suggestions for shaving it all, Telly Savalas like, and the second question: is there some kind of head cover or bandana to wear, to make me look like a stylish cancer patient?" Richie looked at himself in the mirror. He would soon look different. Somehow, a random thought about David Crosby and his freak flag popped into his head. And then he wondered about Nancy. First a worried look, but then he smiled. They had survived a fight and she still cares about him. He imagined how it would feel to have her fingers exploring his bald head.

"Well, we have disposable shavers on the unit and some shaving cream. I'm sure your mom can handle it. There are a few different head coverings available. I can bring you some catalogues. If you find something you like I can order it for you."

"That's great, thanks."

"Anything else? Games?" said Carol.

"No," said Richie, "just the catalogue, I really need to concentrate on school stuff, at least while I'm feeling well enough."

"Right, see you later," and Carol took off.

"I've been thinking that since you're feeling better," said Betty, "I might leave Thursday morning and come back early Friday before your LP. There's stuff at home and I can shop around for a card and a bracelet for Nancy. There's a new jewelry store near the gallery, I can take some pics for you to look through. What do you think?"

"That'd be great, Mom. You know I like it when you're here, and especially if I'm crashing. It really helps to see you in that chair, always nearby, like my guardian angel. I don't know how you do it, I don't think I could. But it's also good for both of us when you can get out some."

"I hope that you never have to find out what it's like to have a child who's really sick like you are. And honestly, I can't imagine not being in this chair next to you. You're everything to me Richie, I've said that before, but sitting here next to you, through your treatments and crises, I know that more surely than ever. Too often, I've taken life for granted, and it's sad that it has taken your illness to remind me how precious life is, and how fragile it can be. The mundane routine of daily life slowly chips away at the wonder of it. It requires an effort to maintain the respect for who we are. I hope that when you're completely recovered, and this is all behind us, we never forget how important that is."

"Gee, Mom, I guess this disease does really affect both of us. I hadn't looked at it that way." Richie smiled a bit, "maybe I need to sit in your chair a bit."

Betty smiled too, "that might work. I guess you should never judge a person until you've had a chance to sit in their chair for a few hours."

"Sounds like a bumper sticker," said Richie, "hey, I see the lady pushing the lunch cart around. I'm hungry."

Betty went over to check and came back with two trays, two small cartons of milk and two bottles of spring water. The food disappeared quickly. After refueling they opened their laptops and went to work. They were so consumed by their assignments that they didn't notice the time slipping by. It was late afternoon when they finally looked up and saw how much they'd accomplished.

From the nurses' station, Betty got a call that a visitor was on the way up. Almost immediately the elevator doors opened, and they watched Nancy start over. Her smile was infectious. As she sailed past the nurses' station, one of the aides reminded her to wear a mask. Nancy complied and although the smile was covered, Richie could still see how happy she looked. "Hi, Ms. Samuelson, so good to see you," she said.

"You seem to be in a good mood, Nancy," said Betty.

"Oh, well I know we had a rough morning," said Nancy, "and there were words, but I know Richie didn't mean them, and well, we all have had more than our share of scares and stresses. Whatever was true this morning, is history now, it belongs to the past."

"You are a special young lady," said Betty, "and I hope that Richie appreciates how lucky he is."

"Ms. Samuelson, I suspect he's learned that," said Nancy. "And I will be quick to remind him if he forgets."

"Hello ladies," said Richie, "I'm actually sitting here, and I can hear your conversation." Richie was playing his assigned role in the banter, but he was overjoyed to see Nancy, and to see her smiling. It seemed that he'd been forgiven.

"It seems time to make myself scarce," said Betty, "is your dad downstairs?"

"Yes, he's in the waiting area, they have some cubby desks with outlets, USB ports, and wi-fi access. He told me I have 30 minutes."

"Yes, I know the area, I'll go down and see how things are. I'll see you later, Nancy." Betty got up and walked toward the elevator bank.

Richie was happy to be alone with his girl. He had apologized on the phone, but he felt that it was important to do it with her right there. He wanted to see her face, know her feelings. "Nancy, I really am sorry about what I said this morning. I've thought about it more and I don't know why I said it. It was mean, but I wasn't trying to be mean, it just came out that way. I guess because I wasn't thinking about it from where you are. But when I finally did, I could see how hurtful it was. You seem OK, even smiley, are you really all right?"

"I think you've squirmed and sweated enough, and I really am OK now," said Nancy. "But you were in deep shit for a while."

"Oh, I don't ever want to be there again. So, I guess I'm on probation?"

Nancy smiled, "Sort of. I'm teasing, you're not really on probation, but what you said hurt, and I know you didn't mean it, but please be careful with me. And please be careful with yourself, I don't want to lose you. I've been happy since we've met. I think about you a lot. And I worry because I care. You know, Dad and I have lived in other places, and we've moved, and then moved again, let's just say it's been a few times. But since I started at Horace Mann, and met you, my life's changed. All those things have happened, all those choices made, and if one of them had been different we might not ever have met. And please don't ever suggest that I would be better off if that didn't happen. You just don't know.

I guess, I'm not supposed to kiss you, at least not on the lips." She came over to him, "I see a little bald spot right on top of your head."

And she pulled down her mask and leaned forward, cupping her hands around the back of his head and kissed him on that bald spot. Her lips felt warm and soft on his head.

"I guess we really can't do anything much in the hospital, Richie," Nancy cooed, her dark sultry voice drew his attention and excited him. She reached for his hand, and kissed him there, soft, tender kisses, her lips brushing each of his fingers.

"It really is too bad that we can't do anything here," she said again.

"Oh, my god Nancy, that was amazing. If this isn't doing anything, I can't imagine what it'll be like when we're doing something."

"See what you'd be missing if you fuck up again."

Richie took her hand and held it. "You know, since this diagnosis and making it through several scary crises, I've thought about my life differently. I guess this kind of thing does that. I've seen that all we have is what's happening now, no one knows the future."

"I have been there too, in a way, and I totally know that too, Richie."

"So, I hope what I say next will be OK," he said.

Nancy held her breath, she was not sure she wanted to hear what he was going to say, but she gave him permission, "I am here."

"I don't know, I've never felt this way, but I think, that I love you," Richie braced himself for her response.

Nancy breathed again, she smiled, ear to ear. She stood up and took a step toward him. "Oh, Richie." She lay down beside him, pressing her body against his. Feeling him next to her. She put her arms around him and kissed him hard and passionately, flagrantly violating the rules. She came up for air, "I've felt that way about you too, Richie, but I was afraid it might freak you out, if I said it. I love you too!"

They rested against each other, smiling and giggling. Richie knew that they shouldn't be doing this, not with zero white cells. Everyone had said that, but he didn't care. They were in love.

There was a loud, "ahem," as his nurse announced her presence. "Let's have a little decorum here. I need you out of Richard's bed, young lady, and to maintain a modicum of space between you. Both masks back on, please." She furrowed her brow and set her mouth in a tight grimace, hoping to deliver a message. "I'm not the love police and I hope that we are not going to need them."

Richie looked up at his nurse Annie, he couldn't help but smile, "Sorry, Annie, we'll try to behave."

"It was my fault," smiled Nancy.

"It looked to me, like you were both, guilty," said Annie. "You two are going to need a full-time chaperone."

When, a bit later, Betty and Walter approached Richie's room, Betty leaned forward guardedly, peeking into his room, not sure what she would see. She was relieved to find that they were laughing and giggling, leaning on each other, talking back and forth, looking as excited as children opening presents on Christmas morning. Betty, announced herself, with a loud guttural, "ahem," she paused, "it looks like you two, are fine."

Nancy looked up and saw Betty and her father standing there. She smiled and laughed, "Oh, yes, Ms. Samuelson, we are fine," and she turned to Richie, "aren't we?"

"Yes, Mom we're fine, we're more than fine," laughed Richie, "in fact, Annie came by and warned us not to be any finer." Nancy rolled over, covering her mouth as she giggled at Richie's comment.

"I see," said Betty, "maybe you two need a chaperone."

Richie laughed even harder, trying to get the words out between guffaws, "you know that's also what Annie said." Now they were both laughing and smiling and exchanging knowing glances.

Betty watched how they looked at each other, and made a mental note, "be careful," she thought, "there's potential danger here."

Walter was watching too. "OK, young lady, it's time for us to get going."

"Yes, Daddy," she said, and leaned over, giving Richie, a warm kiss on his lips, lingering there for several seconds, before coming up for air, "bye, Richie," she smiled, "talk to you soon." Before she disappeared down the hall, she turned, blew a final kiss, and waved goodbye.

Betty was watching Richie. He looked like the cat that ate the canary. She wondered exactly what happened between those two while she was downstairs. It certainly was not a falling out. No, it was not. Betty sensed that there was a change in their relationship, and it was not the change that she had been worried about.

Betty sighed. Was it a tragedy playing out? What could she do, what should she do? Trying to figure it out made her head hurt. She decided she needed someone to talk to. Maybe Madelyn could at least be a sounding board for her. For now she would just wait and see. She would remain vigilant, ready to step in. Hadn't it been complicated enough worrying about her son and his leukemia, now she had to worry about his soul and hers too.

Richie had settled back. He took a break from his schoolwork and went back to his drawings.

He was sketching new green creatures and large turtle people. He was very busy when Carol came over with some pamphlets.

Betty saw her first. "Hi," she said, as Carol approached. "I'll get Richie's attention for you in a minute, but first I was hoping to speak with Madelyn, do you know if she's around? It's nothing urgent."

"I think she's still around, I can let her know that you're looking for her," said Carol. "I have a couple of catalogues showing head coverings for Richie. I'm not sure what he's looking for, but there's a variety to choose from."

"Thank you, Carol," Betty leaned over nudging Richie on his shoulder to bring him back to planet Earth.

Richie looked up and removed his earbuds. Betty couldn't understand how he could listen to music and make those wonderful drawings at the same time.

"Hi, Richie," said Carol, "I have those catalogues you asked for. You can look them over and let me know what you like. I can get them delivered quickly. I'll be back later to see what you've decided."

"Thanks Carol," he took the offered catalogues, "can you wait a sec?" Richie thumbed through them and in about thirty seconds, he had picked out two that he liked. They were black and simple. He let Carol know.

"That was quick, you're sure these are the ones you want?" asked Carol.

"Thank you, Carol, those'll work. Hopefully, I won't be wearing them for too long."

Betty watched as Richie made some quick choices. He seemed pretty cavalier about losing his hair. She imagined that it would have been quite different if it were her with that disease.

"OK, I'll order those for you. That was easy." Carol smiled. She turned and headed back to the Child Life office.

Soon after Carol left, Paul popped his head in, he had finished rounding on the other patients. Betty and Richard were busy at work on their devices. He knocked on the doorway.

Richard had his earbuds in again and didn't look up right away, but Betty saw him, "Hello, Dr. Belkin, are you getting ready to sign out to Dr. Gardner for the night?"

"Yes, how are you guys?"

Betty leaned over to get Richie's attention. She had to push on his arm several times before he looked up. "We've had a good day, Dr. Belkin," said Betty, "and we're hoping to avoid anything like last night. What do you know about Richie's lab tests?"

Paul pulled out his iPad mini and scanned through Richie's lab results. "His chemistries are all in the normal range, his hemoglobin is 8 gm/dL, and his platelet count is 30,000 and of course his white blood cell count is still zero. He won't need any transfusions tonight, I'll order them for the morning. I want his platelet count to be over 50,000 for his LP on Friday, but that's still a few days away. I expect that the next few days will be quiet, but of course there are no guarantees. Any other questions?" When they both shook their heads, Dr. Belkin said, "see you tomorrow," and turned away toward the nurses' station.

While Paul was leaving, Betty got a text from Madelyn, "C U tomorrow unless urgent." And Betty texted back, "2 morrow OK," followed by a thumb's up emoji. Betty had hoped to meet with Madelyn right away. There were so many concerns building up inside, it was overwhelming. But, she would wait, she had to.

29.

Richie was in bed, reading something new he found in the Child Life area. The mother part of her was hoping he would get back to his school studies, but she was content that he was not stuck playing those violent video games. Betty thought about how much time she was spending with him. Their lives were truly connected again. She was able to see little idiosyncrasies that she might never have noticed had they not shared this tiny room for so many days. She watched him read, watched him play games and do his schoolwork, she watched him when he talked to his girlfriend. They shared thoughts and feelings. He had asked for her advice about Nancy. It was an intimacy between mother and son that may not ever have happened. Betty didn't know how she should feel about all of this. She would have done anything, paid any price, made any kind of deal, if she could have prevented that fucking disease. And yet, this time with him was special, she treasured every moment, trying to commit each of them to memory. It occurred to her that she should keep a journal, she couldn't trust her memory. Maybe she could find one in the hospital gift shop, or when she was out doing chores on Thursday. She thought it would be neat to use a fountain pen and ink for her journal entries.

Betty looked at her son, "Hey, it's getting kind of late, do you want to watch something on the tube? I can make popcorn."

Richie looked up from his French lesson, "Gee, Mom, we keep falling asleep before the movie ends and we never find out what happened. How about we find a board game from the Child Life room?"

"Hey, I know, how about a game of cards?" We could play gin rummy, we used to play that when you were younger. I guess it's been a while."

Richie smiled, "that sounds good, I think I still remember how."

"Oh, it'll come right back to you, I'll try to find a deck."

"OK, hey that doesn't mean we can't have popcorn, does it?"

"I'll make some after I find the cards," his mom smiled.

While his mom was gone Richie set up the tray table between them so they would be facing each other when they played. Within a few minutes, there was a steaming bowl of popcorn and Betty was shuffling the cards. She put the deck down, Richie cut the cards and soon they were engaged in a heated game of rummy.

After a couple of hours, Richie and Betty had gone through two bowls of popcorn and several hard-fought gin rummy games. Some of the games were very short, it seemed that after only a few plays someone would yell 'Gin.'

Playing cards with Richie reminded her of home and all the things they did together when he was young. They would go for walks in the park near their little house. In the summer they'd drive over to the nearby beach and camp out under the umbrella. She had images of throwing the frisbee and playing in the surf. Where had those days gone? Betty wondered if they would ever have them again.

Then Richie got a text. Momentarily distracted from the game, he smiled and tapped out a response. Betty knew who was on the other end. Nancy was now a part of her life too.

Betty asked anyway, "Nancy?"

"Yup," said Richie, "what's the score?"

Betty picked up the notepad that was divided in half by a vertical line. She started to add up each side, but got tired after a few moments doing it in her head, "let's just call it a draw, OK?"

"Sure Mom, that was fun, but I'm getting tired. Bedtime, huh?"

Betty got up and feeling like old times with her son, she tucked him in, kissed him on the forehead, and said goodnight.

Richie was skillful at falling asleep. Betty watched his eyes close, and soon heard the steady deep breathing of her sleeping child.

Betty turned over in her chair, she had it extended and was trying her best to fall asleep. Thoughts raced through her head, but she willed herself to quiet them. She imagined a quiet Cape Cod beach, the night sky ablaze with stars painted across the Milky Way, she matched her breathing to the visualized waves lapping at the shore, and pretty soon, she too was able to fall asleep.

30.

The next morning at shift change, Paul and Sandra came to Richie's room and reviewed the unremarkable labs from the night before. No action had been needed.

The white count was still zero, and no transfusions were needed. Everyone seemed happy with the quiet night and the test results. Hopefully, a quiet day would follow the quiet night.

Betty was desperately looking for a quiet day. She had enough crises.

Soon after Paul had moved on, Madelyn stuck her head into the room.

"Hello, guys," said Madelyn. "You both look well rested. How are you, Richie?"

"I'm good," said Richie, "I know there's more chemo and the LP coming on Friday, but mostly I'm feeling pretty good."

"That's great. Is it OK if I talk to your mom for a bit?" asked Madelyn.

"Sure, take her away," he smiled, "I've got work to do."

Betty told Richie she'd be back soon and then she walked away with Madelyn.

"Carol, told me you wanted to talk," Madelyn started, "but she said it wasn't an emergency."

"Thank you for coming over, and it was fine to wait for today. Some things were bothering me, and I don't know if there's an answer, but I thought at least it might help if I said them out loud to a dispassionate professional."

Madelyn smiled, "I'm not sure if I'm dispassionate, but I am a professional, what's up?"

"I'm going to say some things that are confidential, and that Richie doesn't know. I know that what we say between us, doesn't go any further, right?"

"Yes, as long as I don't hear anything about a crime being committed, or someone trying to harm others or themselves, it remains between us."

"Well, you know that Richie is smitten with this girl Nancy, and they, well whatever it means to say for 17-year-olds, think they're in love. They had a fight the other morning and by the end of the day, they were back together. But, I also know, from her dad, that Nancy's mother died of a brain tumor five years ago, and she'd been depressed since then and intermittently in therapy. And now, her dad tells me she's come out of her funk, and she's been happy since meeting Richie. And Richie's happy with her. They're clinging to each other like life rafts at sea. I'm pretty sure that Richie doesn't know all about Nancy's mother, and what it's been like for Nancy. So, here are these two teens, they've found each other and connected. There's the specter of death in both their lives. I'm sure that Nancy's psyche is very fragile. Of course, I'm scared for Richie, what might eventually happen with his leukemia, but I can't do anything about that. I am here for him. Now, I'm worried for Nancy too, and I don't know what to do."

Madelyn listened carefully to the whole story. "So, you're clearly worried about this. The situation is complicated. There are four people involved, two adults, and two nearly 18-year-old adolescents. Your main concern," said Madelyn, "is that one of the kids gets hurt emotionally, and it seems that you have focused on Nancy, because of your perception of her fragility considering her history. It is interesting that you're concerned about what might happen to Nancy if Richard died. You're shouldering a burden that should be borne by her father. One option would be to discuss this with him. What's his name?"

"It's Walter Peters," said Betty, "and I've thought about doing that. I've only talked to him a couple of times so I don't know him well. I think he's a good man and I have no doubt that he loves his daughter, but he seems a bit overwhelmed by the challenges of raising a teenage girl by himself."

"It seems hard to imagine," said Madelyn, "that he hasn't thought about the possibility of Richard dying and how that would affect his daughter. It may also be that, like you, he's not sure what to do about it. Right now, he sees that his daughter is happy, she's coming out of her shell, and he doesn't want to rock the boat. There's potential danger in any action from either of you. Often when a parent intervenes in a relationship, especially involving older adolescents, it results in unintended consequences. In fact, it may lead to an outcome exactly the opposite of what you're hoping to achieve. Richard and Nancy are too old to confront with ultimatums, that would not turn out well."

"What do you suggest?" asked Betty.

"It is hard to know the right answer, but I think that the best you can do, is to make sure that each of them are aware that you're available to talk to, in confidence and without judgement whenever they want. And that you will listen to what they have to say and be a friend that can be trusted."

Betty smiled, "that's what my heart told me, but I wasn't sure I could trust it. Often, I'm alone, trying to figure out how to be a good parent. Most of the time, I think I do a pretty good job without guidance, but I worried, there seemed to be a lot riding on this, and I was scared that, somehow, I might fuck it up, and that I would have to live with the consequences of making the wrong decision. Thank you for listening and being there for me."

"Well, I think you're a very good parent," said Madelyn, "and that's because you love your child, and you're there for him. That's mostly what a parent needs to do, love them and be there. You've done a wonderful job with Richard, it shows. And I'm here too if you need."

Betty stood up, and wiped some tears from her face. She'd been tense and worried, torn between her love for Richie and her perceived responsibility for Nancy. Madelyn had eased at least some of that. Betty thanked her again, and left, trying to make sure she looked OK, for Richie.

Richie looked up from his schoolwork and watched his mom walk back to the room. "Hey, Mom, you've been gone a while, how was your talk with Madelyn?"

"It was fine, sometimes I just need to talk, I'm sure you understand that there's a bit of stress in my life, and it helps. Of course, there's stress in your life too, Richie, and if you ever need to talk about it, I'm here for you. And if you felt it was hard to talk to me about some things, we can get Madelyn or someone else for you."

"Sure, I know that Mom, but what did you and Madelyn talk about?"

"You know, some about my work, but mostly about how I worry about you and also about Nancy."

"Really? I'm not surprised that you worry about me, but you worry about Nancy too. Why is that?"

"Well, she seems nice, and it must be hard coming to a children's hospital to see you and yet she still does. And she's important to you, so that makes her important to me too. You know that just as I'm always here for you, I could be there for Nancy if she needed to talk to someone. Maybe she might want to talk to, you know, a female for some things, I could be there for her."

Richie looked at his mom. "Mom, that's really nice that you think of Nancy like that. You can still surprise me sometimes. And I'm glad that you think about her like that because she is important to me, you know I really like her."

"I know you do, Richie, and it's nice to know that I can still surprise you."

"Mom," Richie started.

"What is it dear?"

"You know that fight, that Nancy and I had the other day, I told you that it was because I said that maybe she would have been better off if she never met me."

"Yes, I remember." Betty looked at her son, it came to her, all at once, what he was going to say, and her heart sank, the color drained from her face. She moved over to sit beside her son on the bed.

"Well, I felt bad, you know, what it would be like for her if I died. That's why I said that maybe she would have been better off if she never met me. I know that was wrong to say. But it helps me, I feel better now knowing that you would be there for her, you could help her."

Tears fell down Betty's face, she made no effort to stop them. She looked at Richie, the words from his lips, said out loud, pierced her veneer of invulnerability, it went straight to her soul, tearing her apart. The walls that she had so carefully put up to protect herself from thinking about her son's possible death, came tumbling down. She pictured her old age, alone in her house with no family. No Richie to visit, no grandchildren to play with. It hurt to even think about it. She sat down with her son, holding him tightly, as they cried together. They stayed like that for a while, Betty cradling Richie's head in her lap, as he curled up beside her.

Betty quietly began to hum a soft melody, one she remembered from her youth, when her mother would comfort her grieving child. If there ever were lyrics, she no longer knew them. Her fingers passed through what hair was left as she gently stroked his head, trying to soothe her grieving child. Before too long, the tears dried, the melody quieted, and as they sought solace in each other's embrace, they were able to find a peaceful place and together, they drifted off to sleep.

They slept like that for hours. The days in the hospital, the stress, the treatments and crises, all had taken their toll. Their only escape was in slumber and their bodies grabbed it when they could.

The day passed slowly, and at least medically, it had been uneventful. The two daily doses of dexamethasone, barely recognized as chemotherapy faded into the background noise of treatment. Without realizing it, the daylight ebbed, and evening brought Paul around to check on them.

"How are you guys?" he asked.

Betty looked up at Dr. Belkin, "I guess we just mellowed out today."

"You're entitled to a day without excitement," said Paul. "From my point of view, everything is going as it's supposed to. His blood cultures are still listed as "no growth to date" and if that remains the same tomorrow, I'll stop the vancomycin. Ceftazidime will continue until his white count begins to recover. Do you have any questions?"

"My plan," said Betty, "was to go home tomorrow morning, and return early on Friday before his LP. Do you think that'll be OK?"

"Tomorrow should be another quiet day," said Paul. "If Richard needs transfusions we already have consents. It should be fine for you to leave."

Paul had EMR notes to catch up on, so he excused himself to work at one of the computer workstations.

They had a few hours to go before bedtime and Betty decided that they should look for a fun movie to help take their minds off all their worries. She asked Richie for suggestions.

"A fun movie sounds good, I have some ideas that would fit the bill, how about *Ferris Bueller's Day Off*, or if you can't find that, then either *Groundhog Day* or *My Cousin Vinny*."

"Oh, those are great, I could watch any of them over and over again, and we certainly could use a day off," said Betty, "I'll be back with one of those and a bowl of popcorn."

A little while later, Betty came back with a DVD, and a bowl of popcorn.

"Which one did you get?" asked Richie.

"I guess we're going to get a *day off*, which we deserve."

"Awesome," said Richie, he popped the Bueller movie into the DVD player, and they sat back to enjoy the show. As the opening scenes started, Richie, who was always full of trivia tidbits, told his mom some fun facts about the movie. "You know, that in the movie, Matthew Broderick's character is seeing Mia Sara's character, Sloane Peterson. And he's always battling with his sister in the movie, cause she's envious that he's taking the day off. He's pretending to be sick, and she's annoyed that everyone keeps wishing him to get well. But off camera, Matthew Broderick is actually having a relationship with Jennifer Grey, his sister in the movie. And the actors, Lyman Ward and Cindy Pickett, playing Bueller's parents in the movie, fall in love during the movie, get married, and have kids together.

Betty had a bit of a chuckle hearing Richie tell what he knew about the movie. That was the old Richie, he would love explaining stuff about the show they were going to watch. It was a bit of normalcy even in the hospital. Betty loved her son even if he was kind of nerdy.

Richie and his mom were enjoying the movie together when Paul came by to check on them one last time before signing out to Sandra. The parade scene in downtown Chicago had just started, and Richie paused the movie.

"How are you guys?" asked Paul.

"We're fine," said Richie.

"Ferris Bueller's Day Off?" said Paul, "I like this movie."

"You know," said Richie, "that on the first day of shooting the movie in Chicago, the director found out that there was going to be a German American parade for Von Steuben Day, they built their own float and kind of sneaked into the parade and filmed these scenes. Of course, they edited the singing of *Danke Schoen* and the girls on their float were actors."

"That's cool," said Paul, "can you start it up, I'd like to watch this part again. Sometimes knowing background stuff spoils the scene, but it can also make it more interesting."

It started again, and they watched the parade scene together. Now Matthew Broderick was lip synching, the Beatles song, *Twist and Shout*. Before too long, Richie felt the urge to stand up and join in. Soon, the nurses and staff, hearing the commotion, gathered around, smiling, and clapping in time to the music as Richie, Betty and Paul lined up, becoming part of the Von Steuben parade, lip synching the words and marching around the unit.

As the movie parade scene finished, everyone on the unit was smiling and laughing. Their audience appreciated the performance and the trio bowed graciously to the crowd. Betty enjoyed it so much, she almost forgot that they were in the oncology unit.

Whoo-hoo, that was great!" The nurses yelled, whistled and applauded.

"Well," said Paul, "I think that from now on, every time I see this movie, I'll remember our own parade. I better leave you both to finish the movie." He smiled and walked on.

Leaving the cares of the hospital behind, Betty and Richie settled in, and enjoyed watching the rest of the movie.

Paul signed out to Sandra, who took over the night duty. It was another quiet shift, and once again, Sandra spent the night undisturbed.

The next day began uneventfully as the medical team stopped at Richie's room. "Good morning, guys," said Paul, "we're hoping for another quiet day. Tomorrow's a repeat of the day one therapy, except the spinal tap will use methotrexate instead of Ara-C. Richard will have a platelet transfusion early tomorrow morning. We'll use the LMX-4 on his back and the Versed to relax him. Do you have any questions?"

"I was hoping that I could be unhooked from the IV pole," asked Richie, "at least for a while today so I can walk around. Would that be OK?"

"We can do that," said Dr. Belkin, "you'll have to stay on the unit and wear an N95 mask when you are out of your room."

"No problem, thanks" said Richie.

"I plan to go home for the day," said Betty, "and return tomorrow morning before Richie's procedure."

"Today should be quiet," said Paul, "it's probably a good day for you to leave."

"Thanks," said Betty, "I know you'll take good care of him."

Betty turned to Richie, "I'm ready. You're still OK, with me taking off, right?"

"Sure Mom, it's cool. Will you be able to hunt around a bit for that bracelet for Nancy, maybe take some pictures?"

Betty smiled, "I'll try, there's a place near the Gallery. We'll talk later and of course you can call me anytime, otherwise, I'll be here early tomorrow morning." Betty leaned over and kissed Richie on the top of his head. It was sparse up there, but she agreed that it needed some work. "See you, bye," Betty turned and left the unit.

Betty stopped at the Target in the mall on the way home. She picked up a few personal items from the pharmacy section. She didn't want to spend much of her day in the store, and fortunately it wasn't crowded this early on a weekday. She looked for the School/Stationery section and browsed through a few journal books, before finding a leather-bound one that she liked. Betty also picked out an inexpensive fountain pen and a bottle of black ink. Walking through the grocery section, she picked up coffee and milk and a few other items for lunch. She'd get takeout for her dinner. While Betty was waiting on the shorter self-checkout line, she was struck by the apparently normal activity she had seen throughout the store. Shoppers pushing carts through the aisles, some dealing with fussy children, mothers deciding which cereal to pick up. She was pretty sure that anyone watching her wouldn't see a woman in distress. Despite appearances it was far from a normal day for her.

At home, she picked up the accumulated mail from the week, sorting out the ads from the bills, tossing the former into the paper recycle bin, and putting all the bills into her "back to the hospital bag" along with the non-grocery Target purchases. She would manage the bills when she was back at the hospital. Betty texted her boss, letting her know that she'd be over at the Gallery at 1. She would take a nice quiet bubble bath tonight, with a glass of wine, but she needed a quick rinse in the shower before heading out to work. Betty was happy to see that she hadn't left any dirty dishes lying around, but she decided a few spots around the house needed the cordless vacuum cleaner before she took her shower. She managed to finish her clean-up chores and her shower before noon, so she still had time for a leisurely lunch before heading over to the Gallery.

31.

It was an eventful afternoon at work for Betty. In addition to her bookkeeping, she was also on the phone, connecting with clients, chatting them up, making sure that she understood what they were looking for, and then figuring out how to provide it. She kept information about all the Gallery's clients, their buying history and what types of art they were interested in. Betty had a knack for anticipating their needs. She knew where they traveled on vacation, she had a good idea of their budgets and what time of year they would be receiving bonuses at work, and therefore when they would be looking to buy. Of course, there was also incidental traffic in the store as passersby came in to browse. Betty always stood up to greet them, offering to help and quietly disappearing if help was declined.

Shelley came over and sat down to chat with Betty. She asked about Richie and about how Betty was managing with everything.

"I'm glad you could come in this afternoon," said Shelley, "I can't even imagine what you must be going through. Yet here you are. You have a remarkable ability to focus on work, even though you must be worried about Richie. I don't know how you do it." Shelley paused a minute and took a breath. "Betty, you're very important to me and to the Gallery and from a selfish point of view, I want you here as much as possible. But I also want you to be comfortable coming here when you can.

Family is more important than anything. So, I don't want you to ever feel that you need to choose between Richie and the Gallery. Your job is safe here. I will always presume that if you are here, it means that Richie is safe at the hospital."

"Thank you, Shelley, it means a lot to hear you say that." Betty knew she needed her job, and on top of everything else, she continued to worry about how secure her position at the Gallery was, it was a big relief to hear the reassurances from her boss.

As Richie returned to his room with his evening movie, his phone rang. It was his mom's ring chime. He punched the phone icon, "Hi, Mom, how's your day been?"

"I just got home from the Gallery. It's been a good day. Shelley had some nice words for me, and I also think I have two new sales. How's your day been?"

"You'll be very happy to know that it's been extremely boring, I spent some hours on school stuff, and I just finished a few laps around the unit."

Betty laughed, "sorry, I guess I am happy that's it's been boring, excitement and hospitalization are words that don't go well together. I also have a couple of pictures I took of bracelets at the jewelry store next to the Gallery. I think you might like something from there. Is there anything else you need from home?"

"I'm good Mom, thanks for doing that. Bath and a glass of wine tonight?"

"Yup, I've earned it. And I started a new book, a romance suspense novel, it should be good reading for the end of the day."

"OK, Mom, sounds good, I'll see you in the morning. Be careful. I love you."

"I love you, too," his mom rung off.

Betty finished a relaxing bath, with her glass of wine, and climbed into bed. She made a few notes in her new journal, trying to sort out the sequence of events as she remembered them. Happy with the first few pages in her diary, she closed the journal and picked up her new novel.

32.

Tuesday morning started early with Carol's appearance in Richie's room. He was feeling better after the uneventful weekend and how well the spinal tap with chemo had gone. Carol handed Richie the packages with the head coverings that had arrived that morning. "I hope these work for you."

Richie thanked Carol and turned to his mom, "let's get the shaving done, OK? There are still a few stragglers up there and now that I have the head coverings, I'd like to try them on."

Betty arranged the shaving cream and the disposable razor. She draped a towel around Richie's shoulders and used a warm soapy washcloth to clean and moisten the top of Richie's head. After shaking the can a few times, she covered his scalp with the soapy cream. Betty decided that he looked a bit like Harpo Marx. Never having shaved a head, she imagined it couldn't be much different than shaving her legs and went to work. She got the hang of it quickly, the few hairs he had left were scraggly and marcescent. When Betty finished, she stood back, inspected her work and was satisfied. Using another warm wet washcloth she cleaned his head, and then dried it all with the towel she picked up from around his shoulders. "Ta da!" she exclaimed, "I guess I can add barber to my long list of motherly roles."

Betty handed Richie her mirror. He reached up, feeling around his head, and then used the mirror to make a complete survey.

Richie had sat through the shave struggling to understand how he'd gotten to this point. He for sure looked like a cancer patient now. He'd been trying to appear positive but inside he was a mess. Dark thoughts swirled around in his head. His junior year at school was gone, as was his summer and track. Would Nancy be gone too? Would he even have a senior year at school? Doubts crept through his head. But he didn't want his mom to worry, so he gave a thumbs up, and made an effort at a smile, "way to go Mom." He opened the packages and tried both head coverings on. "Which one do you like?"

They looked pretty much the same, simple black skull caps with a tie hanging down at the back. Betty, somewhat arbitrarily, picked the one that was the durag, rather than the chemo cap. "OK, that's set. Let me take a picture." Betty pulled out her phone, Richie posed and the moment was documented.

Betty took out her journal and fountain pen. She scribbled something about Richie's shave, and added some private thoughts.

"I see your new journal, what's it like?"

"It's good," said Betty. "I started, last night at home. I tried to remember everything that's happened since you first noticed the bruise. Now, I'll start a fresh page each day, mark the date, and write what happens. I'll try to be objective, but of course, it's all from my viewpoint."

"Is it fun?" asked Richie.

"I would say it's cathartic, it's enjoyable and calming in a certain way. You know, Richie, it's private, I put down my thoughts and feelings about what's happening. Someday, I might let you read it, but for now, I'd rather that you don't try, OK?"

"Sure Mom, I get it. Hey, can you show me the pictures you took at the jewelry store?"

Richie flicked through the pictures of charm bracelets on his mom's phone. He wasn't sure which one Nancy would like. It wasn't like picking head coverings, he needed more time to think about it. He returned the phone, and they both went back to their laptops. Working on his school assignments helped Richie push those dark thoughts back into some hidden corner of his brain. It was a welcome respite.

After working a while longer Richie announced that he was going to call Nancy.

"Go ahead, Richie," she said, "I'll take a little walk, I need some time for myself.

On the phone with Nancy, they would talk about anything, except his leukemia and its treatment. They talked like old friends, it was familiar and comforting. Nancy liked to talk about Ms. Shute and how she enjoyed being on the library committee and Richie talked about Dr. Gardner and how cool she was. They each had their own worlds, and as they shared, they grew closer. They delighted in hearing each other's stories. They were two souls, learning to trust, learning to love, learning about life and who they were. On the phone, the rest of the world disappeared. They were alone together.

They would have talked for hours more if Nancy's father hadn't called out to her.

"Oh, oh, Richie, I gotta go." Nancy kissed the phone, a loud smack, and rang off.

Richie looked around for his mom, but she was nowhere to be found. He vaguely remembered her saying something when he started the call with Nancy. He had a memory of his mom walking toward the elevator, but not much else. That had been a while ago.

Finally, he saw his mom exiting the elevator, returning to the unit. Richie immediately noticed that distant look on Betty's face. He knew it well, her head was clearly occupied with something and they didn't appear to be happy thoughts.

"What're you thinking about, Mom?"

She looked up and half smiled, "well, just you, Richie. That's mostly what I think about. You and your disease. How you've already had a few close calls. I should be paying better attention but sometimes I'm overwhelmed. This place plays games with my head and that's not good." She took a breath, "I have to focus."

"You're doing great Mom. It's all new, and after all the doctors are watching me."

"The doctors are good," said Betty. "I like them. But they might not see everything."

33.

Ritchie woke up and stretched, trying to shake off the cobwebs of sleep. He glanced across the room and saw his mom, already awake in her chair. She still seemed lost in thought. "Good morning, Mom, how'd you sleep?"

"Not so good, I guess. I can't remember exactly what I dreamed, but I seemed to be chasing someone or something and no matter how fast or far I ran, it's always just out of reach. It wasn't a good dream."

"That sounds disturbing. I think I know that feeling."

The medical team was gathered outside Richie's room, reporting to each other. They finished and Betty watched the team as they entered. Usually they'd been chatty, and gregarious. But it was different today, no smiles, and they avoided eye contact. Betty had a bad feeling. It recalled her dreams.

Dr. Stanner began, "we now have the report from the gene analysis of Richard's leukemia cells. Unfortunately, the analysis identified a gene mutation that will require a change in our approach to Richard's treatment. I'll come back shortly, after rounds, to discuss that in more detail."

Betty's mouth went dry. Somehow, the terrible news wasn't a surprise. Hadn't she known that something bad was coming. She summoned all her strength to do what was needed next. Before he could leave, she stopped him to ask the question whose answer she dreaded to hear. "Dr. Stanner," she began, a tear fell, that she did not try to wipe away, "sorry," she stopped again, took a few deep breaths, trying to compose herself, "sorry, Dr. Stanner, I must know, whatever this is, are there still options? Is Richie going to...," she couldn't finish the sentence. "What happens now?"

Dr. Stanner stopped, turned around, he paused a moment and then sat down on the bed, next to Richie, across from Betty, and looked her in the eye, "yes, Ms. Samuelson, we have options, it's going to be tougher than we had hoped, but we have weapons in our armamentarium. There are still ways to treat his disease. We're not giving up."

'OK, Dr. Stanner," said Betty, she wiped the tears with her sleeve, she tried to control her sobs. Just breathe, she told herself. "As long as there's a chance, we can face it and do whatever it takes. We'll be ready to hear your plan when you come back."

Betty let the team go and came over to hold Richie. He looked blank, shell-shocked. Betty wondered what he meant by *treat* the disease. That didn't sound like *cure* the disease. That fucking roller coaster again, she wanted nothing more to do with that fucking ride. She held him. Rocking together, they cried, "it'll be OK, Richie, I promise, it will be OK."

It seemed they waited a while, but it was only a short time later when Drs. Stanner and Gardner came back and suggested that they meet in the parent conference room. They could talk more comfortably in there.

Richie and Betty walked together, supporting each other, across the corridor to the parent conference room. They sat down and held hands. A box of Kleenex was nearby.

"We're ready, doctors, tell us everything," said Betty.

Dr. Stanner began, "one of the bone marrow samples from his first morning was sent for something called *Next Generation Sequencing*, now a routine part of the disease stratification. It's likely that all cancer cells have mutations, that is changes in the DNA from normal. About a million cells in the body are replaced every second. Each cell carries about 20,000 genes. That means that in anyone's body billions of genes are copied each second, and so there are invariably errors. Normally there are mechanisms to repair mistakes, or if they can't be fixed, the cell undergoes something called apoptosis, a programmed cell death. A gene called p53, also known as the so-called suicide gene, is involved in initiating apoptosis. If the mutations in a cell are recognized as being too dangerous or irreparable, a cascade of events in the cell is triggered. A cluster of proteins is then released from tiny packages inside the cell called lysosomes. The proteins include DNases, caspases and other enzymes that begin to digest the mutated cell from the inside. The residual cell carcass will then be devoured by macrophages, scavengers of the body's clean up squad. This surveillance system is designed to protect us. Unfortunately, sometimes a mutation happens in those guardian suicide genes and then when a second dangerous mutation occurs in a cell with an already damaged apoptosis program, the transformed cell can't be eliminated. It continues to grow and divide. And while most mutations are innocuous, some changes lead to a malignant transformation resistant to therapy. That puts the patient into an even higher risk category. We're not always sure why, but we do know which of those mutations are not good to have. Are you following me?"

"Some gene mutations are worse than others, right?" said Richie.

"Exactly," continued Dr. Stanner, "and unfortunately in Richard's gene analysis we found a mutation called MLL at 11q23. MLL, stands for Mixed Lineage Leukemia. This mutation leads to the creation of unique fusion proteins. That means that a fragment of one protein attaches to a fragment of a different protein, creating a sort of Frankenstein's monster protein. That freakish novel protein leads to changes that make those cells unresponsive to the usual cellular controls."

"So, this MLL gene rearrangement, puts Richie into a higher risk category, is that right?" asked Betty. She could hardly get the words out. Her hopes were being crushed.

"Unfortunately, yes, and that means that conventional chemotherapy is less likely to work for him," said Dr. Stanner.

"So, you said there are options," said Richie.

"Because of this new information, Richard's best choice for treatment has changed. His best path forward now will be to undergo a bone marrow transplant," answered Dr. Stanner.

"Transplant!" said Betty. "Shit, I don't like the sound of that." Betty looked at Richie, she was terrified. She pictured a horrific ordeal littered with a series of anguishing calamities. Was this how Richie would die? A desperate attempt that was bound to fail. She wondered what else they weren't saying. "What does this all mean?"

"The transplant process begins with a short course of very intensive chemotherapy," Dr. Stanner explained, "it's designed to eradicate every single leukemia cell in his body. As a result of the procedure, Richard's normal blood forming marrow cells suffer collateral damage and will need to be replaced with a new set of cells from a healthy volunteer donor. But there's a remarkable added benefit. If any malignant cell manages to escape the initial therapy, the newly created immune system from the donor will track it down, consider it foreign and destroy it. Imagine bloodhounds hunting their prey. And that will be crucial for maintaining Richard's remission. In essence, we will have installed a new security system."

"You said we would use a healthy donor, right?" asked Betty.

"Yes, for a bone marrow transplant, we take cells from a healthy donor, who will then grow new cells to replace the harvested cells. We'll need to identify someone who's a match for Richard's blood stem cells. A parent typically would have half of the important match criteria. A full sibling would have a twenty-five percent chance of being a complete match, unless of course the sibling is an identical twin in which case he would invariably be a perfect match. As Richard doesn't have any siblings, we'll have to search the bone marrow transplant registry list to find that person. It's a bit like identifying a blood donor. But instead of just A, B or O blood types, there are 10 genetic spots or loci, that must align with Richard. These loci are part of the HLA system, and we want to find a donor who matches at least 9 of 10 of those antigen spots. Preferably, it would match all 10. The International Bone Marrow Transplant Registry, or IBMTR, keeps a computerized list of many thousands of potential donors, and their HLA profile. We already know Richard's HLA, Human Leukocyte Antigen, typing from a blood sample taken his first day here. We can enter that information into a computer program that will search its base for possible matches."

"So, what happens now?" asked Betty.

"With your consent, we'll request a search of the bone marrow registry, hopefully to find a 10/10 HLA match for Richard. If a match is found, the donor will be contacted to verify that their profile on record is accurate and that they are still willing to donate. Most people on the list are excited to be chosen and offered a chance to help save a life. If all goes well, they'll evaluate and prepare the donor to harvest his or her blood stem cells.

Once harvested, the cells will be sent to PGL, a lab we use in California. They have a unique process for optimizing the cell's performance. From there the cells will be shipped to our blood bank and then infused into Richard, sort of like a blood transfusion. Once the donor cells are in Richie's bloodstream they will find their way to his bone marrow where they will implant and grow. Those stem cells will eventually produce all the blood cells he will ever need.

This will take time to arrange, and so Richard will require interim therapy until the transplant can begin."

"This transplant procedure, the whole thing, it's dangerous, isn't it?" asked Betty. She already knew the answer. Betty couldn't help exploring worst case scenarios and this was at the top of her list.

"There are in fact significant risks, including infection and marrow rejection. There's also something called Graft versus Host Disease, a kind of reverse rejection. Graft vs. Host Disease, or GvHD, occurs when the immune cells of the donor recognizes the host, its new home, as foreign and attacks it. It could affect Richard's skin, his eyes, liver and many other tissues. He will need medications to mitigate any damage from that. But GvHD also has an upside. As I mentioned, any leukemia cells left hiding in Richard would also be considered foreign by the new marrow and would be attacked. And that part is good. So, there's a sweet spot for GvHD. The Goldilocks level of GvHD that we hope to achieve. And that is why it's critically important to carefully HLA match the donor with Richard. This type of transplant is referred to as an allogeneic, matched unrelated donor transplant. Allogeneic means that the infused cells come from a donor, as opposed to an autologous transplant in which a patient uses their own cells for rescue. We'll review all of that in detail over the next several days.

Of course, you can elect to continue conventional chemotherapy and not undergo a bone marrow transplant. We can, and I do recommend that we start the search for a donor. There's no obligation to proceed. But historical data tells us, given the genetic mutation that we found, that Richard's chance of being alive and in remission two years from now, is greater with the transplant than if we continue with conventional chemotherapy. If that were not the case, I wouldn't be discussing this with you."

Betty reached out to hold Richie's hand. They looked at each other, too numb for words. She'd been having bad dreams for days. Deep in her gut, she had known that something bad was coming. And now it was here. There were monsters everywhere.

34.

At the Pharma Gene Laboratories, PGL, in southern California, Drs. Hans Benzi and Jordan Carlson, both Ph.D. laboratory investigators, were leading several animal studies trying to improve the outcomes for allogeneic bone marrow transplant. Their work focused on the effect of genes transferred from one animal species to another.

Dr. Benzi was one of the scheduled speakers at the upcoming annual American Genetics Symposium in San Diego and he was preparing to give one of the featured talks about their lab work. He and Jordan Carlson were huddled in his office, going through the slides for his power point presentation. There would be hundreds of researchers listening and they wanted everything to be perfect.

"So, your first few slides are going to be pretty standard stuff," said Jordan, "pictures of the mice we're using. A slide or two about how they're created without an immune system so we can test our new process. That looks good."

"Yes," said Hans, "and then I'll review the background genetics on the animals we know never seem to get cancer. The slide will show that they seem to be random unrelated species, whales, sharks and tortoises, among others. They have very long lifespans and yet they rarely develop cancer.

"I think this is where we can add some background about the genetics of the woolly mammoth," Hans chimed in.

Together they worked on a slide describing how they used AI programming, to sort through hundreds of genes that might be useful in their research. One of those genes called p53, also known as the suicide gene, because it initiated self-destruction in cells that were becoming malignant, was already known. The woolly mammoth's genome contained dozens of copies of this gene and that likely helped its survival. Well at least against cancer, it clearly didn't work against humans throwing spears.

"Someone in the audience might ask how this work can apply to humans," added Jordan, "you have to be prepared to answer that kind of question."

They worked for several more hours, polishing the presentation until they were happy with the finished packet.

Across campus, a separate division of PGL, the company's current source of revenue, continued to process donor blood stem cells for people who needed a transplant. It turned out that at that moment, in the back corner of the half buried building, the board was deep into their quarterly review of their financials and there were concerns.

The board was discussing one of their recent initiatives to improve profits for their shareholders. They had recruited Drs. Benzi and Carlson from academia, luring them with large salaries and substantial research funding to create an improved marketable product. The board, of course, knew how much money the company had invested in providing their lab with ultra-fast computers loaded with sophisticated artificial intelligence programming. But the only board member who knew the details of their studies was Dr. Brickston.

In preparation for the board meeting he reviewed the latest report from the lab. It read like a medical abstract:

'We are currently conducting a genomic analysis of several species of interest. A full report will follow. It includes DNA analysis of the

following animals: a 100 year old giant tortoise, Chelonoidis abingdonii, found in the Galapagos Islands; an elephant, Loxodonta Africana, with fifty-six chromosomes; and a 200 year old bowhead whale, Balaena mysticetus, with forty-two chromosomes and 3.7 quadrillion cells. Our lab is using these results to evaluate the effectiveness of testing various combinations of their genes. We use the previously reported approach of gene transfer via the lentivirus vector.'

He was only able to understand a bit of what he read. After the company's large investment he was counting on a payoff soon, or he might find himself out of a job.

Drs. Benzi and Carlson's hypothesis was that cancer immunity could only be created by using the correct combination of genes working in concert. That would mean that there would be hundreds of thousands of gene combination permutations possible. Normally it would take thousands of mouse years to evaluate all of the permutations. However, by using AI programming to create virtual models of those gene combinations, they could analyze tens of thousands of permutations in only a few months. The program would then choose a much more limited series of combinations to test in their animal models.

The transfected experimental genes provided the mice with a blueprint to make new proteins with novel functions. The hope was that some of those novel proteins would provide cancer resistance.

Dr. Benzi was in the animal lab discussing the next round of experiments with his lab technician.

"How many mice will you be injecting with the new gene combinations today," he asked.

"I have twelve cages set up this time. There are 6 male mice and 6 female mice." His tech had the cages lined up on the work bench. Each cage was labeled with a code for that gene combination and a date. "We're testing two different gene combinations today," he told Dr. Benzi. Each combination will be given to 3 male and 3 female mice. As usual after 3 days we will inject each one with a lethal dose of leukemia cells. As you know, we obtain blood samples from the tail vein each day to monitor their progress and to analyze any new proteins they might be producing. Every result is carefully documented."

"Maybe we'll get some survivors with this set." Dr. Benzi was hopeful despite the fact that so far none of the gene combinations had protected the mice. They had all died within a week of the leukemia challenge. "Even if some of them live just a little longer, our AI program can use that information to help choose a better combination."

The technician had his doubts, "there's always a chance," he said.

35.

Richie and Betty were back in their room, quiet and lost in thought. Richie was in trouble, but exactly how much was a dark mystery. The real possibility that Richie might die haunted them. Betty and Richie cried. They lay together, silently on the small hospital bed, holding each other. Betty brushed her hand across his head as he lay in her arms. Each knew the other's mind, no words were needed. They rested like that for a long time, and in their quiet contemplation, they mercifully found comfort in sleep.

His nurse, coming by to check on Richie, watched them sleep. She knew about the conversation with Dr. Stanner. Annie was sad too, thinking about what they were going through. As was often the case, on the small pediatric oncology unit, connections were made, and feelings ran deep. Annie would go home tonight and give her children an extra squeeze. She pulled the curtain, and closed his door to let them be, as long as possible.

Sandra came by to speak with Annie, asking about the Samuelsons. Sandra, like the others, had grown close and invested in Richie's fate.

"They're asleep right now," said Annie. "They're having a really hard time. I haven't heard much from the room since the meeting.

What do you think, Dr. Gardner, what are his chances now?" asked Annie.

"That's a bad mutation for him to have, he was already at high risk because of his age, and this, unfortunately, puts him into a very high-risk category. If we find a good donor match for him and he can get through the transplant process, he'll at least have a shot. We'll do another bone marrow exam tomorrow and see how much leukemia is left.

Annie, will you buzz me when they wake up?"

Hours later, Betty woke up next to Richard. She gently disentangled herself, trying not to wake him. Betty walked to the nurses' station and asked for Sandra. She was hoping to speak with her alone.

"Dr. Gardner asked me to let her know when you're up. She's expecting to talk with you. I'll call her."

Betty walked over to the fellow's room, waiting outside. Soon the door opened with Sandra standing in the doorway.

She opened the door a bit wider and invited Betty in.

For the first time, Betty saw their inner sanctum, it was spartan. She saw the lockers, the single cot, the door to the bathroom and the computer stations. There were reminder notes taped around the computer. It was a clean space, but by no means tidy. It seemed to Betty that the invitation to come inside arose from a mixture of intimacy and compassion. It was comforting and unsettling at the same time. Betty and then Sandra sat down in the small room.

"I wanted to talk to you without Richie," said Betty. "I know that he has been in on all our conversations before, but it seems different now, perhaps this is more about me. I need to hear answers, while I'm alone, and I can feel and react without constraint. I need to know what he's up against."

"Of course, I understand," said Sandra, "the finding of the MLL gene rearrangement puts Richard at a significantly higher risk. He needs more intensive treatment to have a shot at a cure."

"Yes, that's what Dr. Stanner said, but what are his chances now?" She took a deep breath, steeling herself to ask the ultimate question, "Dr. Gardner, is he going to die?"

"I am sorry for you, Betty, I can't begin to imagine what you're going through," she answered, "but he really does have a chance with the bone marrow transplant."

"Yes, but what chance, Dr. Gardner? Is it one in a million, one in a hundred, I need to know."

"Do you really want a number? Those are statistics, and it usually comes from data that's at least 5 years old, it also doesn't include people who've received this new antibody. And in the end, for Richie, it can only be 0 or 100%. He's not a statistic."

"I have to know, please tell me." Betty would not be put off. Despite her persistent queries, she still feared the answer she might get. Beads of sweat formed across her brow and she felt her heart pounding in her chest. She tried to brace herself for whatever answer was about to come.

Sandra looked at her carefully, she took a breath, "OK, you could look it up, so, I'll tell you that based on older studies, his 5-year survival with this mutation and the bone marrow transplant is expected to be about 25%. Those are population statistics. Richard is unique, he's not a number and honestly, we don't know. My guess is that his real chance may be better than that."

Betty sat there thinking about the number she just heard. She turned it over in her head, she weighed it carefully. Finally, Betty stood up, "thank you Dr. Gardner," she said, "if we do the transplant, Richie will be in that 25%. I know it!" And she walked out of the room.

Betty went back and sat down in her sleeper chair, waiting for Richie to wake. She reviewed everything that she'd been told since Richie's diagnosis. It was all very complicated, a fucking roller coaster. She hated that damn ride.

Richie soon began to stir, groaning a bit as he woke. He looked exhausted though he had slept for hours. With an obvious effort, he pushed himself up into a sitting position. Richie looked over and saw his mother watching him as he tried to shake off the effects of hours of sleep. He chased her out of the room so he could pee.

Betty came back when he was done. "I guess you've been thinking about what Dr. Stanner told us," Richie said, "and you've considered the options, no doubt, so what have you decided?"

"I can't decide anything without you, Richie."

"OK, what have you thought?"

"I have some thoughts about this, Richie, but I'd rather hear what you think, before I say anything."

"I guess you've struggled with this," said Richie, "but to me it's simple, I need the bone marrow transplant, and I just hope they can find a donor, soon. I want to live."

Betty smiled at hearing the words from the mouth of her baby. "It's true, I have struggled with this. And while you were sleeping, I had a chance to talk with Dr. Gardner."

"Mom, I don't need to know the details. Did she think I should have the transplant?"

"She thought your chances would be better with the transplant, but she didn't really make a recommendation. And as we spoke Dr. Gardner answered some questions I had."

"So, Mom, what's the bottom line?"

Betty took a big breath, "I had decided to support your decision, whatever that was going to be."

Richard smiled, "I guess I shouldn't be surprised. So, transplant it is," he got up and hugged his mom. They stood that way, holding each other. When they let go, Richie looked at his mom and said, "I'm really hungry now, what can we eat?"

Betty laughed, "way to cheer up the crowd with a critical question. Let me check, maybe the gang is ordering, and we can piggyback in on their plan." Betty walked over to the nurses' station and indeed, they were getting ready to order out, but hadn't decided where to get food from, they were open to suggestions. Betty's idea was pizza and that seemed to get a general nod of agreement. She gave them her order and some cash to cover the pizza and delivery.

Betty texted Sandra, "pizza coming, U R invited."

Sandra came over a few minutes later, "how'd you know I was hungry?" she asked.

"Richie is kind of the canary in the coal mine, so if he's wanting something, I know," said Betty. "I wanted to let you know that Richie and I feel that we're in good hands here, and if you and Dr. Stanner think that transplant is the right choice, we're ready to follow your advice. You're planning a bone marrow exam for tomorrow, is that right?"

"Yes, I've called Dr. Street to provide anesthesia, it'll be like Richard's previous bone marrow exam. It's important to know how much leukemia is left, that's his residual disease. We know that there will be some disease, but how much gives us valuable prognostic information. Richie will need a platelet transfusion in the morning before the procedure. Dr. Stanner has already requested the HLA search in the bone marrow registry, and we'll likely hear something tomorrow afternoon. He'll also be speaking with you more about the transplant. Potentially some interim chemotherapy might start on the weekend. Dr. Stanner will decide about that. The transplant could begin as early as next week. That'll depend on finding a donor, his or her availability and preparing the donor for harvest. Whatever blast cells remain in Richie's bone marrow will have survived the initial therapy, and so they will be the hardest to treat. We'll need something different, strong and soon."

Richie, Betty and Sandra sat around the unit day area, quietly eating the pizza. Betty watched as they ate in silence. The scene would have seemed surprisingly normal, but inside Betty it was anything but. Thoughts swirled in her head, endless possibilities presented themselves and then quickly vanished. She had no way to sort them out. In the end, all she had was hope.

36.

Back at PGL, Dr. Carlson got a call from his lab tech, who wanted to show him something in the animal room. Bill, the technician led Dr. Carlson back to where hundreds of cages housed the experimental mice. As they entered, Dr. Carlson reached for the light switch, but Bill stopped him. "Leave the lights off, just listen for a minute."

Dr. Carlson listened. At first, he didn't hear anything, but Bill signaled for Dr. Carlson to be quiet and wait. After a few moments, he heard a distinctive whirring sound. Bill already knew where it was coming from. He quietly led Dr. Carlson, in the dark, over to that cage. Reaching up, he pulled it off the shelf, and carefully laid it down on a table in the aisle. The mouse was hurtling along, making the exercise wheel spin. They remained quiet for a few minutes, watching in amazement. Bill carried a flashlight, which he turned on, and pointed at the mouse. Immediately, the mouse scampered off the wheel and cowered in the cage's corner.

Bill said, "this one doesn't like the light at all, but in the dark, he's got tons of energy. And whatever I bring it to eat, he wolfs down immediately. And no matter how much it eats, it never gains weight. Wearing a glove, he carefully pulled back the top grill, just enough to avoid giving it an opportunity to escape, but enough to be able to catch it. Bill held the mouse upside down, extending his gloved hand toward Dr. Carlson, so he could get a good look. Bill simply said, "see!"

At first Dr. Carlson didn't notice anything unusual. But then something caught his eye, something *was* different about this mouse. Finally, he saw it, the tail was different, it didn't look like a mouse tail. It was short and stubby, conical, not long and thin as it should be, and the tail's skin was hard and scaley, covered with geometric shapes. Dr. Carlson was curious about it, but not overly impressed.

"Now," said Bill, "look at the label on the cage." Every cage was labeled, with information identifying the animal, the experiment number and important dates.

Dr. Carlson read the information on the label. Finally, Bill had his full attention, he was transfixed. This mouse was injected with leukemia cells three and a half weeks ago, and it still looked strong and healthy. Dr. Carlson was immediately excited, but then, he shook his head, "there must be some mistake, the label has to be wrong." he said. "Bill, you screwed this up, didn't you?"

Bill put the mouse back, covered the cage and returned it to the shelf. He had recorded the mouse ID number, and they could later check in the lab logbook. "Follow me," said Bill. He led Dr. Carlson over to a different part of the animal room, and located another cage, also with a very energetic mouse inside. Bill pointed out the date on this label. This mouse was also injected 25 days ago, and its tail looked like the one on the first mouse. Bill had recorded the ID number from this mouse as well.

"How could these mice be alive this long and you're only now bringing it to my attention." Dr. Carlson didn't know whether to be angry or thrilled.

"There are so many animals here and so many cages, we had to use some high school students. They're doing some of the care and feeding. These two seemed to have been fed and placed back on the wrong shelves, alongside more recently injected mice. When I came by earlier today, I noticed that the codes on these cage labels didn't match the others on the same shelf. And when I checked the lab logbook, these two mice, now housed at different ends of the animal room, were each transfected with a lentivirus carrying exactly the same combination of tortoise and bowhead whale genes. They both have transformed tails, they both have a high metabolic rate and they both cower in the light. And of course, they are both alive."

"Holy shit, Bill," said Dr. Carlson, "that's amazing!" Dr. Carlson became quiet, he seemed to be calculating. This was his dream to find a set of genes that would protect against cancer. He felt a rush of adrenaline as he realized the significance of what he was seeing. Dr. Carlson closed his eyes and slowed his breathing, he had to think. What's next? "We'll need to repeat this with a new group of mice to verify the result. A dozen mice will receive the same gene combination as these two, and another dozen mice should be given various other gene combinations. It must be blinded, so you don't know which mice are injected with which set of genes, until of course, the code is broken. You'll have to use someone else to inject the lentivirus with the gene combinations, so you don't know which mice are in the control group and which ones get these same genes. I want daily pictures of each mouse. We need to document any physical changes. Each mouse will have its own logbook. All the data, how much they eat, daily weights, how long they sleep, we need everything. Bill, this has to have the highest priority, start tomorrow morning, OK? This needs to be quiet, no one else can know about this."

Bill smiled, "yes, sir."

"And Bill," said Dr. Carlson, "don't let any high school students near these mice, I want you to personally supervise this."

37.

Earlier Friday morning, Richie finished receiving the single donor platelet transfusion.

After his procedure, Sandra came over to let Betty know that the exam went well, and that they had all the samples needed. It would be a few days before they'd know the results. The technology used SNPs (single nucleotide polymorphisms), which would match unique mutations in the DNA from Richard's original leukemia with today's aspirate. Any cells sampled in today's exam that had the same mutations found in his first marrow, would be residual leukemia. It would be best if that were less than one in a thousand cells.

Sandra also told Betty that Dr. Stanner was hoping to have information about the donor search later in the afternoon.

Betty had no further questions. Sandra walked off, while Betty sat, watched Richie, and worried. Betty browsed through her phone while she waited for him to wake up. She came across emails from Nancy and Shelley directing her to a video posted on social media showing their Ferris Bueller parade around the unit, it made her smile despite all that was happening.

Back across the country in the PGL lab, Bill and one of the other lab techs were preparing two dozen mice for testing according to Dr. Carlson's instructions. While the lab assistant was injecting the mice, Bill used the time to meet with Dr. Benzi, and explain what they found and what Dr. Carlson had asked him to do.

Dr. Benzi, had a similar skeptical response, "is that real?"

Bill explained about the two separate mice and the new experiment now being set up to confirm the result. Bill could not come up with an alternative explanation consistent with the findings, "I think it's real," he said.

"Dr. Carlson was right of course. It's critically important to begin this new set of experiments to verify the results," said Dr. Benzi. "However, best-case scenario, we're still looking at years of work before this could be used to help people, or that we can justify our work to the company."

Dr. Benzi paused, he stood with his arms crossed over his chest, his folded right hand laying across his chin, and his raised forefinger tapping slowly against pursed lips. He seemed far away, his eyes unseeing, unblinking, trance-like, his voice was lower, softer, almost a whisper as he spoke, "but we also need to do more than that, Bill." Dr. Benzi's face was blank, he stared off into space. He seemed to be talking to someone that Bill couldn't see. He haltingly sketched out a plan.

Bill was shocked, he couldn't believe that Dr. Benzi would even think about doing anything like that. "Are you sure that's a good idea, Dr. Benzi? Maybe we should think about this for a few days."

Dr. Benzi was lost in thought, now biting his fingernails, the hitch in his left shoulder was acting up. Absentmindedly he rubbed it. "I'm sorry, what did you say Bill?"

Bill started to answer, "well, I was wondering..."

Dr. Benzi interrupted him, "no, it's OK, Bill, that was just a thought, of course, don't worry about it, just set things up the way Dr. Carlson instructed you."

Bill watched Dr. Benzi. He was trying to decide if he should be worried. Finally, Bill decided that it must have been as he said, just a thought experiment. No one would actually do what Dr. Benzi had just suggested.

Betty watched Richie as he began to stir and look around. He stretched his legs, he groaned a bit and reached for his backside. "I guess I've already had the bone marrow exam, it's sore. Did they get the samples they needed?"

"Dr. Gardner thought she got what they needed. Is it bad?" asked Betty.

"Naw, not too bad, it's more stiff than anything," said Richie.

Betty came over to show Richie what she found while browsing her phone, "Nancy and Shelley sent us some links to a video of our Bueller parade."

"Oh, I guess I need to tell Nancy about the mutation and the transplant, I'm not looking forward to that conversation," said Richie.

"I get it," said Betty, imagining how difficult that conversation might be, "but she needs to hear it from you, just tell her what the doctors said. The longer you put it off, the harder it'll be."

"I know you're right," said Richie, "I'll wait until she's finished with today's classes. Maybe we'll also have some information about the donor by then."

Just then, Dr. Stanner and Sandra knocked on the door.

"We just got back from the pathology lab, looking at Richard's marrow slide," said Dr. Stanner, "and as expected, there aren't many cells to see. As is typical at this point in his treatment, his marrow is fairly empty. We didn't see any lymphoblasts. That's good news of course, but it's also not very sensitive given the few cells remaining. We need to wait for the molecular studies to get a more detailed analysis of the marrow's residual lymphoblast content. We're sure that the molecular studies will identify some remaining leukemia cells, the important question is how many.

There is more good news, we have identified a donor who is a 10 of 10 HLA match, we know it's a male and he's 36 years old, so all that's good."

"That's great news about the donor, Dr. Stanner, so when can we start?" asked Betty.

"Well, we know the donor is from one of the Scandinavian countries, but not which one. The local chapter of the bone marrow donor registry will contact the person identified from the match. They'll make sure he's healthy, available and still willing to be a donor, so that'll take a little time. We have some back up donor choices identified, but this one's the best, so, we'll keep our fingers crossed. If everything goes well, because of the time difference, we should know by Monday. If he still wants to donate, he'll be referred to a specialized center where he will have medical and psychological evaluations. The next step would be to prepare him to have his blood stem cells harvested. He'll need IV access, it's like donating platelets at the Red Cross. The cells will then be packaged, and express flown overnight to the lab we use, PGL. There they'll be processed for Richie's infusion. It will look like a platelet transfusion."

"So, when do you think Richard could start?" asked Betty.

"We start numbering the transplant days like a rocket launch countdown, with minus numbered days, counting backward until the day of the cell infusion. It will start on day -8, when he gets his first high dose chemotherapy agent, and then the preparative chemotherapy regimen continues, with medications given on each subsequent day: -7, -6, and continue until the last chemo dose on day -2.

Day -1 is a rest day. No transplant medications are given, the day is used to wash those drugs out of his body. The following day will be day zero, on which Richard will receive the donor's blood stem cells as an intravenous infusion. After that we count positive days, the first day after the stem cell infusion would be day +1 and so on. The first of his new blood cells could appear as early as day +14, but it often takes longer than that.

So, if the donor is located on Monday, and he's available, and agrees, he could be evaluated and start the preparation within the week, and harvest cells five days later. All told that would make Richie's day zero 15 days from now, and his treatment would start 8 days earlier."

"What happens until then?" asked Betty.

"So, for now, since under the microscope we didn't see any leukemia, we can continue his current treatment regimen, at least until sometime next week when we know the results of today's MRD test. We can then decide whether to change his therapy to include a cycle of high dose methotrexate or to just stay the course with his current treatment until his transplant preparative regimen can start.

For now, we'll keep him on schedule, and he'll receive his conventional day 8 drugs, the antibody, inotuzumab ozogamicin and his IV vincristine, today."

"I guess that means, we're not going home anytime soon." said Betty. She already knew the answer. She had counted the days on the calendar, and couldn't find any time for them to go home. She asked anyway.

"Sorry, yes that's right," said Dr. Stanner. "Before the transplant starts, we'll move Richard to a different room here on the unit, our transplant room. It's a bit larger. It has a HEPA filter, to clean the air he breathes, thereby reducing the risk of infection. That'll be important during the transplant, when, for a time, he'll have no immune system at all. The door of the transplant room will remain closed. Everyone coming in will need to mask and glove. A small consolation, Betty, you'll at least have a real bed in the transplant room in addition to your recliner chair. Any questions?"

"I'm sure we'll have more questions later," said Betty, "but for now, I have enough information in my head. It might explode if anything more goes in."

Betty watched Dr. Stanner and Sandra walk away. "How are you Richie, you've been unusually quiet."

"I'm kinda numb," said Richie, "it's hard to describe. I thought things were going well, you know the white count went down to zero for a while. I felt that I knew what to expect, and I had accepted it. Now, the whole journey's changed. I've lost all direction. It's disorienting, like someone turned off all the lights and I'm walking in the dark."

"Richie, I'm sorry this is happening, I wish I could do something to change it," said Betty. She'd been watching her son. Up until now his mood had swung wildly from abject fear to acceptance and resignation. There were even moments of laughter in the face of his diagnosis. But Betty could see how different he was now. Abruptly all of his hope had been dashed. He seemed depressed and dejected. Betty didn't like what she saw. She tried to comfort her son. "I'm here for you Richie, and always will be. I promise we'll get through this. It's going to work. Every one of those fucking leukemia cells will be destroyed, and this nightmare will be over." Betty went over to lie down with Richie and hold him while they wept together. This was not what they had bargained for.

For several hours they slept, a dreamless sleep. Richie's scheduled chemo started while he was asleep and he awoke with that chemo taste in his mouth. He didn't need to look at the bag hanging from the IV pole, he knew the antibody was being infused.

Sandra came by to check. "It looks like you both took a needed nap. What are you feeling?"

"We've been having a hard time," said Betty. "My head's spinning. We're trying to forget what's happened and just look forward, but it's not easy.

Dr. Gardner, all that Richie's been through, I keep wondering if he was put in danger, subjected to days of a drug assault and anguish, and if that was all for nothing."

Sandra sat down, "I can see why you might think that. But no, none of this was wasted. We couldn't wait for information about his mutation before we started his therapy. When he arrived here his leukemia was progressing rapidly. We can only judge what was done based on the information that was available at that time. Secondly, his first marrow exam showed that it was packed with leukemia, and it was likely infiltrating other organs, like his kidneys and liver. We have the microscopic results of today's bone marrow exam, and we don't see any leukemia cells. My guess is that when we have the MRD results, we'll find that he still has some lymphoblasts, and probably more than we would have hoped for. But the fact that we don't see any under the microscope means that we have destroyed more than 99.9% of those cells. For a cure, it means getting rid of that last tenth of one per cent. That's nearly a billion cells, and that's the hardest part. The rest of his therapy will be focused on the eradication of those remaining cells. But we couldn't get rid of those last cells, until the vast bulk had been managed, and we've done that. Starting the transplant in a visual remission is the first essential step. So, no, this wasn't wasted, but it does mean that we must change our treatment strategy to finish the job."

Betty and Richie sat for a while, they thought about what Sandra had just said, and they could see the events of the previous couple of weeks with a better perspective. It didn't change anything that happened, of course, but it helped to know that the treatment up until then had been important and that there really was no way, at the start, to have known how to do it any differently.

"That fucking roller coaster," said Betty, "I really hate that ride now. I hope I never ever see one again!"

Richie smiled for the first time today.

"Thank you, Dr. Gardner," said Richie, "that helps. I'm glad you're my doctor."

"It's nice for you to say," said Sandra, "and much appreciated, but you have other doctors and nurses and the rest of the staff caring for you, I'm just one person on your team."

"Yes, that's true," said Betty, "but we still like you. So, what should we be looking for in the next few days?"

"Richard finished his vincristine, and he's finishing his antibody now," said Sandra. "He'll continue the steroid doses. The weekend should be quiet, and hopefully uneventful. Hopefully, by early next week we'll have secured a good donor, and we can plan the transplant. We'll also have the MRD results, so all the information we need to make the next decisions will be available.

Is there anything else I can answer for you?"

"I guess that you and Dr. Belkin will have a weekend off again this month?" asked Betty.

"It'll be the following weekend. The same doctors that covered us last month will cover us in June. And, you know that there will be new fellows in July, but Dr. Belkin and I will still be around."

"I was thinking about that," said Betty, "and I must say that it doesn't make me happy."

"All over the country, medicine programs switch on July first. Because of that the more senior doctors are on high alert, and I know that the new doctors coming are excellent. Richard will be in good hands."

"Thanks, but we'll miss you, I hope that we'll still be seeing you some," said Betty.

"I'll certainly be coming by to check in on you guys after June," said Sandra, "you'll never really be far away." She turned and walked away.

Betty turned to Richie, "you've been unusually quiet, young man. What's going on inside that noggin of yours?"

"Well, Dr. Gardner's explanation did make me feel better, more hopeful and less focused on the last few weeks. I know the past can't be changed, and I need to let go of it. It's the kind of stuff my coach always preached, don't be looking back at whatever just happened on the track, that's done and gone, don't beat yourself up for the past, it won't help. Just think about now, that's all there is. So, I'm ready for what may come. In fact, I'm feeling pretty good again."

"Well, track as a microcosm of life, whaddya know?" said Betty. "I feel better after listening to Dr. Gardner, too. I'll miss her come July."

"I hope we're not here in the hospital too long in July," said Richie. "She'll have a clinic and I expect that she'll still be my doctor.

Betty had been trying hard not to focus on the future. Thinking about the summer and Richie's senior year next Fall, and all those years to come, was too much for her. There were so many things that could go wrong. It hurt to think about it. The only way that Betty could function at all was to manage the next few moments of their lives. And even that felt like jumping into a den of monsters.

Hey, Mom, I know you were planning to go to the Gallery this weekend, there's no reason that you need to change those plans, I'll be fine here, OK?"

"Richie, you are something," Betty said, "I was just thinking of calling Shelley and telling her that I needed to be here."

"You don't have to, Mom. You know, I was bummed for a little while. Pretty obvious, I guess. But when I needed you, you were here. I'm really OK now. And honestly, I feel better when I know you're doing what you need to do and not canceling because of me. I don't want to be an albatross."

Betty laughed, "you don't look anything like an albatross, I doubt that anyone would confuse you for that bird. But, if you're sure, I'll keep the plan and leave tomorrow morning, there are things I should do, including some time at the Gallery."

"It'll be fine, nothing has really changed for this weekend, we can still talk on the phone, and I know I can get you if I need to. I'm good. You always seem to come back rejuvenated, so go for it."

"Aren't you the observant one? I worry about you when I'm gone, but I also feel good about getting some chores done, and being at the Gallery, so, if you're OK in the morning, I'll keep the plan."

"Sure, it'll be fine, and I may also have a visitor tomorrow."

"I see, there are machinations going on inside that noggin. You probably should speak to Nancy today, before she gets here, I don't think she'll be happy if you keep this new information to yourself, even for a day. I'll call Shelley now."

"Sure, Mom, will do. Did I mention being hungry?"

"Let's make the phone calls, first and then I'll go rustle up some grub."

Betty walked out of the room to call Shelley. It would be brief.

Richie punched Nancy's speed-dial.

Nancy picked up right away, "Hey, Richie, I was just thinking about you. I'm missing you, lots. How are you?"

"Nancy, I miss you too, it's hard when you're not here, I want to hold you, and never let you go."

"Ooh, that sounds nice, I want that too," said Nancy, "I'm going to be there tomorrow, so we can do some holding," she giggled.

"I can't wait for that. I close my eyes and I can imagine you're in my arms. I can feel you next to me. I can't help but wear this nonstop grin.

But, Nancy, I need to tell you something, and we can talk about it more when you're here."

"I'm not sure I like the sound of that," said Nancy.

It wasn't easy for Richie to tell Nancy, but he knew it was the right thing to do. And as his mom told him, he had to do it now. So, he bit his lip and began, "Dr. Stanner, my doctor, talked to us. They got back some information from the bone marrow test they did when I first got here, and, well, they found some mutation in my leukemia cells, that he's worried about. It's not good."

"Fuck, Richie," she said, "what does that mean?"

"Well, they did another bone marrow test today, to see how much of the leukemia is left, they hadn't planned to do it this early, but they needed to know because of this mutation. And Dr. Stanner now thinks that regular chemotherapy isn't going to be enough, so I'll need a bone marrow transplant."

Richie was not sure what to expect. The phone was silent for a while, but then it was filled with a shocking string of expletives.

"Fuck! Shit! Fuck," Nancy started to cry' each time she started to speak all she could do was sob.

Richie had braced himself for whatever was to come. But Nancy was way more upset than he imagined. He had mixed feelings. He didn't want to be the reason she was hurting, but he knew her anger at the news was because she loved him.

"I don't know what to say, it's too fucking scary, Richie. I wish you were here with me right now and we could be together. Fuck, Richie, I am... Wait, I keep talking about me, I'm so sorry. How are you, Richie? What you must be thinking, I can't even imagine. It must be awful for you."

"When I first heard it from Dr. Stanner, I sort of fell apart, I couldn't say anything at all. Mom asked all the questions and I just sat here. I really didn't hear anything more after he said *transplant.* But my other doctor, Dr. Gardner, talked to us after Dr. Stanner left, and she has this calming way of talking. I heard everything she said, and well, I feel better. I hope it will be OK, but I guess, I'm not leaving the hospital anytime soon."

"Shit, Richie, I'm so sorry, maybe I can come tonight."

"It's OK Nancy. Mom will be at work tomorrow, I would really like it if you could come tomorrow, all right?"

"Sure, Richie, I'll be there tomorrow. Is there anything you want? Can I bring you anything?"

"Bring your lips."

Nancy giggled, "that's my Richie, I'll bring more than that! I'll see you tomorrow."

"Nancy?"

"What," said Nancy.

"I love you!"

"Me too!"

Out in the hallway, not long after she'd hung up with Shelley, Betty heard her phone ring and saw that it was Nancy calling. Betty answered on the second ring.

"Fuck!" said Nancy, "sorry, I just talked with Richie, and he told me about the mutation and the transplant. He scared the shit out of me, and I don't even know if he's told me everything." Before Nancy could say anymore, she started to cry again. She sobbed, quiet gasping sounds.

Betty heard her trying to compose herself. "It's OK, Nancy, take your time. I feel the same way. It's not easy."

Finally, Nancy was able to continue, "I think that sometimes he feels that he's protecting me by not telling me everything, so, Betty, I trust you to not hold anything back. Please tell me, what the fuck's happening to Richie."

"You know he does really care about you," said Betty, "you know that right?"

"Yes, Betty I know, and I love him, but right now I can hardly think, so please help me, I need to know everything, and I need to know if I should come right now."

"Nancy, he's fine right now, he's no different than when you were together a few days ago. What's changed is the news we got and how it's going to affect how he gets treated later on. You're planning to see him tomorrow, and I know he's looking forward to that. He always loves seeing you and tomorrow will be fine. Honestly, I don't think I can tell you much more than I imagine Richie's told you. It was only a few hours ago that we heard about the mutation in the DNA of his leukemia and what that means. Unfortunately, he has one of the not so good mutations." Betty went on to explain about the risk factors and how they thought that with this DNA mutation, he was better off with the transplant. They needed to find a donor. They were hoping to start the transplant medicines in a week or so.

"But a transplant, that sounds so scary," sobbed Nancy.

"I know, we feel that way too, we're both scared."

There was a pause, then, "I don't know if I should ask you this," said Nancy.

"Honey, it's OK, you can ask anything you want, whatever is on your mind, ask it."

"Is Richie going to die?"

Betty took a breath, "I wonder that too, Nancy, and it scares the shit out of me that a question like that even pops into my head." That question was, indeed, taking up space in her head. The thought had been there since the diagnosis, but it was now all she could think about, it wouldn't go away. It persisted, it ate at her, kept her awake and haunted her. She didn't like the smell of it or the taste of it. She desperately wanted to bury those ugly thoughts. "I don't know the answer. But the doctors are hoping that the transplant will work, that it will kick the damn leukemia's butt. They say that he could walk out of here in five or six weeks without disease. So, that's what I believe too."

"I pray that they're right," her sobs under better control. Betty heard her take a few deep breaths.

"OK, I'll be strong for Richie. Betty, thank you for talking with me, and you know, not treating me like a kid. I know that you won't be at the hospital tomorrow, are you OK if I come visit Richie?"

"Yes, of course, dear, you make him very happy, and frankly, I kind of think he has good taste in girls."

"Well, he better not be tasting too many girls, he doesn't want to find out how that would work out."

Betty could hear a little relief in her voice.

"Betty, will you be at the Gallery tomorrow?"

"Yes, in the afternoon."

"Would it be OK, if I visit you there tomorrow?"

"Sure Nancy, I would like that, maybe we can have lunch. Just text me a time when you know."

"Betty, I feel better, thank you. I do love your son. Bye," and Nancy disconnected.

Betty now had two kids to worry about. But Richie was number one, and she had to rustle up some grub, so she went down to the café to find something at least halfway decent.

She was soon back, with turkey club sandwiches.

Betty watched Richie eating. He looked comfortable, happy even, and anyone watching him right now would not have any idea how sick he really was. "Amazing," she thought. She took solace in his serenity.

Sandra, getting ready to go home for the night, came by to check on Richie. "I see you found something to eat, and Richie looks like he's enjoying it."

"I was hungry, and it's not bad," said Richie.

"Well, Richard's blood count is pretty good, his white blood cell count is up to 0.5 and the cells are all neutrophils, so that's good news, his hemoglobin and platelets are stable, so I don't think he'll need any transfusions this weekend. Do you guys have any questions?"

"So, can I be unhooked and wander around the unit?" asked Richie.

"Sure, I'll ask your nurse to hep-lock your catheter and you can walk around. I've stopped the antibiotic, you've had enough days of treatment. Some normal white blood cells are growing again, so it's all good. I expect that you'll have a quiet weekend, and we can even give you the steroid doses orally, so you can stay free of your friend the IV pole."

"That's great," said Richie, "and that IV pole is not really my friend, just so you know."

"Dr. Gardner," said Betty, "I plan to leave tomorrow morning and I'll be back on Sunday. It seems to me that it should be safe to go. Do you agree?"

"Richard should be fine, "answered Sandra." I don't see any problem with you leaving for the day. We just don't want Richard getting any infections now, before the transplant. So, it's better if he stays here. I know you'll be at the Gallery. You may consider wearing an N95 mask while you meet with the public. That would reduce the risk of picking up anything. You can get a couple from here in the unit before you leave."

"That's a good idea, Dr. Gardner," said Betty, "thanks, I haven't thought much about my own health. I guess I need to be more careful." It gave her pause. Another thing to worry about. She pictured all those people passing through the Gallery. Some of them sick, some coughing, they were walking Petri dishes, ready to spread germs to anyone nearby. She shuddered at the thought of all that bacteria waiting for her. She'd have to bring a supply of masks, and hand sanitizer.

"Have a good night. I'll see you in the morning," said Sandra as she walked off to check on the other patients before signing out to Paul.

Betty looked at her son, remarkably, he seemed happy. For sure, the problem hadn't disappeared. She knew it still bothered him. It had to. It was disturbing news. But he'd been able to set it aside, to tuck it away in some corner of his mind, wrapped up, covered with happier thoughts, a temporary band-aid. But she also knew it would come out again especially once the transplant started and he felt worse. His defenses would slip, and the angst would resurface. She needed to remain vigilant, as always, watching her son like a hawk, ready to step in and protect him as he surely would need her to do. What were all the bad things that could happen? She sorted them out in her head, best to worst, likely to rare, examining each one, trying to plot a path around each obstacle, and how to achieve the best possible outcome.

Lost in her reverie, she snapped back into focus to find Richie watching her expectantly. "What do you want to do for the evening?" asked Betty.

"I really don't have much schoolwork left. Junior year is pretty much done. How about some cards, that was fun last time."

Betty set up the table between them and found the deck of Bicycle brand cards she'd stashed away from the last game. She shuffled the deck. "OK, what's it to be?"

A bit of poker, he decided. They played for a few hours, it was very competitive. There was lots of shouting and cheering and moaning as the games wore on. They used Cheerios from the kitchen pantry to bet with. And the winner wound up with a nice bedtime snack.

Finally, they turned out the lights and settled in for the night, and before long, they were sleeping peacefully.

38.

After an undisturbed night of sleep and an uneventful morning check-in from Sandra, Betty departed. Arriving home, she went through her check list. She had a routine now, managing a week's worth of inattention. Sort the mail, vacuuming a bit, straightening up. There was relatively little to do for a house that was not lived in. While she toiled with the few chores she received a text from Nancy, who hoped to come by the Gallery at 2 if that was OK. Betty responded affirmatively. She decided to arrive at the Gallery a bit earlier, just after 10, so she could have lunch with Nancy. She texted Shelley about her plan.

Before long, she was on her way to the Gallery, it was a beautiful warm day, with a brilliant blue sky, not a cloud to be seen. She realized that while she was in the hospital, she hadn't noticed the weather. It felt good to be out in the world, and while she enjoyed the change, she also felt sorry that Richie couldn't be with her. Betty made a note to stop in the jewelry store next to the Gallery for the bracelet that Richie finally picked. She'd also get some take-out for dinner. The good weather brought out lots of street traffic, and so when Betty arrived, the Gallery was busy with people browsing the works of art.

Within minutes, Betty had settled in and was working the crowd. Despite her worries, the mask she wore was readily accepted. She mingled with the people and could quickly pick out the serious from the gawkers. She was very good at this, she felt at home, and for the moment anyway, the hospital seemed far away. Betty focused on the serious and noticed which pieces drew their attention. She would quietly approach and offer detailed information about the work and its artist. The pieces were not marked with the price, and so, if Betty discerned a true interest, that would become part of the discussion. She soon had two sales being negotiated.

The busy morning went by quickly, and it was just after 2 when Betty saw Nancy walk into the Gallery. At first, she just wandered around seeming to admire the art.

Betty came up to greet Nancy.

"Wow Betty," said Nancy, "I had no idea what your place was like. It's really beautiful. It even smells good in here."

Betty smiled. It was part of the milieu created for the customers. "Are you hungry, there's a nice little bistro just around the corner, we can get some lunch."

Nancy hesitated a second, and Betty added, "my treat."

"Sure, that sounds great, I'm hungry."

Soon they had a corner table. Exploring the menu they found a healthy veggie sandwich on whole wheat with sprouts, along with a fruity blended drink.

The drinks came over quickly, with recycled paper straws, it was that kind of place.

"Thank you for taking time for me today, Betty, I really wanted to talk with you. I guess since you're at the Gallery, Richie must be OK for now, but all the news has me worried. I have these bad dreams. I had one last night. I was in this dark winding alley, with gaslit streetlights. I had trouble walking, I kept slipping over wet cobble stone pathways, strange things were lurking all around. There was a creature, hunched over and scaly, following me. In the dream, I'm lost and panicky. When I woke up, I was breathing hard and covered in sweat. It took a few moments, but I was very relieved when I realized it was just a dream, but I just don't know, it seemed real. Silly, isn't it?"

"No, it's not silly, and I'm scared too," said Betty. "You know, I've had some bat shit scary dreams too. I could see creepy stuff and even smell rotten odors. They're freaky. Your dream was eerily similar to mine. I wanted to talk to someone about them, but I was afraid that if I mentioned it at the hospital, they might tie me up and lock me in the looney bin." Betty reached out to hold Nancy's hand. "I'm glad we're talking. It can be our secret."

Nancy looked at Betty differently, they held hands. "It's Richie that connects us. I feel it."

Betty smiled, Nancy was right, they were connected. "Listen Nancy, does your father know that we've been talking? Does he know you're here with me now?"

"No, I drove over myself, he thinks I'm just out meeting friends. He knows I'm going to see Richie later. Sometimes I talk with Aunt Ruth, his sister, but I haven't said anything about you."

"I think you should tell your father. You and Richie are special together. Richie loves you and thinks about you a lot. I know that you feel the same way. You're both young, but this isn't a typical high school romance. There are all kinds of complications, and ways for you to get hurt. I care about you, and no matter what happens, I want to be there for you Nancy. But it can't be behind your father's back. Are you concerned about telling your dad?"

"Maybe, he tries to be my dad and my mom too, and I worry he may think it's his failure if I'm talking with you. I think he likes Richie, but I'm not sure he would be happy knowing how much I really care for him. He worries about me, and what would happen if something, well, you know."

Betty squeezed her hands. "I know," she said. Both shed tears, they both loved that boy, and harbored fears about what might be.

"I know what you are thinking, Nancy," said Betty, "but that's not going to happen, he'll get the transplant and he will be rid of that fucking monster. I know that he'll get through this."

Nancy, still crying, wiped her tears, and said, "yes, I know that too."

"But I need you to tell your dad that we talked, OK? Whatever he hears, it's better if it comes from you. It may be difficult, but it will hurt him more if he finds out from someone else and you've been deceptive. Truth shines."

"You're right Betty. I'll tell him."

The sandwiches arrived, and they were scrumptious and healthy. They ate in silence, minds busy with their thoughts.

All finished, Betty paid the check and as they got up to leave, Nancy came over and wrapped her arms around her, holding her for several moments. "Thank you."

Betty kissed her on the forehead, "It's I who should be thanking you, Nancy. Be careful on the road, I know Richie is looking forward to seeing you."

Nancy went to her car. As Betty walked back to the Gallery she thought about Nancy and Richie, and everything that might go wrong. Betty's maternal instincts were being summoned, and they were not just for her son.

Over at the hospital, Richie was reading an old book about travel to the Moon that he found in the unit library. Nancy snuck up behind him, and reached around, covering his eyes with her hands. She leaned in, and whispered in his ear, "guess who."

Richie knew of course, he knew her touch, her smell and her voice. A smile broke on his face as he turned to greet her.

"Gosh, Nancy, you look awesome."

"Oh, I didn't even do anything," she shook her hair out and tried to see herself in Richie's mirror as she came over.

"It doesn't matter what you do, you always look awesome."

She smiled, "I guess you're right," and without slowing a bit, she kissed him, quickly summoning the passion of their last visit. Young and in love, their kisses were hot and fervent, there was nothing timid as they came together. Had they been alone in the backseat of a Chevy, that kiss would surely have led to much more.

Nancy sighed and sat down next to him on the bed, her hand resting in his lap. "How are you, Richie, really? I'm still shaken from the news about the transplant. Shit, Richie, it sucks."

"I was worried before, you know, but honestly, you make that all vanish. When you're here, I can't think of anything else. I guess, maybe you need to be here all the time."

"You're already in my head all the time, Richie, but I still miss being with you like this. I think of us together sometimes. I imagine you're not sick, and it's just us, no one is watching, and we can do anything we want."

Richie reached down and moved her hand up higher on his leg. "I think about that too, Nancy, all the time."

She left her hand there, feeling his response, she leaned over, and they kissed again. "I think we'll both need showers after I leave," she said.

"I don't want you to leave," said Richie.

"Hmm, I'd like to stay here with you." They sat together for a while, just holding hands.

Nancy turned to him, and gently traced her fingers across his face, gazing at him, "don't let anything happen to you, Richie, I couldn't stand it if something happened to you."

"I won't," he said.

"I'm scared, Richie."

"I won't let anything bad happen, Nancy, I promise."

"You better not. I do love you."

"I love you too, Nancy."

"I know you do, Richie." She gazed at his face, and then she seemed to move a little bit aside. She drew her hand away, joining her other hand clasped in her lap. Richie watched as she looked down. "Richie, can we talk a little?"

"Of course, Nancy," Richie was anxious. He watched her fidget and knew that whatever she was going to say would be difficult for her. "You can say anything you want, Nancy. I'm here for you."

She cleared her throat, and continued to look down, "I went to the Gallery today and met your mom. We had lunch together." Finally, Nancy looked up at Richie.

"I see." Richie was surprised and not sure where this was headed. He watched her for clues, he was confused and worried.

"Your mom's great, Richie, I really like her. And, by the way, the Gallery is impressive, I had no idea."

Richie waited for her, he figured she was getting up the courage to say whatever it was.

"We talked for a while, and of course most of it was about you." She paused for a moment, and sighed. "I told her that I was really scared about what might happen to you. And I described the bizarre, dark dreams I'd been having. Crazy stuff with monsters, and being chased and how I'd wake up in a sweat, breathing hard and anxious. It would take a few moments to realize that I was in my room, and it was just a dream. Betty, your mom told me to call her that, said that she was having crazy dreams like that too." Nancy looked up at Richie. "It was very weird, the same dreams. It's freaky, I don't even know what that means. Richie, I do love you, but I'm scared. Thinking about what might happen, it's been so hard. And it brings up memories that I'd rather had remained buried."

Richie reached out. He placed his hand over hers, "I'm so sorry, Nancy. I don't know what to say."

"I can't help how I feel right now," said Nancy, "I want to be with you, but I can't. It's upsetting to think about everything. I gotta go, now, Richie, I'm sorry, but I just gotta go."

"I wish you weren't so worried, Nancy. Can't you stay?" Nancy leaned over, she kissed him again, and quickly turned and hurried away. She seemed overwhelmed with feelings.

Richie watched her walk out, trying to understand what had just happened. He was pretty sure that he hadn't said or done anything wrong, and yet, it was his fault. Richie wanted her to come back, to sit and talk. He wanted to hold her and make it all better. But he worried that wouldn't work, not here in the hospital. He might not ever be able to make it better while he was here.

Richie thought about calling his mom, but she was at work. He would wait until she was home. It sure was hard to figure out girls sometimes. He imagined maybe they had trouble like that with boys, although he kind of felt boys were simpler.

He had put the book away, and there wasn't much more schoolwork left, his junior year was basically done, it was time for summer vacation. He grimaced, some summer vacation he was having, not anything he'd wish on his worst enemy. He worried about Nancy. It was this shitty, fucking disease. He tried to imagine what it would be like if that had never happened. If he woke up and this was all a bad dream.

Richie needed a distraction. He was free to roam around the unit. and without many options, he walked over to the Child Life Room to find something. There were lots of choices for little kids, less so for the older teens. He picked out a couple of DVD movies, and an Xbox One, so he could play War Thunder. He was into it. It was one of those video games his mom would rather he didn't play, but it was just a game, and she wasn't here. It would help, he didn't need to think about anything else while he was online trying to navigate its challenges. All set, Richie walked back to his room. He figured he had enough stuff to keep him busy until dinner, when he could check in with Mom. He texted his friends to let them know he was going online to play.

Richie was immersed in the game, and with no parental unit hovering over him, he was transported, unencumbered, into a virtual space along with many other players. Time stopped. It was only when Sandra came by on her rounds that he realized several hours had passed. He paused the game, flexing and stretching his aching fingers. Maybe it was time to sit back and watch one of the DVD movies.

"How's the game going?" asked Sandra, she had been watching for a few minutes, unnoticed, before announcing her presence.

"I guess I've been playing for a few hours without realizing it. You know, it distracts me from the real world, which helps, at least for a while. But I need to stop. I've also got a few movies that I picked from the Child Life room."

"I expect tonight, and the rest of the weekend should be quiet. I'm guessing your mom went to work today and she'll be back tomorrow. When you talk to her, you can tell her that everything's fine. I'll see her tomorrow. Do you have any questions for me Richie?"

"No, I hope you get some rest tonight."

"OK, Richie, see you tomorrow."

Richie went over to the kitchen area and put one of the popcorn bags in the microwave. Before too long, he was sitting in his room watching *Close Encounters of the Third Kind*, with Richard Dreyfus, one of his favorite early Steven Spielberg movies.

Just as Roy and Jillian were scrambling up Devils Tower, skeptical of the announcement of a toxic nerve spill, Betty called. Richie paused the movie and connected with his mom. "Hey, Mom, how's your day been?" he asked.

"It was fine, Richie. Very busy, the good weather brought the hordes out, and a good many of them came into the Gallery. I had another sale. I'm back home now, and I've got take out Chinese. I was just too tired to make a meal. How about your day?"

"So, you still have the bubble bath and wine to do?"

"Yes, I'm looking forward to that bit of decadence."

"Well, I'd like to talk to you about Nancy, she came to visit me, and she was upset when she left."

"What happened?"

"We can talk about it more tomorrow when you're here, it's kind of hard to explain over the phone. But I don't think it was anything I said or did. I think she's just freaked out with the transplant thing and she's worried. Seeing me, seems to have ratcheted up all kinds of scary thoughts. And then I didn't know what to say. She did mention that she met you at the Gallery."

"Oh, yes we had lunch. But you're sure you didn't say anything to upset her?"

"Shit, Mom, I'm not sure of much, but I don't think it was anything I said. She started talking about some nightmares she had, and soon, she got up and left."

"I see," said Betty. "I think I understand, we can talk about it tomorrow. I bought the charm bracelet you picked out. That might help, but she's still going to find that her feelings for you are difficult to manage. Is everything else, OK?"

"Sure, I played some video games and I'm watching a movie. Dr. Gardner came by, and it's all good. Nothing to worry about."

"Then I'll see you tomorrow," said Betty.

"Yep, see you tomorrow. I love you Mom, drive carefully and of course, don't let those bedbugs bite."

"Love you too," and they disconnected.

Richie was ready to restart the movie, when his phone rang again, it was Nancy's ring and he picked up right away.

Nancy sounded like she'd been crying, "I can't talk too much now, Richie, but I wanted to tell you how sorry I am about this afternoon. I love being with you, and you didn't do anything. It's just me. I can be complicated, for sure. Sometimes my mind gets messy, and I worry about you because I care, and sometimes, like today, I get so emotional that it's hard to think straight. There's more, and some time I want to tell you. I know there's a lot that you're worried about, but you don't have to worry about me. I still love you and I hope that you can forgive me."

Even with the distractions he hadn't been able to stop thinking about her visit. Suddenly, Richie felt a huge weight lift and the tension ease. He smiled. "Nancy, there's nothing to forgive. I'm glad you called, I've been worrying about you. I know that you think that you're complicated, well I'm sure I am too, and with everything that's going on, I can imagine it must be hard for you. I think that you are the most special person, ever."

"Oh, my God, Richie, you still like me? Really?"

"I do, Nancy, and much more than that."

"I wish I were there right now. I'd squeeze you and shower you with kisses. I'd never let you go."

"I guess we're just a complicated duo, fighting for love, justice and the American way!"

Nancy giggled, "Richie, I'm just so happy right now. I thought I might have fucked it up and scared you away. But you're still there, and that's all I care about. I have to go. See you soon." Nancy kissed the phone and disconnected.

Richie thought about the call for a while. He was happy, and he smiled thinking about Nancy. He didn't understand everything that just happened, all he knew was that Nancy still liked him. He wondered what else she had to say. What more was there still hiding in her head. He recalled his mom saying how relationships and people are complicated. She was right, for sure. Richie figured that the conversation he would have with his mother tomorrow about Nancy was going to be different from what he had feared, and that was a good thing.

After a few minutes of contemplation, he leaned back and hit the play button on the DVD remote, Richard Dreyfus and company were still making their way up Devils Tower to meet the aliens.

39.

He slept like the proverbial log, immense alien spaceships, hovered over him, their deep bass sounds shook the Earth. His eyelids fluttered, he groaned, and began to stir. Consciousness emerged and he realized that his mother was rubbing his shoulder, and calling his name, "Richie, wake up dear, it's after 10. Time to rise and shine."

"You're not an alien spaceship?" said Richie, he yawned and stretched.

"What? No, I'm not an alien spaceship," said Betty, "but I did bring breakfast from another planetary sector. I've been sitting here, watching you sleep for a while, and I decided that you should be awake by now. I've already had my coffee and ate my bacon, egg, and cheese English muffin sandwich. I can warm yours up, along with the hot chocolate."

"Hmm, that sounds good. I'll go pee while you're doing that," he was still trying to shake off slumber as he shuffled off to perform his morning ablutions.

A few minutes later, "Hmm, this is good, Mom, thank you," he said, as he attacked the meal, washing it down with the hot chocolate.

Betty marveled at the gastric capacity of a teenage male. "Maybe I should've bought two for you."

Although his mouth was still partially occupied with food, he answered, "no, it's fine, this is all I need."

Betty waited until he was done before asking about his day. After a few minutes, when the sandwich and beverage had been consumed, and his mouth seemed empty, she could finally ask.

"Well, for me, medically, it was a nicely dull day. Nothing much happened, I was free from the IV pole all day, I got two doses of the steroid, by mouth. I had to swallow some nasty tasting pills, but it was fine. I played some online games. And then, there was the visit from Nancy."

"I'm glad to hear that the day was medically dull. I was thinking about Nancy and what you told me last night, and..." Betty was a bit hesitant to broach the subject, she was not looking forward to refereeing a dispute between the lovebirds.

"Wait, before you say anything, there's more," said Richie.

"OK," said Betty, cautiously.

"Well, just a little while after I talked with you, she called me, and basically, she said she was sorry about how she was, and she was worried that I might be angry with her. But of course, I wasn't, and we talked for a while and in the end, it was all fine. She said things were complicated, that sounded like you. She said there was more, and she would tell me some day. I wondered about that."

"I see," said Betty. She wondered how and when the things she knew would come out. She had watched how Richie was handling this awful disease and his new relationship. Betty hoped that Richie would be understanding about how complicated things were and how difficult it might be for Nancy to tell him everything. "That's good, I'm happy that you guys were able to work things out, again. It makes for a stronger relationship when you can resolve the inevitable rocky patches. I'm impressed with the amount of maturity that you both seem to have, beyond your years."

"What were you going to say, before I told you we talked again?"

"It doesn't really matter now," said Betty, "but just that lives can be convoluted, it's hard to know what is going on in another person's head. Listening to each other goes a long way toward keeping a relationship healthy."

She came over to him, rubbing her hand over his smooth head, like she was wishing for good luck, and then gave him a big hug. "Listening is always good. Hey, I got the bracelet you picked out, I think Nancy will like it. Want to see?"

Betty watched as Richie opened the box and looked it over. It had a heart charm and a dangling key trinket. He smiled as he took it out, turned it over and carefully examined the attached heart and key. Betty sighed. This was his first gift for a girlfriend and she saw how much he wanted it to be right. He was growing up, and she would have to share his love with another female. She knew it would happen one day, but things were happening too fast. Betty watched as he carefully wrapped the bracelet in the gift paper.

"Thanks Mom, this is really nice. Do you think she'll like it? I hope so." Richie didn't wait for a response. "But I really need to think about what I should write on her card. I don't want it to sound too sappy, but something she'll like."

"Just write something from your heart. She'll like it because it's from you."

As Richie was finishing, Sandra came by, she seemed happy. She was still wearing scrubs, appropriate and utilitarian apparel. "How's everything?" she asked.

"I would ask you that, Dr. Gardner," said Betty, "but Richie seems fine, and I guess yesterday was thankfully uneventful."

"Yes, all good," said Sandra, "his WBC count improved again yesterday, and the rest of his labs have been stable. We won't need to check them today. I'm expecting another quiet day."

"Great, we'll try to keep it that way," said Betty, "I guess that we'll see you tomorrow night. You and Dr. Belkin will be swapping shifts again."

"Yep, I'll have to reprogram my body clock again, thankfully not too many more times," said Sandra. "I'll check with you later," and she walked off to check on the other children.

Betty and Richie kept a low profile, and as promised, the next two days were thankfully dull.

Tuesday morning, Dr. Stanner came by. They were happy to see him smiling. "I had good news yesterday from the IBMTR. They've contacted the donor, and he's looking forward to helping. They should be completing an evaluation today, and it's possible that by tomorrow, they'll begin the process of preparing him for harvesting stem cells. He'll receive the first of five days of twice daily G-CSF injections. That means there could be a collection this coming Monday. We could start Richard's transplant preparative regimen as soon as we confirm the timing."

"That's great news," said Betty, "and scary too. But we're eager to get going."

"I'll keep you posted. Do you have any questions right now?"

"What were the results of the last bone marrow test?" asked Richie.

"Technically, you're in remission, and that's good. So we would be starting the transplant in what's called a CR1, first complete remission. However, there were still more lymphoblasts in his marrow than we hoped to see, the result was less than 1% residual disease."

Richie wondered, "that sounds OK, but it doesn't seem that you were happy with that result."

"Well, less than one percent doesn't seem like much. Only 20 years ago, we would've been very happy with that number. However, with more sensitive detection techniques, and data from our protocols, we now know that it would be best with an even lower number. Along with the mutation, the residual disease result supports our decision to go to transplant," said Dr. Stanner. "Starting in a clinical remission is much better than trying to do this after a relapse and with a marrow full of disease."

"OK, so how long do you think Richie will be here?" asked Betty.

Dr. Stanner explained, "once the transplant preparative regimen starts, that's the chemotherapy to ablate his current marrow and prepare his body to receive the new blood stem cells, it should be a minimum of 3 weeks, probably more, before we can expect to find the first evidence of marrow engraftment, usually neutrophils. The whole process, start to discharge home is typically six to eight weeks, at best."

Betty listened to Dr. Stanner as he seemed to matter of factly describe what she thought was a very risky procedure. She certainly hoped for the time when she'd be able to look back at the whole transplant as routine.

"What is the most dangerous part of the transplant?" asked Richie.

"That's an interesting question, and probably not everyone would agree on the answer. The medications will begin on day -8, and by day -4, all your white blood cells will be gone. With the complete loss of your immune system, you'll be vulnerable to infections. And later, when the white count recovers, and the donor marrow tries to adjust to its new home, it brings a new set of problems, including the potential for Graft vs. Host disease. Even after the new white blood cells start to flourish, the risk of infection continues because you'll be taking immune suppressing medications. You'll need red cell and platelet transfusions during the transplant, and there can be reactions to those. Moreover, some people become sensitized to blood transfusions and then it can be hard to locate a blood unit that their body will accept. Unfortunately, there are myriad dangers along the way. But we have decades of experience handling these and there are established responses to each of these challenges. In fact, Transplant Medicine is a science and art in itself."

"I guess Yogi Berra would say, it ain't over til it's over," said Richie.

"I think that sums it up pretty well," Dr. Stanner smiled. "We'll talk more. I'll make sure that Valerie, our transplant nurse, comes to speak with you. She'll provide you with a complete set of printed material that should cover most everything, OK?"

"Thanks, Dr. Stanner," said Betty.

"And me too, thanks," said Richie.

As Dr. Stanner walked away, Richie turned to his mom, "that's a lot of stuff, Mom, and I guess he wasn't even nearly finished. It's scary."

"I'm scared too, Richie, but we've managed scary stuff together, and we will again. It's the old saying."

"What? Shit happens!"

She looked at Richie, "no, we'll face this *one day at a time.* It's too much to worry about everything that can happen during six more weeks in the hospital. Breaking down the tasks into smaller chunks always helps, *one day at a time.* It's less frightening. We can mark off a success after each day, and then look to the next one. I've done that in my journal. Each entry is one day and it helps."

The next days went by slowly, they concentrated on staying strong, eating well, and reading about the transplant. Priority one was to avoid any infection before the transplant started, so they were scrupulous about handwashing and wearing the N95 masks. They used the thermal thermometer scanner on anyone coming into Richie's room. All the staff had been thoroughly vaccinated and they masked for each visit. If any of the staff had a family member who became ill, they were reassigned.

By Thursday, they knew that Richie's donor's evaluation was fine. The donor's twice daily G-CSF injections had begun, and he would soon be ready for his blood stem cell harvest.

As the start day of the transplant loomed closer, it was hard to avoid the rising anxiety. They talked with Madelyn about their fears. Madelyn had a great deal of experience with families before, during and after the transplant. She never dismissed their worries, but tried to contextualize their concerns and reviewed the tools they needed to properly assess and prioritize the risks.

Valerie, Richie's knowledgeable and patient transplant nurse, spent time with them, too. She reviewed the transplant process in detail. She explained the medications, their side effects and what to expect. She described how Richie would feel on a day-by-day basis, and what the team would do to mitigate the possible problems.

Valerie described the preparation for the transplant as like removing everything from a sold house, and creating an empty place, so the new owners could move in. And to protect Richie from the damage that could happen as the new owners moved in, he would receive insurance, Graft vs. Host Disease (GvHD) prophylaxis, and in case the new owners carried diseases, he would be given antibacterial and antiviral medications to reduce the risk of infections.

Once the required number of cells was collected from the donor, they would be flown overnight, in a special container to PGL where they would be processed and prepared for infusion on Richard's day zero. That special container kept the cells protected and at the optimal temperature, just above 0° Celsius. After the cells arrived at PGL, and were processed, they would then be shipped to the hospital for the infusion. The product would arrive at the hospital the following morning and then be given to Richie later that day. It required the execution of a well-choreographed dance.

Betty tried to think. She'd been overwhelmed when Richie was first admitted to the hospital and she had to learn about the standard chemo. This transplant stuff was a whole nother level. Finding a donor, matching a donor, medications to ablate the marrow, making room for new cells, Graft vs. Host Disease, it was too much to sort out. She felt like someone shoved her through a hidden portal and she landed in an alternate universe. She'd just been getting used to the first world when she was forced to learn a new set of rules for this one. Despite the help, it was confusing and scary. It was like her dreams, she was lost in dark halls filled with monsters.

40.

At PGL, Bill was working in the animal room, making sure the mice were fed, the water bottles filled, and the cages were cleaned. The wood chips at the bottom of each cage were changed every few days to maintain sanitary conditions. He also carried the logbook, making entries next to each mouse identification number. Bill had set aside one of the shelves in the large room, to house the two dozen mice, now being used to test the latest findings. The twelve experimental mice were randomly mixed on the shelf along with the twelve control mice. And so, without breaking the code, Bill couldn't definitively identify which mice received the same set of genes as the two long surviving mice and which were the control mice with the random gene combinations. However, Bill saw that half of them were not well. Five days after the injections of the malignant cells, twelve of the mice weren't eating. Many of them lay at the bottom of their cages, pale and panting, teetering on death's doorstep. On the other hand, the other twelve mice were active, eating and drinking. They ran on the exercise wheels. They appeared healthy and vigorous. But Bill saw the other changes too, the active ones had thick new hair and their tails were different, not like mouse tails. Bill thought for a minute, it came to him, the tails appeared reptilian. As he shone his flashlight toward their cages, the mice would retreat to the furthest corner, and begin digging at the walls of their enclosure, desperate to escape from the light. He took pictures to document the changes which were then pasted into their logbooks.

Bill would have bet a week's paycheck that he'd be able to correctly identify which mice had received the same combination of tortoise and whale genes as the previous two long surviving mice. And, in fact, when he checked on those two original mice, they were still alive and active, but their appearance was dramatically different. It would be hard to identify them as ever being part of the BALB/c strain of mice.

Meanwhile, back at the hospital, Betty was sitting in her chair while Richie played video games. He wore headphones, so although she could see the military vehicles engaged in battle, to Betty it was a silent movie. Tank cannons spat out artillery, but all Betty heard was silence. She could see Richie shimmying around, leaning one way then the other, working the game controller buttons and joystick.

Betty focused on her journal book, using her fountain pen to enter all the latest information. She added quotes from the staff and whatever details she could remember. She also jotted down her private thoughts. While she was busy working on her journal, her phone, which she had been set to silent/vibrate, began to buzz. She looked at the screen and saw that it was Nancy. Betty put down her journal and walked out of the room as she answered the phone.

"Hello, Betty," Nancy started, "are you at the hospital with Richie?"

"Yes, I've been here," answered Betty, "right now he's busy on a video game."

"Is he OK?"

"He's fine," Betty replied.

"I guess he told you about my visit on Saturday and what happened."

"Richie called me that night, and we talked about it, but that was before you called him back."

"I think about him all the time. But everything I hear scares the shit out of me. And I've been reading stuff online about leukemia and mutations and bone marrow transplants. It's all so confusing. I'm a fucking mess. It reminds me of my mother and how I was back then."

Betty sighed, she worried about Nancy. But she was emotionally spent and didn't know if she had enough strength left to help her too. "I can't even imagine what you're going through. Have you spoken with your father?"

"No, I don't know what to say. I rehearse the conversation in my head, but it doesn't ever seem to come out right."

"Nancy, I'm here for you. But it's important that you talk to your father, please. Believe me, it doesn't matter what you say, just tell him what you're feeling. He loves you. You're only alone if you don't share. Trust me, I know what it's like, it will be OK."

"I don't know."

"Are you home now, is your father there?"

"Yes, he's downstairs."

"Don't think about it anymore, take a few breaths and go talk to him. I guarantee that you'll feel better after you do that. Call me after, if you want, OK?"

"Betty, thank you for everything."

"Are you going to talk to your dad?"

"Yes."

"Promise me, just do it now."

"OK," said Nancy.

"I want you to promise."

"I promise," said Nancy.

Settling back into her chair at Richie's bedside, Betty found him still online with his multiplayer video game, wearing his headset, completely immersed in a virtual world of battle. Betty thought about all the ways that he tried to escape from the real dangers he faced. What did he use? Battling an onslaught of unfeeling, unending columns of soldiers, a perpetual supply of enemies in an imaginary war. She wondered if it was wrong that he hid inside those alternate realities. Was it healthy to wrap up the thoughts of what might actually happen and stuff them in a box, in some corner of his mind? Were men basically different? Had tens of thousands of years of war and battle, mostly fought by men, selected a certain gene pool? Even in the animal kingdom, it was often the male that did battle and the female that selected the victor. What sort of mindset would allow a person to willingly march onto a field of death? Was Richie practicing for that with his video games? And the women, often left to clean up their messes, and ensure the survival of the next generations. What biochemicals, what DNA changes were behind all that craziness? How much could be changed? How much was already programmed in? Thoughts swirled in her head.

Suddenly, Richie threw down the game controller and pulled off his headset. "Shit!" he shouted.

"Maybe give it a rest for a while," offered Betty, "I imagine those battles can be enervating."

"Yeah, you're right, Mom. Sometimes I can't tell if playing the games makes me feel better or worse."

"Why don't you put away all the electronic stuff, and just dial back to the golden olden days? We can talk or play some simple board games, I bet they have a bunch of those in the Child Life area that we could choose from. Hey, how about Scrabble? That could be fun."

"Scrabble it is, Mom, that's a great idea."

Pretty soon they were deep into the game. There were cheers and groans, but it was all fun. They wound up playing two full games, and although some words were challenged, and found wanting, it passed the time wonderfully, winding up with a split decision and the promise of a rubber match to follow.

The next several days required some creative entertainment to keep the time moving along without becoming too mired in worry about future events over which they had no control.

Betty had a couple of long phone conversations with Nancy who was grateful that Betty had pushed her to speak with her father. She and her dad were now having adult conversations, they were emotional and frank, pouring out long held fears. Both Nancy and her father had been trying too hard to protect each other and wound up bottling up their feelings. Since the death of Nancy's mother, Walter's wife, they had both worried that the linchpin of their family was gone, and their world might unravel. They tiptoed around on eggshells, afraid to say what was in their hearts. Walter worried that he was an inadequate parent, and Nancy thought she was a disappointment. The truth was far different. That woman was gone, yes, but Walter and Nancy were still a strong family, and they viewed each other with pride and respect. Nancy talked a lot about what a good father he was, providing for her, and protecting her. Walter spoke of how strong and resourceful Nancy was, and how much she reminded him of his wife. He saw his wife's spirit living on in her.

Nancy also talked about how much she cared for Richie and how worried she was about what might happen. Finally, she revealed how Richie's mom had been nice to her and how close they'd become over their connections with Richie. It turned out that her dad was happy that Nancy had a woman she could talk to, a motherly friend. After opening themselves up to each other, she found herself closer to her dad, it was easier to talk to him and that was good.

Meanwhile, Betty and Richie had several sessions with Valerie, reviewing the details of the upcoming transplant. They were moved into the larger transplant room with the HEPA filter.

As Valerie described, the transplant preparative medications were each different from his previous cycle of drugs. There would be three medications to prepare his marrow for the infusion: busulfan, fludarabine and etoposide. There would also be medications given to mitigate some of the transplant complications. For GvHD prophylaxis, he would receive three medications. A small dose of cyclophosphamide would be given on the third and fourth day *after* the stem cell infusion. The two other medications, tacrolimus and Cellcept, would be given daily over an extended period. They would also watch for damage to his liver, and he would be given a prostaglandin to provide protection against the possible development of dangerous obstructive hepatic blood clots. Finally, infection was the bane of every transplanter, and both anti-viral and anti-fungal medications would be given prophylactically while waiting for the donor cells to engraft. The donor cells would be infused through Richard's central catheter. They would circulate for a while before being drawn to the marrow like moths to a flame. Once there, they would settle within the marrow cavities, adhering to the cellular lining. They would implant, grow, divide, multiply and produce all the blood cells Richie would ever need and they would carry the DNA of the donor. Richie would be a hybrid, a chimera mix of two sets of DNA.

After what seemed like endless days of anticipation, finally on the expected day, Dr. Stanner received word that enough stem cells were collected from the donor and stored safely away. And so, they had the go ahead to begin Richie's transplant. Day minus 8 would be tomorrow.

As the sun rose on the appointed day, the transplant team was busy. Richie was in his hospital bed with his head raised. He'd been well hydrated through the night. Before the chemo began Richie was given the triple antiemetic cocktail that included fosaprepitant, palonosetron and dexamethasone to help mitigate the expected severe nausea. Soon, the busulfan was hanging from the IV pole, waiting for the pump button to be pushed, thus initiating the transplant preparative regimen. Stacy was there, the label was triple checked. His nurse, Stacy and Paul all verified the drug, the dosage and the recipient, Richard Samuelson. The label was scanned and verified with Richie's wristband.

Betty stood by her son, holding his hand. She was anxious, worried about all those drugs, but she was also hopeful. She tried to block her memories of those awful dreams. Her mind was scrambled, here was a chance for cure and the possibility of death. Which path were they on? An image of Richie's video games flashed in her head.

All were gathered, with Richie as the focus, in a somewhat ceremonial way, like the launch of a new battleship. Paul panned everyone assembled, getting nods from Stacy, the nurse, Betty, and of course, Richie. Once the transplant medicines were given, there was no going back, his marrow would be ablated and he would require the stem cell rescue to survive. Finally, Paul said, "let's get this going. Steve, start the busulfan."

Steve pushed the pump start button, and the medication began to flow. Despite the pomp and circumstance, the start was anticlimactic, the busulfan infused like any of his previous medications. Richie and his mom had been through this many times now. They had to wait to find out if this was the beginning of an ultimately victorious battle against the monstrous malignancy that had until now refused to surrender.

The busulfan infused in over an hour. It was followed by the fludarabine through the same lumen of his catheter. To assess the drug levels for the next day's busulfan dose, blood samples were drawn from the second lumen of his catheter, the one that had not been touched by any busulfan. There was a designated target level to achieve, and the following day's dose would be adjusted to stay within that target. This would give Richie the most effective dose while minimizing its toxicity.

The crowd around Richie thinned out quickly once the infusion began, only his mom and his nurse remained at his bedside.

Although there'd been some tension earlier, by now, the routine of chemotherapy administration had returned, and Richard and Betty had settled into their usual state of been there, done that complacency.

With the drama passed, they looked for something else to do for the rest of the day. And as if she had brain radar, Carol came by at that moment to see how things were. She had an e-tablet with her. Carol asked how the infusion went and mostly got back, "no biggie."

Satisfied with that answer, she brought up her tablet and showed Betty and Richie some social media posts about Richie and his treatments and the support they were receiving from the community. Betty had seen some of this, but Carol had more details.

"It seems that someone at Horace Mann, someone called Franny? posted items about you and Nancy."

"Franny? She's the social butterfly at school," said Richie. "I first asked her about Nancy, way back then."

"I guess she has a following and posts stuff online," said Carol. "It talks about how everyone at your school is thinking about you. It also says that at their recent prom, you and Nancy were given honorary special Prince and Princess in abstentia awards. Someone even used AI to photoshop pictures of you and Nancy dancing at the prom. It shows Richie dressed in a tux and Nancy in a very cute dress, with spaghetti straps. You guys are wearing a crown and tiara. I even found a posted video of your Bueller parade at the hospital."

"That's kind of weird," said Richie, "can you send those to us?"

Carol had a thumb drive that she handed over.

"I also wanted to tell you about an inquiry I received," said Carol. "A reporter, from AP News, picked up on all of this. I think she was intrigued by the use of AI and Richie's diagnosis. Somehow, she got my name and contacted me, trying to get follow up on Richard. She wanted to know how he is and what's happening. She asked about *the girl.* Of course, I told her that all that information is confidential. She sent me her business card and asked if I would pass it on to you." Carol gave Betty the card. "Of course, it's up to you to decide if you want to do anything with it."

"Thanks Carol," said Betty, she looked at the card, *Hannah Darrow, AP News.* "That's pretty strange," she thought. Her emotions were raw. She was consumed with her son's disease, his battle, her work and yes, even with Nancy. That was her world. She couldn't imagine sharing it with anyone else. She tucked the card away.

"Anything else I can get for you guys?"

"Thanks, Carol, you've been great, but we're OK for now." said Betty.

The next few days continued with the planned infusions. As expected, the busulfan dose had to be adjusted downward on each of the subsequent days.

By day minus 5, Richie was no longer interested in food. His nurse recommended that he listen to his body. It was time to stop eating. Steve relayed that to Paul, who ordered the IV nutrition to start.

Day -5 was also the last day of his busulfan. The etoposide would begin the following day. Unlike his induction cycle, this chemotherapy was extremely intense and unrelenting. During standard induction, the goal was to kill as many leukemia cells as possible without compromising the marrow's ability to later recover normal cell production. Not so during the transplant. The aim was to completely destroy all the leukemia cells with no concern about the marrow's ability to recover. New cells would have to come from the donor. Richie's normal marrow elements were untargeted collateral damage. Also, induction therapy was given with the intention of having it followed by many more cycles of therapy, up to three years' worth. The seven days of therapy during transplant was now or never, going for broke. A level of therapy conventionally given over many months was packed into seven extremely intense days of treatment.

As the etoposide began on day -4, they also learned that the donor stem cells were being shipped across the Atlantic, with a brief stop at Kennedy airport and then across the country to PGL. Once the lab did its part, the cells would be sent to the blood bank at Memorial. The planned infusion would be on day zero. So far, the carefully choreographed process was unfolding as intended.

Richie was not feeling well at all, the intensity of the treatments was overwhelming. He was too sick to do much of anything. Even trying to pay attention to a movie was difficult. He had no energy. He would often doze off and wake up lost and confused. One day blurred into the next.

Betty watched him carefully. Although Richie's demeanor was just as they had described in advance, she still worried. She remained vigilant, on guard against, well she wasn't sure what, but she wouldn't rest. She wrote in her journal, recording the drugs, Richie's reactions and how she felt. The notes from those days described a living nightmare, it was a battle each day for her to remain positive. Betty did her best to encourage Richie and to present an optimistic front that she didn't feel.

Reading online postings, she imagined that anything that could go wrong would. At least she thought she had it all covered. Betty spent time while he slept talking with Madelyn, maybe that helped. Still her gut ate at her, it became more difficult to put forth a brave face. She went through boxes of Kleenex, it was the hardest thing she ever had to do.

Betty spent time on the phone with Nancy and together they commiserated about Richie's daily travails. Maybe not so unexpectedly and without much fanfare, Nancy and Betty had grown very close. It was too hard for Nancy to be at the hospital and watch Richie but she could use Facetime to be with him at those moments when he was awake. Even then, he might fall asleep in mid-sentence.

For Richie, day -3 brought the same etoposide and fludarabine treatment as the day before.

The nightmares that Betty had been trying to forget were more disturbing than ever. They punctuated her sleep, dark and foreboding. Monsters that had been chasing her were now after Richie. He tried to run. In her dream, she wanted to shout and warn Richie, but when her mouth opened she had no voice. And just as they were about to pounce, she would wake, covered in sweat.

41.

It was Saturday night, actually very early Sunday morning, when the donor stem cells arrived at PGL, the tech assigned to accept the package, filled out the paperwork. He signed multiple documents attesting to receiving the shipment. He inspected the exterior, documenting no evident damage and that the temperature monitor was functioning correctly. Once the package was safely stored in the cold room, his job was finished, and he left for home.

The cell processing division of PGL was carefully arranged to be independent, a silo, separate from the experimental animal division. By design, there would not be any communication between the two. Dr. Benzi should have had no business in this arm of the PGL corporation. But for several days he had surreptitiously accessed the cell processing division's intranet, monitoring the site for news about any arriving product and had found what he was looking for. He had a plan.

Later, the morning of the product arrival, the full cell processing team arrived. Their first order of business was to download the temperature log to verify that there were no red flags, the stem cell product had arrived safely. The cells were then processed according to the PGL proprietary protocol. A very small, 0.25 mL sample was withdrawn from the unit to be analyzed. Cell viability was documented. The entire preparation took four hours and twenty minutes. That was documented in the log that would accompany the product when it was shipped to Memorial Medical Center later the following morning. Satisfied with their work, the unit was packaged again and returned to the cold room. The team, with no other products to work on and finished with their task, left in the late afternoon.

Dr. Benzi waited until after 1 AM, very early the next morning, his ID gave him access to the main entrance, but not the processing room. He was dressed in black, even donning a black stocking cap. He carried an Igloo ice bucket containing a very special sample from his animal lab.

He had made two trips earlier in the week, casing the unit and asking questions for a so called report he was preparing for one of his upcoming lab inspections. He expected that his story would address any curiosity the processing team had about his inquiries. He asked about how the processing was done, where the cells were stored, and under what conditions. Dr. Benzi inquired about the shipping process for the completed unit. He added several extra questions, whose answers he didn't care about but which he thought would help support his charade. He also took note of where the employee lockers were. A needed trip to the men's room allowed him to briefly check the lockers. The security was not very tight. At least two lockers had no padlocks, and when he looked inside, he found security badges clipped to lanyards hanging on hooks next to white lab coats.

It was 1:30 AM. He entered the processing building. He had planned exactly what needed to be done. He slipped on a pair of blue nitrile gloves and walked quickly along the corridor just outside the entrance to the unit. The second locker he tried had what he was looking for. As before an ID badge hung from the end of its lanyard looped on a hook. He expected that the temporary use of the badge wouldn't be noticed and it would give him the needed access to the work area and the inner cold room where the cells would be waiting.

He had to work quickly, the guard would soon be rounding the corner. Once inside the cold room, Dr. Benzi opened the shipping container and withdrew the transfusion bag holding the precious processed cells. Using the alcohol pads he brought, he cleaned the self-sealing membrane at the end of the infusion spike. He then opened the Igloo ice chest, and removed the 20 mL syringe filled with a solution of 500 million lentivirus particles carrying the unique combination of experimental genes still being tested in his lab. He attached a sterile needle to the hub of the syringe. Holding the IV bag in his left hand, he gripped the barrel of the hypodermic with the other and pushed the needle into the infusion spike, piercing the membrane. Steadily advancing the plunger he injected the contents of the syringe into the suspension of donor cells destined to be infused into some waiting transplant recipient. He withdrew the needle and syringe and dropped them into his Igloo, along with the used alcohol wipe and its torn wrapper. He inverted the stem cell bag several times, to be sure that the viral particles were well mixed within the cell suspension. He returned the bag to the unsealed shipping container and put everything back as he found it. He picked up his Igloo and done with his task, he started toward the cold room door.

About 10 minutes before, a silent alarm alerted Bobby Reynolds, the head of security, that something was happening in the PGL processing center. He got up and turned to a group of monitors hung on the wall. There were cameras mounted throughout the cell processing lab and a person dressed in black showed up clearly on multiple screens at security headquarters. Bobby watched the figure, something seemed familiar about the intruder, but no one belonged there at that hour. He studied the prowler as he entered the cold room. Bobby was trying to figure out who he was and what he was up to. Something about the way he moved, and a gesture he made, triggered a memory.

Bobby called his contact on the PGL Board of Directors.

Dr. Brickston of the PGL board picked up the ringing phone by his bed. He'd been in deep REM sleep, and it took a moment to be awake enough to answer. "Yes."

"Sorry, to call you at this hour, sir. It's Bobby from security, I'm watching the monitors and there's an intruder in the processing lab."

Dr. Brickston was annoyed, "Bobby, I'm sure you know what to do about an intruder, why are you fucking calling me at, what time is it? Oh, almost 2 AM."

"Well sir, I'm not sure what he's doing there, but I'm pretty sure that it's Dr. Benzi."

Dr. Brickston sat upright. He was fully awake now. "Fuck, show me what you have." Dr. Brickston turned his phone over and opened the security app. He could see what Bobby was seeing. He watched for a couple of moments. It could have been Dr. Benzi.

"Bobby are you sure it's him? What's he doing?"

"I'm not sure, sir. He hasn't looked toward any of the cameras, but it sure seems like him. He did something in the cold storage room, and he's just coming out now. In about two minutes our guard will be coming around the corner, and he's sure to see Dr. Benzi. What do you want me to do, sir?"

Dr. Brickston continued watching the video stream. Suddenly, he saw it, the intruder had a tic, he saw the hitch in his left shoulder as he crouched. It was him. What the fuck are you up to, Hans?

John Stevens scanned the large windows, searching with his flashlight.

Back inside the lab, Dr. Benzi crouched behind a table as the beam of the security guard's flashlight swept across the room. When he saw the guard reach for his key ring, he knew he had to act. He ran through his options. There was little choice, and so crouching low, he ran toward the emergency exit door, the ID badge held up in one hand, the Igloo, down at his side in the other. He wasn't sure, but he hoped that the ID badge would allow him to leave without triggering the alarms.

Watching it all unfold on the security monitor, Dr. Brickston worried about the implications of a lab breach. He had been instrumental in recruiting Drs. Carlson and Benzi to PGL. He received regular reports from Dr. Benzi updating him on their progress toward identifying a gene set of interest. A lot of money and PGL's future was riding on their success. "Listen, Bobby," said Dr. Brickston, "I don't want Dr. Benzi stopped. I don't know what he's doing there, but it could be trouble if he's caught. I don't want alarms to go off or the police to be poking around. I don't want anyone to know about this. I don't want any record of this. Can you fix it so he can get out without being caught?"

"Yes, sir," said Bobby, "I'll make it so."

Dr. Benzi opened the exit door and was out of the lab. He ran to his car. He sat inside waiting. He heard no blaring alarms. That was the good news. The bad news, the "borrowed" badge was still hanging from the lanyard around his neck and it needed to be returned.

He didn't want to, but he had to go back. Dr. Benzi left the car and waited in the shadows, near the building. He remained alert, watching for any response to his incursion. He imagined the guard talking to his boss about the breach. Dr. Benzi slowed his breathing, he'd take his time. He'd be patient. Thirty minutes, then an hour passed, and still there were no alarms, no security searching around, no police appeared. It was as if nothing had happened.

Dr. Benzi made sure the guard was not near the lobby when, two hours later, he carefully stole back inside the building and headed to the corridor where the lockers lined the walls. Wearing his gloves, he lifted the badge and its lanyard from around his neck and hung it back on the hook in the locker. He was soon back in his car, driving home.

It had not gone exactly as planned, but still five hundred million viral particles were mingling in the suspension with the donor's stem cells. During the night, they would latch on and then enter those cells delivering the experimental genes they carried. And before long, the intended recipient would be given those transformed blood stem cells.

Dr. Benzi was sure that the patient would be cured of his or her disease, in a dramatic fashion. That had been his lifelong dream. It was why he studied medicine and worked to have his own lab. It would be a new way to cure cancer patients without those awful cycles of chemotherapy. If only that had been available to his mother, or his sister. Well, now at least it would be available to others. After a few months, when the patient was deemed to be cured of his disease, Dr. Benzi would reveal how it was his work that led to the remarkable recovery of that lucky patient. He would claim credit. He would be awarded patents for his discovery. Dr. Hans Benzi would become famous for his contribution, and very rich. He could imagine it all, he might even win the Nobel Prize in Physiology or Medicine. That would be a just reward indeed.

42.

Monday was day minus one of Richie's protocol in preparation for the stem cell infusion the following day. Today was a *rest* day, the treatment medications were finished. His body would have time to clear the transplant drugs so they wouldn't harm the new donor cells when they infused.

Richie was exhausted. Fortunately, on day -1 at least, he would have a respite from the very strong toxic medications. Richard and his mom were anxious, but they were also eager to receive the stem cell infusion and begin the road to recovery. They learned that the cells would arrive in the hospital blood bank around mid-morning tomorrow. Once they were checked out and deemed to have completed the journey safely, the cells would be sent up to the unit to be infused through Richie's central line.

Throughout the night Richie and his mom slept uneasily. Richie woke several times. He had bizarre dreams. He remembered how he felt, the details were vague. He was chased by something dark. The creature had multiple large, yellow, glowing eyes. It blocked his every effort to escape. He woke up with a start, breathing hard and dripping with sweat. His mom tried to be reassuring. It was only a dream.

At last, early that afternoon, Drs. Stanner and Gardner approached their room. She carried a small ice chest. "The cells are here," Sandra announced.

Steve had everything prepared. His medications and nutrition fluids had been stopped. Only a saline drip kept his central line open and accessible.

Sandra hung the stem cell bag from the IV pole. The standard IV pump advanced fluids by squeezing the tubing, like kneading a tube of toothpaste. To avoid any damage to the cells, there would be no pump, the suspension would drip freely using only gravity. Everything now depended on the success of those cells. He was too tired to think about all the possibilities. His whole body hurt. He only had enough strength to hope it would work. Steve connected the bag to Richie's central line via the stopcock. On the signal he turned the valve, and the stem cells began to flow, down the tubing, through Richie's central line and into his subclavian vein. The journey would eventually end in his bone marrow, where the cells would settle and grow.

Betty sat with Richie, holding his hand as they watched the steady drip of cells. It didn't look like much, another bag of fluid among the hundreds he'd already received. But this one was different, so much rode on its success. It took twenty minutes for the bag to deliver its precious cargo. Once the flow stopped, Steve added more saline to the bag, inverted it a few times, picking up any cells that might have stuck to the sides of the bag, and then he let it flow once more. And it was done. The cells were in. There were no fireworks, no bells ringing, no drum roll, no explosions, it was just a quiet coda to his treatment.

Steve was prepared with a dose of solumedrol in case of any untoward reaction. Within minutes, Richie began to feel a bit edgy and tremulous. He wasn't sure how he was supposed to feel but everyone kept telling him to speak up if something seemed different. So he did and Steve added the steroid to his saline solution.

Richie had been anxious and jittery as he watched the infusion finish. Once he received the solumedrol his anxiety abated, and he fell asleep.

Betty remained at attention, watching. Her eyes darted back and forth from her son to the vitals monitor. She was alert for any reaction, any change, a mother guarding her child, ready to take on any danger. But all was quiet. In the end, as Richie might have said, "it was no biggie."

Once completed, Steve took down the empty bag. It would be packaged and labeled, then sent to the blood bank, where it would be kept in the cold room for 48 hours, available for potential analysis, if needed. If there were no adverse events, the label would be removed and pasted into blood bank logbook as a record of the infusion.

Nancy called. She had waited until she knew the infusion should be completed. Betty answered, "it's all done, it went smoothly, now we just wait."

She had held her breath until she knew. Now a sigh of relief, "I'm so glad. I imagined all sorts of things going wrong. I guess it's just me, and my paranoia. Can I talk to him?"

"He's sleeping now, but I'll let him know when he wakes up. I'm sure he'll want to talk to you."

"You've been so nice Betty, thank you. Do you think I could come visit tomorrow?"

"That would be great. You'll have to wear a mask while you're here, you know, no fluid swapping."

Nancy giggled, "sure I know, I promise to be good, no matter how much he begs me. See you tomorrow," and Nancy punched off.

Having finished the stem cell infusion nominally, Betty began to think that maybe this would be OK after all, perhaps her worries had been unwarranted. As the day ended, Betty settled into her bed, still on alert, but with some easing of her wariness. She was able to gently drift into a comfortable, restful sleep.

43.

Day plus one of his transplant started quietly, it was his third day without chemotherapy. The newly infused stem cells were being drawn to his marrow by invisible signals from the cells lining that cavity. They would soon settle and begin to grow.

The acute effects of the treatment had begun to fade. The fog of chemo brain began to lift and he could feel some of his strength returning. He had slept most of the last 36 hours and it took a few moments to shake off all that slumber. Richie sat up and rubbed his eyes trying to clear his vision. He was surprised to see his mom still asleep in the nearby bed. He remembered that there was no therapy planned for today. He was happy about that. On days +3 and +4, he would get small doses of cyclophosphamide but that was not to treat his leukemia, it was designed to blunt the activity of the donor T lymphocytes that would be responsible for GvHD.

Paul came by to check on Richie, it was the last week of his first year of fellowship. This coming weekend, on Saturday, July 1, two new doctors would begin their training to become pediatric oncologists. One weekend a month, he and Sandra would be covering the service, so it wasn't goodbye, but it would be a big change. As an outpatient Richie would be followed in one of Sandra or Paul's clinics. Richie thought the timing was lousy. He was convinced that his fate was tied to the doctors he had grown close to, especially Dr. Gardner.

"How do you feel today?" asked Paul.

Betty began to stir when she heard his doctor's voice. "Oh my, I guess I slept well, for a change."

"I feel better," said Richie.

"It should be a quiet day for you," said Paul. The parenteral nutrition will continue, it's better if you don't try to eat for at least a few more days. It's OK to drink bottled water or chew on the ice chips that we've made from purified water. Please don't use the ice or water from any of the machines. We need to minimize exposure to any microbes until the new cells begin to engraft and proliferate. We should also limit your exposure to foreign proteins, and minimize blood flow to your gut by avoiding all food, at least for a while. That's another way to moderate GvHD."

"I guess you must be excited, you'll be finishing up year one," said Betty.

"Yes, it will be a new chapter for us, Dr. Gardner and I are looking forward to the change."

"We certainly appreciate everything you've done for Richie, and both of you will be missed," said Betty.

"I agree," said Richie.

"Thanks, that's very sweet of you to say," said Paul. "The new fellows are excellent, and you'll be in good hands. I'll check in again with you guys later."

The next two days were quiet. Friday was day plus three and he received the first of two, post stem cell Cytoxan doses, as part of the GvHD protocol.

Later that day, Richie began to develop mouth sores, severe mucositis. Richie knew they'd be coming, but being told was much different than experiencing them. He could trace the holes in his mouth with his tongue. It was much worse than he expected. As he took a breath, the air passed across the sores, making them cry out in pain. It hurt to swallow his own spit. His oral secretions mostly wound-up dripping down the sides of his mouth. He knew it would happen, but it was still embarrassing to be drooling like a baby. His nurse informed Paul, who ordered the first dose of intravenous morphine for the pain. Initially, his morphine was given intermittently, every 3 to 4 hours. Pretty soon that wasn't enough. The intermittent therapy was converted to a continuous drip, employing PCA, patient-controlled analgesia. Richie could give himself rescue doses of the pain medicine by pushing a button on a remote device. The pump was programmed with lockouts to prevent an overdose. It would not respond if he asked for too much morphine. Richie pushed the button whenever the machine let him. The IV morphine, like the natural endogenous version, helped ease the pain. He wasn't euphoric, it just helped him get through the severe pain of mucositis.

It wasn't long before Richie developed chills and fevers. Blood samples were sent to the lab for culture. The sample would incubate in special vials that could later be used to identify any growing organisms.

With his new fever, treatment was aggressive. Richie received the broad-spectrum antibiotic, ceftazidime. Vancomycin was added to cover a possible gram-positive staph. He also received an antiviral medication, ganciclovir, and the antifungal medication, Ambisome. He would remain on these anti-biologics until his white blood cell count recovered.

With the new fevers, Paul examined Richie frequently. He listened to his lungs, percussed his chest, and palpated his abdomen. He looked for any decreased peripheral perfusion. He pressed on Richie's fingertips to assess the briskness of his capillary refill. If his fingertips were not receiving adequate blood flow, that was also happening elsewhere in his body. And that would suggest that internal organs such as his liver and kidneys could be in trouble.

For now, Richie's vitals were stable, but that could change quickly. When Paul queried Richie about what might be bothering him, Richie mentioned that his lower back itched. He pointed to his lower spine, near the coccyx, his tailbone. He said it felt like he had a new pimple down there.

That was a classic site for a possible herpetic outbreak. It wouldn't be surprising given Richie's stress, and his immune status. But when Paul examined the area, he didn't find any vesicles or pimples that would typically accompany a flare of herpes. There was swelling at the end of the coccyx, but it wasn't inflamed or tender. As he pressed around the site, it was firm, not fluctuant. It almost seemed as if something was growing there, under Richie's skin.

Paul wasn't sure what to make of it. He took a picture with his phone and sent it to Dr. Stanner to get his impression.

Over the next six hours, with Tylenol and several doses of antibiotic on board, Richie's fever began to ease. His breathing became more regular. He was less tremulous. The low-grade temperature continued, but there were no new fever spikes.

It was getting to be late in the day on Friday, June 30, and soon Sandra would be covering the unit for her last regular shift.

All of a sudden there was a bit of commotion at the end of the unit. As everyone in the nurses' station turned toward the noise they watched an animated group of folks exit the elevator and walk onto the unit. The nurses recognized Drs. Stanner and Gardner, but the other two were new. After a few moments of laughter and chatter, they turned toward Richie's room, taking on a more serious professional look. Betty stood up as Dr. Stanner led them into the room.

"This is Richie and his mother, Betty," Dr. Stanner introduced them to the group. "Of course, you know Dr. Gardner and Dr. Belkin very well. I want you to meet the new fellows. Drs. Miriam Lester and Roland Reed, they will have their first day in our program, tomorrow, July 1."

Everyone had donned a mask, and as part of the standard infection control protocol, there was no handshaking, just a nod of their heads. Dr. Stanner continued, "Drs. Lester and Reed have been briefed about Richard, and his current therapy. Just to be clear, and likely to the reassurance of both the new fellows and our patient and his mom, throughout July, this first month of the fellowship, either me or one of the other attending physicians will be overseeing every part of Richard's care. Despite the notoriety of a hospital visit in July, it is one of the safer months. Everyone is being extra vigilant.

Tomorrow morning I'll be on rounds along both Drs. Reed and Lester and with Dr. Gardner, who'll be finishing up her first year of fellowship. After rounds, Dr. Reed will leave for the day, to come back later that night for his first evening coverage.

They both have excellent credentials from their pediatric residency programs, and I'm confident that within a few weeks, they'll be up to speed and terrific members of our team."

"I'm sure they will be," said Betty, "we've been happy with Dr. Gardner and Dr. Belkin, we wish them all the best. Of course, we understand, but we also hate to see them go."

"Thank you, for the very kind words," said Sandra.

Despite the game face she put on with Richie and Betty, Sandra worried. Dark images nagged at her too. She would trade the sweet thoughts for a guarantee of his good outcome.

Dr. Stanner and the soon to be fellows had left. Sandra caught up with Paul in the fellow's room as he was getting ready to leave.

Sandra asked, "how do you think Richie will do?"

"I don't think you'll have any problems with him tonight, he seems stable enough," said Paul.

"No, I don't mean tonight, I mean do you think the transplant will work for him?"

"I don't know," said Paul, "the odds are not that good, but he could make it, I hope so, he seems like a good kid. Hey, sometime tonight, look at his lower back, will you, it was itchy and there's something there, I'm not sure what it is." He showed her the picture on his phone, but it was hard to make out much from the grainy image. "It's like there's something growing under his skin."

"OK, I will," said Sandra.

Paul left and Sandra put her stuff away in the locker, fastened the combination lock and walked onto the unit to check on the kids. She wondered what Paul had seen on Richard's back. His description didn't seem to fit with anything she knew about transplant and the picture Paul showed her was fuzzy.

Sandra went over to Richie's room, and they chatted for a few minutes. She had checked the EMR, and the blood cultures were still "no growth." The labs didn't tell her much that she didn't already know. The white blood count was zero as expected. As she approached Richie in his room, she asked if that spot was still itchy. He said it still was, but maybe not as much.

Richie removed his shirt so she could examine the area. As she looked it over, she tried to picture the details from Paul's phone and visualize the landmarks for perspective. There'd been nothing abnormal at that site recently, for sure, she would have noticed it during her exams. What she saw now seemed bigger than she'd expected from the picture. On exam it was firm and neither tender nor inflamed. The skin over it was slightly scaly. When she squeezed it, it felt firm, but not hard. She took out a marker and drew some lines on the growth. The first line was a circle around its base where it seemed to emerge from his lower back, the other line, using a paper tape measure, was exactly one centimeter, less than half an inch, from the base circle she had just made. She took another picture. And then one more, this time asking Betty to hold her finger next to it, as a reference. As Sandra finished, she rubbed the top of his head, and noticed that he already had some peach fuzz growing back. That was unexpected.

After she finished, Betty asked her what it was. But Sandra didn't know. She'd been a fellow in oncology for a year, but she had never seen anything like it. Still she wasn't particularly worried. Although it looked odd, it didn't appear to be very concerning. She'd go to Google and see what she could find. She advised Betty to be sure that Dr. Stanner got a look at it when he made rounds in the morning.

Sitting down, back in the fellow's room, Sandra looked closely at the pictures she had taken. It seemed that there were two fingers there now, one was Betty's, and the other was growing from the end of Richie's spine. She texted Paul, asking him to send her the picture he took earlier. She went to Google with AI, searching for answers, which she did not find.

She could only imagine that it was somehow related to the transplant, perhaps some type of Graft vs. Host Disease, but not any kind that she'd ever heard of. And anyway it was pretty early to be seeing much of that, there shouldn't be enough donor T cells circulating yet to cause GvHD.

It was early Saturday morning when Sandra woke up. She was surprised that she hadn't gotten any calls during her last regular night of coverage. Sandra spent a few minutes in the bathroom and then came out to the unit. Dr. Stanner and the new fellows were at the nurses' station, no doubt learning details about the overnight and what concerns they might have for the day.

"Welcome to Fellowship 101 guys," Sandra greeted the new docs.

Miriam and Roland smiled and thanked her.

"I don't have much to tell you about the overnight, it was quiet" said Sandra, "I'll be packing up and leaving soon. But I want to come with you as you examine Richie. He has a physical finding that I've never seen before. I'm not sure what to make of it. I'd like to know what you think, Dr. Stanner."

Sandra had her phone with the pictures from the day before. She would show them after they examined Richie. She carried a paper tape measure and a marking pen. The team gathered around Richie, asking the usual questions.

"I'm feeling better today," said Richie, "no more chills, and I slept well. You can turn down the pain medicine, my mouth feels better, and I'm hungry. Oh, and I still feel that thing on my butt, it's kind of annoying when I sit on it. What is that?"

"I am glad you're feeling better," said Dr. Stanner, "I don't want you to eat for at least another day or so and then we'll see. We would like to examine you now if that's OK?"

Each of them took turns examining Richie. Dr. Stanner described what they were seeing and what they should be on the lookout for. GvHD of the skin could start with itchiness and a red splotchy rash. There was no rash of any kind. As it could affect other organs, there might be changes in the laboratory results, but there was no evidence of that. When Dr. Stanner examined Richie's mouth, he was impressed that the sores seemed to be healing already. They completed the remainder of the usual physical exam, listening to his heart and lungs, pushing on his abdomen, and finding nothing remarkable. Dr. Stanner asked Richie to remove his shirt and turn so they could see his back.

The change was obvious. There was something at the base of Richie's spine, and it was nothing that Dr. Stanner, with his decades of experience, had ever seen.

It was bigger at the base and tapered toward the tip. The girth at its base was comparable to Dr. Stanner's little finger. It was covered with scaly skin, in geometrical shapes, like tiny stop signs. He noted the two lines that Sandra drew the night before and asked if she had measurements. Dr. Gardner handed him the paper tape measure by way of answering his question. Dr. Stanner measured the distance between the lines she had drawn. "I get 2 cm."

Dr. Gardner showed him the pictures she had on her phone including the one that Paul had sent. "It was only 1 cm between the lines yesterday."

Dr. Stanner was stumped. "Richie will be getting his second dose of Cytoxan today, for GvHD prophylaxis. I recommend adding a generous dose of steroid, to reduce any swelling and help mitigate any potential GvHD. Let's start with 40 mg of IV solumedrol. As to the new growth, I'm not sure what it is. Let's ask Dermatology for their assessment. General pediatrics should have a set of ring sizer gauges to measure diameters. Let's get that up here to keep a record of its girth over time. I'll contact some of my transplant colleagues around the country to get opinions. Anything else?"

There was no reply.

"Let's keep tabs on this," said Dr. Stanner. "Review this with the nurses so they can chart their findings, at least twice per shift. Also, I'd like pictures.

Dr. Lester I'll be checking in with you this afternoon, but please call me sooner if anything changes."

"Dr. Stanner, what does this all mean?" asked Betty. She could only imagine the worst, but she couldn't even put a name on what that might be. And what scared her the most was that no one else seemed to be able to do that either. A creeping doubt began to grow.

"Richard seems otherwise fine, his blood tests are appropriate for now, his vital signs are stable, and he seems rather comfortable. We'll continue his antibiotics. It's encouraging to see his mouth sores beginning to heal and his appetite improve. Overall, I would say Richard has tolerated the transplant better than expected. The swelling at the base of his spine doesn't seem to be causing any harm or posing any threat at this time. Frankly, I'm not sure what to make of it. It raises concern for GvHD, but it doesn't seem to fit with any manifestations of the disease that I'm aware of. It's also too soon for GvHD. I'll need to investigate further. With your permission I'd like to circulate pictures among some of my colleagues. It may come to an MRI study and potentially a biopsy. However, to start, I'll ask Dr. Lester to order an ultrasound. That's the least invasive and it can be done with a portable machine. It'll be safer if Richard doesn't leave the unit."

"Of course, do what you feel is necessary. As you might imagine," Betty continued, "the unknown is unsettling and frightening. Do you think this could be his leukemia coming back or some sort of new tumor?"

"I don't think this is his leukemia," said Dr. Stanner. "If an ultrasound showed lymphoid tissue inside that might be worrisome. We could biopsy the tissue, but let's wait before we take that step. The ultrasound will also show if there is a cystic structure inside, a bubble of fluid which could be sampled with a simple needle aspiration. As to the question of a tumor, the ultrasound should show the internal structure of the growth and help us identify it. But it's not like any tumor that I've ever seen or heard of. Reemergence of his leukemia only in this growing protuberance and not in his blood seems unlikely. I'll let you and Richie know whatever we find."

"Thank you, Dr. Stanner," Betty was not very happy with his non-answer. "I'll be here, of course and definitely worried until we can figure this out," said Betty.

"I understand. I'll make sure that you know as soon as we do." With that, the doctors moved on to the next patient.

Betty turned to Richie and asked him what he was thinking.

"I'm not sure what to think," said Richie. "It's hard to see it myself, except with a mirror. Of course, I can feel it. The pictures look weird, for sure. On the other hand, I feel OK, in fact, I feel better today than I have since the transplant started. That must count for something."

"I don't like whatever it is," said Betty. "Something's rotten in the state of Denmark."

"What?" said Richie.

"It's from Shakespeare's Hamlet, it implies that something is amiss."

"Oh, okay."

"Well, it doesn't seem like much, but no one seems to be able to make any sense of it. That can't be good."

Richie's phone buzzed and he looked at the screen, "It's Nancy, she's coming up."

"She's so sweet," said Betty. "OK, I'll just say hi to her and then make myself scarce."

"Thanks Mom, you're swell."

"Swell? Have you been watching Mickey Rooney movies again? Really, swell?"

"I guess I could say cool, but that's so mundane."

"Well, I wish that more things around here were mundane," said Betty.

Pretty soon, they saw Nancy skip out of the elevator and walk over to the nurses' station. She picked up an N95 mask and put it on as she came over.

"Hi Betty, hi Richie," she said, she seemed bright and cheery. Richie's spirits rose as she entered his room. She was a breath of fresh air that seemed to wipe away the layers of tension that had been building. She had her hair up in braids, like the first time he saw her. She wore a bit of rouge, a touch of eyeliner, but mostly she looked just radiant on her own. She wore flared jeans and a floral white lace peasant blouse with a string tied in a bow at the top. She looked like summer just walked onto the unit.

"Hi Nancy," said Betty, "you're looking good."

"Thanks, Betty, I feel good, and I hope that Richie's good too."

"Ah, yo, ladies, I'm right here, by the way," said Richie, "and yes, I am feeling pretty good. And, by the way, you look unbelievable, Nancy."

"Well, hmm, I'll give you two love birds some space," said Betty, "I think I hear someone calling me from the lobby." Betty smiled and left with the unspoken invitation to spend some time elsewhere.

Both Richie and Nancy kept their promise to wear masks, but no one said they couldn't embrace. They did, and held each other, closely, warmly, sharing that moment together as best they could. It was an intimate communication of bodies and souls. After a while, they parted, still holding hands and sat down together. It'd been more than a week since they'd been together, physically, but their bodies remembered. As they held each other, they connected again.

"Richie, I've been scared for you. Ever since I heard that you needed a transplant my anxiety has gone through the roof. I've told you about my nightmares. They're worse now, more vivid. I wake up in a sweat, breathing hard and I have to take a minute, looking around my room, to be sure it was only a dream and that I'm truly alone in my bedroom. Do you think it means something? Richie, do you think I'm crazy?"

"Those dreams sound frightening." Richie didn't know what to make of them. But he was worried about her. Those dreams must have been disturbing, interrupting her sleep, amping up her anxiety. He wanted to calm her fears. "I'm so sorry that you're going through this. I know it's because of me. You're definitely not crazy, Nancy." He wanted to hold her, to reassure her. "But I feel pretty good now."

Nancy smiled and gently rested her warm open hand against his cheek. "You do look good, Richie. For a while I was afraid to come see you. I'm sorry. I couldn't help how I felt. I tried, but the thought of seeing you so sick was too much. I wish I could have been stronger."

"It's OK, Nancy," said Richie, "please don't feel bad. You're here now, and that's what matters. I love you."

Nancy looked at Richie, "I love you too, Richie. I can't wait until you're out of here and we can be alone together." She looked at him, "we have a lot to make up for."

Richie imagined what it would be like to be with her. The vision excited him. "I think about that all the time," said Richie. "I hope that'll be soon. It's kind of weird how good I feel. They were saying that wouldn't happen for a while.

I feel stronger, and I'm hungry now. I could do with a big cheeseburger, fries and a chocolate milkshake. I haven't even thought about food in a while, but it's like I'm famished. You know, I've always felt at ease here, they've taken such good care of me. But now I'm starting to feel caged in, like I need to get out and start running, like back on the track."

"I don't know, Richie, maybe you should take it slow."

"Hey, Nancy, I got something for you." Richard handed her the wrapped box, tied with a ribbon and a bow. He had the card too.

Nancy looked at Richie as she held the gift. She wiped a tear from her eye. "Oh, Richie, I can't believe it, that's so sweet."

"It's just a little thing," said Richie.

"Oh no, it is not a little thing. It's wonderful."

"Well, you haven't even opened it, Nancy."

"Yes, but it's still wonderful." She opened the card and read:

"To my girl, you've always been here for me, and I'll always be there for you. All my love, Richie"

She looked at him again. "It's so special. I wish that I could hold you and kiss you. And we could be together." She looked at him, tilting her head just a bit. A sly smile crossed her face and he saw a twinkle in her eyes, "that will happen, Richie."

His heart beat a little bit faster. "Open it."

Nancy tore it open and saw the bracelet. "Oh, Richie, it's perfect. Can you help me put it on?"

Richie fumbled a bit but did the best he could. Finally, he got the clasp closed and sat back as she smiled. She wiggled her wrist, and the trinkets danced and jingled on her arm. She played with it, and a sparkle of light reflected off the charms. A small tear fell down her cheek.

Richie watched, anxiously at first. It was his first gift to a girl and he wasn't sure what to expect. But it was soon pretty obvious that she was happy. She liked it. He was overjoyed.

"Oh, Richie, it feels like you're wrapped around my wrist. I love it." She looked at him, "and you."

Nancy ran her hand along his arm, caressing him. At first it was just a loving touch, but it soon became more exploratory. Her smile changed to a look of concern.

"Your arm seems different. The skin feels, I don't know, tougher. It's like you're wearing one of those wet suits, like divers have." Nancy looked perplexed. "Richie, your mom said, there was something on your back."

"Yeah," said Richie, "everyone seems very interested in it and puzzled."

"Can I see it, Richie?"

"It's kind of near my butt."

Nancy smiled, she was determined, "I'm sure you have a very cute butt."

He smiled at her. He wanted to show her everything, he wanted to feel her hands on him. For the first time in weeks, he felt those stirrings again. Richie stood up, facing her and then he turned around. He slipped his scrub pants down, just a bit, exposing the top of his behind, and the lower end of his spine. He felt her hands touch him there. It was electric.

"Ooh, Richie, you do have a nice butt," she said, as Nancy first explored a bit more than seemed absolutely necessary. Richie didn't complain. Then she focused on the new growth, touching it, moving it around, playing with it. It was different when Nancy did it, it wasn't clinical like the doctor's exam. Maybe it should've been embarrassing, but it wasn't. It was exciting and titillating. He felt her touch, and the heat as it spread through his body creating changes on the other side.

"Richie, you have a little tail back here. You know, when I was little, I had a pet turtle, and it kind of looks like his back side."

After a minute or so of her inspecting his backside, Richie turned around again, facing Nancy. It was immediately clear that her explorations in back had an effect in front. She reached up and touched him there, her hand folding around him, smiling, "I don't know about the backside, but I do know how to manage this side, Richie."

"I wouldn't mind being your pet turtle," said Richie, he looked down at her, enjoying her touch.

She smiled up at him, it was a wanton gaze. He couldn't look away. She kept her hand there for a few more moments, and then withdrew it. She stood up and reached around him to pull his pants up to their proper place. Her face was so close. "Maybe," she said, "we should wait until we're alone." She patted him once more.

"Oh, Nancy, that was incredible. But now I'm in desperate need of relief."

Nancy seemed sympathetic, but at least for now, he would have to manage that on his own.

"Richie," she said, "what are they going to do about your turtle tail?"

"I don't know, Dr. Stanner's going to ask his colleagues about it. He thinks it may be some sort of reaction to the transplant, but he's never seen anything like it."

They talked for a while longer and they were still talking excitedly when Richie noticed his mom approaching.

Betty was happy to see Nancy and Richie together, giggling. "You guys seem to be getting along quite nicely."

Nancy looked up at Betty, with an ear to ear smile, "we're fine. I guess you probably knew about the bracelet." She extended her arm for Betty to see. "I love it." Nancy paused, "Richie showed me his tail, what's that all about?"

Betty shrugged her shoulders. It caught her attention that Nancy called it a tail. "They're trying to figure it out, it seems to have stumped Dr. Stanner."

The three of them chatted a while longer, mostly avoiding the elephant (or turtle) in the room. They talked about what Nancy had been up to since school ended.

Nancy glanced at her phone to check the time. Her dad would be waiting, and she had to leave. She stood up to go but asked about the changes again. "Betty, you know those dreams we've had. Something's wrong. And his doctors don't even know. What the fuck, Betty. It gives me the willies."

Betty had been worried about the changes, but as Nancy voiced them out loud, her worry deepened, a sense of dread was growing. His doctors seemed to give it little weight, but maybe that was just for show. The more Betty thought about it, the more distraught she became.

"Betty, I have to go," said Nancy, "and don't forget to ask Richie about his skin." Nancy looked at Richie and blew a kiss. She smiled and turned toward the elevators.

"I guess you and Nancy had a good visit," said Betty.

"It's always nice to see her, Mom. Did you notice how pretty she looked today?"

"She's a very nice girl, Richie," said Betty, "she really does like you. Be careful with her, Richie. And yes, she did look pretty today. And I noticed she had the bracelet on her wrist when she left."

"I think she really likes it," said Richie.

"I'm sure she does. But what was she saying about your skin?"

Richie stretched out his arm, offering it to his mom. Betty was immediately apprehensive. She reached out, tentatively exploring his changing skin. Her fears deepened, she was now sure that something was wrong. Betty was happy that her son was feeling better, but her head was spinning. Strange things were happening, the post stem cell infusion period was not going as the doctors had described. Something was wrong, and it was all moving much too fast.

Roland was making the evening rounds. He stopped at Richie's room, and they chatted for a minute before Roland examined Richie thoroughly. When he came to Richie's back side, he pulled out the paper measuring tape. Richie's tail was now 3 cm between the lines that Sandra had drawn the night before. It was growing very quickly.

Betty, always on alert for any changes, also noticed that his eye color was different, it was a lighter blue. Was it related to the other changes? She asked Roland what he thought about his skin, the protuberance and the new growth of hair on his head, though she didn't expect that Roland would have an answer. He didn't. She asked Roland about the results of the ultrasound, but Roland told her that he hadn't had a chance to see the pictures yet. He was planning to head down to Radiology and review the imaging with the radiologist. He would report back to her later.

Down in the hospital basement, Roland sat with the radiologist and presented Richie's medical history, his diagnosis and the course of his recent bone marrow transplant. He described the changes they were seeing including the finding that led to the ultrasound order.

The radiologist nodded and turned to read the ultrasound image on her high-resolution monitor. She described what she saw, a conical structure, widest at the base and tapering toward the distal end. The computer program would measure its three dimensions, and that would be included in the report. Internally, it was composed of a pair of parallel muscles, running the length of the structure, she saw blood vessels and lymphatic drainage. There were no cystic structures or lymphoid tissue. At the base of his spine, she pointed to his vertebral bones. The upper and mid vertebral bones were normal, but she also pointed to a small additional bone, below the coccyx. That was unexpected. She asked Roland more about the structure, and if Richie had any symptoms from it.

Finally, the radiologist gave her impression. It looks like a tail she said. "There are about 40 reported cases of infants born with tails, they're typically nonfunctional, and they can be surgically resected without any neurologic deficits. Normally, in humans, when a tail is found, it's a vestigial organ, and though it exists during embryogenesis, it normally involutes before birth. I've never seen one develop in an adult. The structure itself has no associated pathology, but obviously doesn't belong there. I recommend that you order an MRI of his lower spine for further evaluation. That will all be in my report. Any questions?"

Roland had no questions and thanked her for her help. He went back up to the unit and called Dr. Stanner from the fellow's room. He reviewed everything he had learned about Richie. Dr. Stanner asked him to order the requested MRI and a dermatology consult for Monday, no need to stress the staff on the weekend. It would require some coordination to get Richie safely to radiology while minimizing his exposure to potential pathogens. Likely, they would do his scan as the last one of the day, after all the other patients were finished and gone. Roland ended his discussion with Dr. Stanner and then went to tell Betty and Richie about the findings, the plan for further imaging and the requested Dermatology consult. Roland watched Richie and Betty, trying to gauge their reactions. He was a new fellow, but he had a few years as a pediatric resident and that included experience with sick children and their parents. He could tell they were still anxious, and that his explanations had not helped much. Frankly, he knew that nothing he had just told them explained very much. He then went back to the fellow's room, logged onto the computer workstation and dove in to see what else he could find about a turtle tail as a finding after a bone marrow transplant.

Bill was in the animal room at PGL, taking care of the mice. From the cohort of two dozen mice, in the mini trial that Dr. Carlson had requested, 12 were dead and the other dozen were thriving. Each of the surviving mice seemed fine, except for some obvious transformations of their tails, their enormously increased metabolism and avoidance of light. Bill had photographs documenting the daily changes for each of the 24 mice. Each of the dead mice had undergone a postmortem examination and they were found to have widespread leukemia. It was obviously in their blood, but it was also everywhere else, infiltrating their livers, kidneys and brains. It was time to break the code, revealing which mice received the same specific combination of tortoise and whale genes, as the two previously long surviving mice had received, and which ones had different random combinations of genes. It was no surprise to Bill, once the code was unsealed, that all the surviving mice had received that same successful combination of genes as the two previous survivors. The result was fantastic and indisputable. They had identified an array of genes that together worked to eliminate an otherwise lethal dose of leukemia. There was much work to be done. They needed to find out which of the genes were essential for the outcome, which could be discarded. Would this work for other cancers? The genes would need to be tested in other animals, eventually, unfortunately, monkeys or pigs would be used to document safety and efficacy. There would be years of testing ahead and many obstacles to overcome before this could be tested in a human. But these were exciting first steps. He carefully organized all the data to bring to Drs. Benzi and Carlson for review. Bill was sure that the doctors would immediately prepare to submit an article for publication in one of the top medical journals and begin the patent applications to protect their work. This was big news.

44.

Betty watched her son as always, but she wasn't sure what to think. Richie seemed as healthy today as he'd ever been. His color was good, his fevers had resolved, and he was hungry. He was asking to eat and be more active. All that was positive and reassuring. But the tail lent an eldritch atmosphere to his recovery. No one seemed to know why he had those changes. Betty had done her own digging online and could find nothing. And of course, it was not just that weird appendage, his skin was different, his eyes were changing and all that new hair on top of his head. Dr. Stanner was thinking about GvHD, but Betty found no description of GvHD that matched those manifestations, anywhere. And as far as she could tell, it was too early after the stem cell infusion to see any effects from GvHD.

She began to suspect that that idea was really a wild shot in the dark, grasping for straws. In fact, she was pretty sure that they had no fucking clue about what was happening to her son.

"Richie, how do you feel?" she asked.

"I feel great, Mom, the best I have in weeks," said Richie, "and I'm hungry."

"What about your back?"

"It's definitely weird Mom, but it doesn't hurt or anything. And you know, I was able to wag it a bit, if I concentrate, I can make it move."

Betty wasn't sure she liked that. Things were getting weirder by the minute.

"You know, when Nancy was here, she asked to see it, and you know what she said?"

"I'm afraid to ask," said Betty, "what did she say?"

"Nancy said that when she was little, she had a pet turtle," answered Richie, "and she thought that my thing looks like a turtle's tail!"

Betty never had a pet turtle, but she had seen large turtles when she had snorkeled in the Caribbean. Of course, she could always Google images of turtle tails. She went over to look at Richard's back again, and sure enough, it had a reptilian appearance, it might look like a turtle's tail. "Show me, Richie, show me how you can move it."

Richie concentrated. It was like trying to extend your pinky toe.

But then Betty saw it move, side to side, just a bit.

"Can you move it up and down?" she asked.

"No, it doesn't work like that, I've tried, I can only move it side to side."

This was definitely freaky, she thought. What the fuck was going on here? Dark thoughts churned in Betty's mind. Indeed, none of what was happening was listed as a possible side effect of a bone marrow transplant. Something was not right. She would find out what it was. Grabbing her phone, she stepped outside the room to text Sandra. Betty was freaking out and she needed help.

Sandra read the text from Betty. A while back, when Richie was first diagnosed, she had given Betty her cell phone number in case she ever needed to talk to her, but Betty had never used it, until now.

"Please call when u can, I'm worried," was all it said.

Sandra dialed Betty's number. "What's going on?" asked Sandra. Betty had answered after the first ring.

"Dr. Gardner, thank you for calling back," Betty began, "I know it's July and well maybe you're not Richie's doctor anymore, but I'm not sure who else to turn to."

"It's OK, Betty, I'm still Richie's doctor, what's happening?"

"I'm worried that there's something seriously wrong with the transplant. It's not any of the shitty complications we were told might happen, this is completely crazy, fucked up stuff. And I'm scared."

"Is this about the growth on his spine?" Sandra asked.

"Yes, and more than that. It's bigger. It's knobby and pointy, it looks like a fucking turtle's tail, and he can wag it. The skin on his chest is also different, it feels like he's wearing a diver's wet suit, and his eyes are changing, he avoids the light. No one seems to understand what's happening. It's like, I don't know," she took a breath, "OK, it's like he's been invaded by something. I'm pretty sure that sounds crazy, but he's different."

Sandra didn't know what to make of any of it. Betty sounded desperate and scared and a bit wacky too. But there really had been something strange at the base of Richie's spine. "What does Dr. Stanner say?"

"He doesn't know, he ordered a dose of solumedrol. Richie's had an ultrasound, and they ordered an MRI for Monday. Dr. Stanner said he would consult with his colleagues. But I can tell that he has no fucking clue!"

"How does Richard feel, Betty? Does he have pain or chills and fevers? Does he seem sick? Tell me more," said Sandra.

"That's the other weird thing, Dr. Gardner, he feels great, he says. He has no pain, the morphine dosing was cut way down, and they're going to stop it altogether soon. He's not drooling, his mouth sores are nearly healed, there are no chills or fevers, his heart rate is low, like 60 all the time. He says he's hungry and needs to get exercise. He seems strong too, he doesn't look like someone who's just had a bone marrow transplant. At least not what I would imagine he should look like.

Dr. Gardner, I don't expect that you would know the answer, but something's happening, something very bizarre, and Richie needs help. I don't know how, but it's not going to come from what they're doing."

"OK, Betty, first off, I don't know what's going on either. Of course, I've only been doing this for a year, but those things certainly seem strange. I'm going to talk to Dr. Belkin and see what he thinks. I'll get back to you, I promise, OK?"

"Thank you, Dr. Gardner, I know that you don't have to this, but I am counting on you," Betty disconnected.

Sandra put the phone down. She was disturbed by the call. It made no sense. Betty had always seemed stable and level-headed, not easily rattled. She kept herself together during the tumor lysis and sepsis crises. But she was different. After all, for weeks, she'd been confined to that small space next to her son who's being treated for a life-threatening illness. No easy feat for any parent, let alone a single parent. Over time, the continuous assault could result in post-traumatic stress disorder, and that could take many forms. It could certainly make someone batty and imagine all sorts of things. And yet, Sandra had also seen something on Richie's back. She tried to visualize it. Could someone think it looked like a turtle's tail? Bizarre, wasn't it?

It was just an hour later when the nurses on the unit all turned to look at each other as they saw Paul and Sandra step out of the elevator and walk towards them. It was quite surprising to see them on a Saturday evening, in July, when they weren't scheduled to be covering the service.

Annie stood up as they came near, "well, doctors, to what do we owe this unexpected pleasure?"

"Well," said Sandra, "we were in the neighborhood to get something to eat, and we thought we'd come in and see how Dr. Reed is."

"You guys haven't even been gone long enough to say we missed you, but it's nice to see the old folks back. I think you'll find Dr. Reed in the fellow's room."

Sandra thanked her, they walked over to the room, knocked on the door and went in. Roland was surprised to see them, but also seemed happy to have some friendly faces to talk to.

"Hey, guys, is something wrong? What's going on?"

"Nothing's wrong, Roland," said Paul, "we wanted to see how you were, and if there's anything we could help you with. And to be honest, Richie's mom called Sandra. She's concerned about him."

"I'm glad to see you guys. It's July 1, and I'm a newbie, of course, but this stuff is pretty strange. I can't seem to make any sense of it."

"Let's see what you have," said Sandra.

Roland reported all the notes, the labs and the ultrasound findings.

After reviewing everything, Sandra asked Roland what he thought.

"I don't really know, and I'd rather you just look at him and tell me what you guys think before I say something. Frankly, anything I say, would sound rather wacky."

Wacky, it sounded like what Betty had said. Sandra had a bad feeling about this. She couldn't put the pieces together, nothing made sense. What else had Betty said? He had been invaded by something. What, a strange virus? She shook her head. Something gnawed at her. There must be an answer, but whatever it was eluded her for now. Richie needed their help.

The three walked over to Richie's room and Betty came out to meet them. She looked worn. She'd lost weight. Her walk was without that confidant look she used to have. She was slouched over and her face was crisscrossed with worry lines. "I really wasn't expecting to see you tonight, but I'm very glad you're here. I'm hoping that after you see Richie, you'll just think that he has a looney mother."

They went in together to see Richie. Roland stepped back, letting Sandra and Paul get close.

"Hey, it's good to see you guys," said Richie. He looked from one doctor to the other, "I'm guessing my mom called you."

"I did," said Betty, "I'm worried and these doctors know you pretty well, so I was hoping they could help."

"OK, I guess it's kind of weird, I know that I'm not supposed to but I feel good," said Richie.

Betty offered to step out of the room so the doctors could examine Richard.

Sandra borrowed a stethoscope from the room and listened to his heart and lungs. She examined everything from his head on down. She used a penlight to look in his mouth, and the ophthalmoscope to examine his eyes. The bright light seemed to bother Richie more than expected. It took several tries before he could keep his eyes still enough for Sandra to see the fundus. She felt around his neck, above the collar bones and wherever he might have enlarged lymph nodes. She pushed on his abdomen, and examined his groin, testicles, and legs. She tested his reflexes at the elbow and knees. She asked him to flex his arms at the elbow. She directed him to keep his arm bent and resist her attempts to straighten out each arm. Though Sandra used both her arms, and leveraged her weight, she couldn't force his arm to straighten. She paused her exam for a moment and asked Paul to help test his arm strength. Sandra watched as Paul strained to straighten out Richard's arm. It seemed hard to believe that he couldn't.

Sandra hesitated, but she went back to her exam. She ran her hands over the skin of his chest, back and arms. Finally, she examined the base of his spine. She tried to remember everything she saw so she could document it all later. She created a visual memory that she could access when she needed. And, with Richie's permission, Sandra used her phone to take several pictures.

"Richie, there are certainly things I see on your exam, that are unusual, and unexpected. Obviously, the growth on your spine is not a usual finding. Overall, despite the unusual physical changes, you look very strong and healthy. Would it be OK, with you if I talk some more with your mom outside the room?"

"I guess that would be OK, but I want someone to tell me what's happening," said Richie.

Sandra could see that he was becoming annoyed with all the exams, and no doubt the lack of answers. "I promise to let you know, when we know," said Sandra.

Leaving Richie in the room, they stepped out to join Betty. She looked at Sandra expectantly.

"First off," said Sandra, "I don't think you're a loon. There's no doubt that there are changes that I can't explain. I see that the growth at the base of his spine is bigger. By ultrasound it has muscles and a blood supply. It does look reptilian, as you say, like a turtle's tail. Which, of course, just by itself is pretty weird. I see that he's lost pigment in his irises, the color is now a very light blue, and he seems particularly sensitive to light. His skin has changed too. You've described it as having the feel of a diver's wet suit, which is an interesting interpretation. As crazy as it sounds, I'd say that it feels like the skin of a marine mammal, like a dolphin or a seal. And he's clearly very strong. I agree that he doesn't look like someone who's just had a bone marrow transplant. And none of this makes any sense to me. Dr. Belkin, do you have anything to add?"

"I think that you've given an excellent detailed summation of the transformations that we're seeing. The changes are astounding and so far, unexplained. Temporally, they seem to be related to the transplant. And the only aspect that is unique to this transplant is this donor-recipient combination. Something is different about how these donor cells have reacted with Richard's body. Many other transplantees have had identical treatments, but no one else has received cells from *this* donor. So, I think we need to look there."

Betty scanned their faces. "That all sounds very clinical, but that's my son, what the fuck is happening? What are we going to do?"

"I think Dr. Belkin is right, we need to trace those cells from the donor," said Sandra, "we'll start by contacting the International Bone Marrow Transplant Registry, the IBMTR, and find out what we can about his donor."

"How long will that take?" said Betty, "he keeps changing and so far, we don't really seem to know much. It's like some freakin' horror show."

"We're going to figure this out," said Sandra. "And Richard seems OK, at least for now. Let us work on this."

Roland, Sandra and Paul sat in the fellow's room. "That's some crazy shit," said Roland.

"I think we have to figure this out quickly," said Sandra, "those changes are progressing, and I'm worried about what could happen."

"So, you've scheduled the MRI for Monday night after hours, right?" said Paul.

"Yes, that's correct," said Roland.

"OK, tomorrow you'll be drawing some blood for testing," said Paul, "we'll see his CBC, blood chemistries and liver tests. Monday morning, I suggest some additional blood testing."

"What do you have in mind, Paul?" asked Sandra.

"We need to send a protein electrophoresis panel, a chimerism study and a genomic microarray analysis test. When dermatology sees Richard on Monday, we need them to send a skin scrapping for chromosome analysis as well."

"The chimerism will show how much of the blood is Richard's and how much is the donor's right?" said Roland.

"Exactly," said Paul, "and the protein electrophoresis will report a panel of proteins from his blood and may help identify a potentially unique subset of them. The microarray test could reveal any new mutations in his circulating DNA."

"And we need to contact the IBMTR, on Monday also," said Sandra. "We need to track down his donor and find out more about him. I'm not sure how much time we have to do all this. Those changes are happening quickly."

"Tomorrow is day +5," said Roland, "and things are happening for sure. He'll start the GvHD prophylaxis with tacrolimus and Cellcept. Maybe that'll help."

"I think we have some time," said Paul, "but there's lots of work to do if we're going to figure this out. The microarray test could take a while and we need to find a way to expedite that result."

The three doctors looked worried and grim, but at least they had the beginnings of a strategy. They had no idea how this was going to work out for Richie. Although they wanted to be, they were not particularly sanguine about his prospects. Before leaving, Sandra and Paul made sure that Roland had their cell numbers on his speed-dial. They'd resolved to talk again after the team made rounds in the morning.

Paul and Sandra wound up in a corner at Pat's Tavern. It was, of course, their go-to place when they needed somewhere to sit and think. They ordered a couple of the local draft beers from the day's specials listed in chalk on the large blackboard, and a bowl of peanuts and pretzels. They weren't particularly hungry but munching on something seemed to make it easier to focus on the problem. They appeared somber and deep in thought as they sat quietly together. For a while, neither of them spoke.

Finally, Sandra said, "I feel bad for Betty, I can't imagine what she must be going through."

"Yeah, I know," said Paul, he had finished his first pint, and was looking for a second. "Let's think about this. He had his cell infusion four days ago, no hint of craziness before that, right. So, now he has, what a turtle tail and dolphin skin, what can that mean?" He paused a moment. Sandra could imagine his wheels turning. "It's got to be some like errant DNA. Somehow, his stem cell product was contaminated."

Sandra looked at him, "what are you saying Paul, how could that have happened?"

Paul started his second pint. He was listening to Sandra, and then he sat straight up, his eyes widened as he looked at her. "You're right, Sandra, but the real question is not how it could have happened, but *where* it could that have happened!"

"OK," Sandra was thinking, "so, it could have happened during the collection in whatever center the donor was at on the day of his harvest," said Sandra, "it could have happened in our blood bank, before the bag came up to the unit."

"Or," said Paul, "it could have happened at PGL, where the product was processed before it was shipped to us."

"Holy shit, Paul," said Sandy, "do you really think that it could have happened there?"

"I have no idea, but I can't think of anything else, it makes sense, it fits what we know."

"We can look at PGL online," said Sandra, "and find out if they've had any violations, they must be required to undergo routine inspections. The FDA would be doing that, and FACT, the Foundation for Accreditation of Cellular Therapy, so there should be some reports available that we can check."

"OK, that's a great idea Sandra, let's try to find out everything we can about the lab."

Paul and Sandy sat quiet again, but their demeanor had changed, there was now a focus to their plan. They would begin to track it down and hopefully find a way to help Richie.

Moments later, Paul was still thinking about the stem cells. "I was thinking," said Paul, "that maybe we should explore this idea a little more before we mention it to anyone. What do you think?"

Sandra tried to imagine how that conversation with Dr. Stanner might go. He might think they were a bit nutty, and she didn't want him to think that. "Yes, I think it would be a good idea to do a little more of our own research before we start discussing an idea that we came up with over a couple of pints at Pat's tavern."

Paul smiled at her phraseology. "Just so," he said.

45.

The next morning, Roland was stunned when he saw that Richie's white blood cell count was now up to 0.5, it had been zero for more than a week. That would either be a remarkably rapid recovery by day +5, or the first indication of a leukemia relapse. But the differential report showed that the white blood cells were all neutrophils, not lymphoblasts and that made the 0.5 very good news indeed. His hemoglobin was also good, up to 10 gm/dL and his platelet count was 50,000. He expected that everyone would be happy about the recovery. The Sunday team would be ready to round soon. He reviewed all the information so that he was prepared to report. Everything about Richie was crazy, but he definitely didn't want Dr. Stanner to think he was crazy too. That would be a very bad first impression, and he'd been told by his mom many times about first impressions. He would make sure that his presentation was complete, objective and professional. And, given all the circumstances, he was prepared to answer, '*I don't know*' to some of Dr. Stanner's questions.

Dr. Stanner and Miriam arrived before the others. They had both checked the EMR and had seen the lab results from the morning. Dr. Stanner suggested that they go down to the heme lab and review the blood smears before starting rounds.

Down in the heme lab, Roland located Richie's slide from the morning pile, and carried it over to the multi-head microscope. He handed the slide to Dr. Stanner who positioned it on the microscope's stage and secured it with the clips. Dr. Stanner switched on the light, squeezed a drop of oil onto the slide, and then rotated the 100 X objective into place. First using the coarse focus, then the fine focus, they all watched the blood cells as they came into view. Dr. Stanner moved the slide around using the stage controls, viewing multiple areas of Richie's blood smear.

Finally, he looked up at each of the fellows, and he took a breath. "These cells look completely normal. His own cells could not have survived the recent week of very high dose chemotherapy. These must be the donor cells. But it's unheard of to see such an early stem cell engraftment and the appearance of neutrophils." He took a breath and stared out into space, searching for an explanation. He could find none.

"OK, let's go up and see the patients."

Drs. Stanner, Reed and Lester along with the senior pediatric resident, Dr. Lyons, Richard's nurse, Annie, and the weekend pharmacist, Laura, were all gathered for rounds. Roland briefly presented a history of Richie's disease and his current status. He reviewed the unusual physical findings, the ultrasound report and the morning's blood test results. He added that the morning's blood sample was reviewed by Dr. Stanner under the scope, and remarkably, the cells appeared to be normal. Roland added that Richie's mother, Betty, was concerned about the physical changes and has been looking for answers.

Laura stated that Richie was slated to begin his oral GvHD prophylaxis: Cellcept 500 mg, 2 tablets, twice daily, and tacrolimus 1 mg, also 2 tablets taken twice daily. And now that his marrow seems to be producing cells, he should restart his PCP prophylaxis with the Bactrim tablets.

Miriam thanked her and made sure the orders were entered into the EMR.

Dr. Stanner added, "there are several important points to keep in mind about this transplant. First, it's good that it started while he was in a visual remission, rather than in response to a relapse. Second, his white cell count has begun its recovery by day +5. Lastly, he has physical findings, that while they don't appear to be harmful, at least for now, they are nevertheless unexplained. Any questions?"

There were none.

Betty watched as they gathered in the corridor outside the room. She watched their lips move and their body language trying to discern what they were saying. She was anxious about what they might say when they finally entered.

"Good morning," said Roland, "How are you today?"

"I feel pretty good," said Richie, "and I'm kind of hungry."

Roland smiled, and said, "well, we have some good news for you." He reported the blood test results and that they had reviewed the cells in the lab. They were satisfied that they represented a recovery of normal bone marrow.

It was stunning and unexpectedly wonderful news. Tears flowed down Betty's face, she was overwhelmed. "Really," she said, "you saw normal cells, there's no leukemia?" It was hard for her to imagine. The surprisingly great news chased away all of her doubts. And at least for now, Betty was ecstatic.

She turned to Richie, overcome with joy, they embraced and held on. Weeks of tension seemed to melt away. The chemical assault he had endured, now finally seemed to be paying off. No words passed between them, but they were certainly communicating.

"It certainly is good news, but there's a lot left to do," said Dr. Stanner, "please, let me examine Richard."

He checked him thoroughly. There were no mouth sores, no enlarged organs or lymph nodes. He noted the lightened eye color. As Dr. Stanner ran his hands across Richie's skin, he felt it to be smooth, without rash or lesions. He tested the range of motion in each extremity, which were normal. And of course, he examined the base of his spine. The growth was still there, although it hadn't changed significantly since the last exam. On measurement it was still 3 cm, just a bit over an inch long.

Dr. Stanner stepped back. "Mostly, I'm pleased with the findings. The blood results are exciting, and I hope they continue to improve. Richard seems otherwise well. As far as his skin exam, it may be related to a kind of skin GvHD. I must admit that I'm not sure what to make of the protuberance at the base of his spine. But overall, things are moving in the right direction."

Roland added, "Richard will be starting the medications for GvHD prophylaxis. It's typically early to see much graft versus host effect, which depends on a growing population of donor T cells. But, Richard's marrow is recovering at an unexpectedly rapid rate, so we need to be prepared for a different time course of events. We'll be watching carefully over the next several days. Laura, our pharmacist for the weekend, will talk to you more about the medications."

He turned to Dr. Stanner, "his mouth seems much better, can we try something enteral?"

"Yes, I think that'd be OK," said Dr. Stanner, "let's start with just water and clear juices, like apple or cranberry juice, if that goes well, we can advance his diet. Slowly. And we can stop his pain medications." Dr. Stanner smiled, "since his ANC is 500, we can also stop all the antibiotics except the Bactrim."

"Can I walk out of the room, if I wear a mask?" asked Richie.

"Let's not rush things. We'll see how things look tomorrow," answered Dr. Stanner, "if it continues to go well, that might be OK."

"What about that thing on his back? And his skin?" asked Betty.

"Tomorrow evening he's scheduled for an MRI of his lower spine. We should have more information from that. Also, tomorrow is Monday, and I should be able to reach out to some of my colleagues around the country. As to his skin, I think we need to give the new GvHD medicines a chance to work. I might add a few extra doses of solumedrol to further reduce any inflammation that may be contributing to the problem. Dermatology will be coming by tomorrow and we'll have their opinion. I want to wait a bit, before getting too much more aggressive."

"Sounds like a plan," said Richie.

Betty was mollified for now, the latest blood count was encouraging, and she started to wonder if she'd gotten too freaked about the other stuff. Perhaps she had overreacted. Laura stayed behind while the rest of the team moved on. She reviewed the role and possible side effects of tacrolimus, Cellcept and Bactrim.

After Laura left, Betty and Richie were alone. Each waited for the other to say something. They had certainly received good news and now they seemed afraid to jinx it by saying too much. A battle was won, but there was still a war to fight. They'd never been here before, and still after weeks on the unit, they really didn't know the rules to this game of cancer. They hadn't asked to play, somehow they'd stumbled into it. All they wanted was to take their ball and go home. In the end, neither of them chose to speak, they weren't sure what to say. Sitting together in that room, for so many weeks, they had learned to appreciate the quiet moments.

Betty opened her journal, reading some of her older entries and then updating it with the latest news. She drew a picture of what had been the focus of much attention. She added arrows, labeling what she considered to be significant features of Richie's tail. Meanwhile, Richie picked up the book he had recently started, he needed something to take his mind off transplant.

Richie and Betty kept themselves occupied until the evening, when Betty suggested that they find a DVD movie to watch.

"Mom, you pick out something," said Richard.

Betty was gone for a little while. Finally, back, she had selected two old time favorites, *Inherit the Wind*, with Spencer Tracy, and *To Kill a Mockingbird* with Gregory Peck. Betty left it up to Richie to pick between the two. He went with the Gregory Peck movie. He liked the idea of a bildungsroman unfolding around the life of Atticus Finch's daughter, 6-year-old Scout, narrated by her older self. They stayed awake through the entire film. And while Betty saw that Richie seemed to follow the story, she was often distracted. She couldn't help thinking about the day. Even the good news about the count recovery began to take on a sinister aura. She thought about his tail, the skin, his eyes, all unexplained. And those recovering blood cells. They weren't supposed to be there yet. What was it about those cells? Despite the apparently good news, she had a frisson of dread. And though she slept, her nightmares hadn't gone away.

Richie was antsy throughout the night. It wasn't just his body that was changing. Stuff was going on in his head. Something was telling him to search for food, to eat more. He pictured plates of food, piled with all kinds of stuff, unrecognizable red meats, and mostly uncooked. Richie also felt an urge to be on the move. He could feel his rapidly changing body urging him on. He was strangely more comfortable in the dark, the daylight bothered him, the night beckoned. He was stronger. Looking in the mirror, he could see the beginnings of a healthy, rosy color to his cheeks. He felt this was the Richie he was supposed to be. His heart was strong, his pulse was full and steady. He had unexpected energy. The weeks of confinement in the hospital seemed to be closing in on him. He needed to be out of his room, on the go, and running free.

He looked over and saw his mom sleeping, she seemed comfortable. He needed to be doing something. He thought about firing up his War Thunder game, but it didn't feel right. Instead, he pulled out his college lined composition notebook and began writing. He wrote about being diagnosed and how that felt, about receiving chemotherapy, and about Nancy. He wrote what he was thinking, and what he needed to do. Putting his feelings on paper was cathartic, the incessant buzz within his head softened. The urgency to get up and move abated a bit. Before he realized, more than twenty pages were covered with his scribbled words. He could rest. He closed the notebook and quietly tucked it under Betty's mattress, being careful not to disturb her. It would be safe there. All at once, he felt as if someone had pulled the plug and his energy was swirling down the drain. His eyelids became droopy. It was as if a hypnotist had dangled a medallion in front of him and suggested sleep. He couldn't keep his eyes open. His respirations slowed, deepened, and then, thankfully, he too was asleep.

On Monday morning, Sandra called Miriam, who would be covering the day shifts this week. She wanted to make sure that the lab tests that they had discussed had been collected.

"Richard seems to have had a quiet night," Miriam told Sandra. "No fevers, no chills, his vitals have been stable. He drank clears all day yesterday, and he hasn't suffered any problems from that, at least so far. No diarrhea, no bloody stools, no abdominal cramps. So, it's all good."

"That sounds great," said Sandra, "and all the blood tests we talked about were drawn?"

"Yep," said Miriam, "looks like the CBC is back, but the differential isn't in yet. Get this, his white blood cell count is up to 1.5, his hemoglobin is 12 gm/dL, and his platelet count is 70,000. Hopefully when his blood smear is reviewed those will turn out to be normal white blood cells, but this looks incredibly good."

"It sure does," said Sandra, "but it's not supposed to look this good so soon. What about the tail?" she asked.

"It hasn't changed much since yesterday," she said. "Richie looks good today, he seems strong. He wants to eat."

"That'll be up to Dr. Stanner, but he's scheduled for the MRI of his lower spine tonight, right?"

"Yes, that's been ordered," said Miriam.

"I'm itching to see what we find out from that and the gene microarray study," said Sandra. "I have a feeling that those results will help us figure out what's happening. Listen Miriam, you can call me anytime if you have any questions or just want to run something by me. I'll let you go now. You've probably got lots to do."

The full team was gathered for rounds Monday morning, day +6 of Richie's transplant. As they discussed the new lab results, Dr. Stanner remarked on how quickly Richie's marrow was recovering. He was perplexed, but it seemed to be good news for Richie. So far, at least they were normal appearing cells, it wasn't his leukemia roaring back.

Among the tests being sent for analysis was a chimerism study which would analyze the DNA of the white blood cells and report the percentage of cells that matched the donor. They would hope to find more than 90% of the cells to be from the donor, and that percentage should continue to climb over the coming weeks, eventually rising to more than 99%. If, on the other hand, that percentage began to drop, it would mean more cells were coming from Richie's own marrow, and that would most often indicate that his disease was relapsing.

Dr. Stanner, along with Miriam, examined Richie. Overall, he seemed healthy. His heart, lungs, and abdominal exams were normal. But the growth at the base of his spine was larger, almost 2 inches long now, and though Dr. Stanner was not convinced, Miriam might have described it as reptilian. Curiously, as they closely examined his skin, particularly important for someone post-transplant, they found no redness or splotchiness, none of the inflammatory changes that one might associate with GvHD. In fact, Richie's skin was smooth, there were no lesions, no bumps, no wrinkles. He had no hair on his arms or chest, although it was growing on his scalp. And, while Dr. Stanner noticed some normal moisture across his brow, his chest, back and arms were distinctly dry.

As rounds were finishing, the differential report appeared in the EMR, and it showed that his cells were indeed normal neutrophils. No sign of his leukemia. Results of other tests, including his chemistries, LDH and uric acid, were also normal. Based on his continued recovery, Dr. Stanner agreed to ease up on Richie's restrictions, allowing him to eat toast and jelly, dry crackers and some clear broth. Dr. Stanner also gave instructions allowing the nurse to saline lock Richard's central line so that he could be unhooked from his IV pole when he was brought downstairs later in the evening for the after-hours MRI.

With permission, Dr. Stanner took pictures to use as he conferred with colleagues about Richie's very curious "turtle" tail. Dr. Stanner's own online research had not shed any light on Richie's metamorphosis.

Betty was anxious. It was clear that neither Dr. Stanner nor anyone else around Memorial Medical Center had a clue about the cause of Richie's changes. She hoped to have some answers after Dr. Stanner consulted with his colleagues, but she had creeping doubts. Dark thoughts slunk through her head, and a sudden chill sent shivers through her body. Betty tried to keep a brave face for Richard, but that was becoming harder to do.

Richie was happy enough. He enjoyed whatever food he got, and asked for more. No longer needing the morphine and no longer tied to the IV pole, he had some freedom to move about. Before lunch, as he was strolling around the unit he noticed the display of hospital maps and picked one up to further explore the facilities.

As requested, a doctor from Dermatology came by in the early afternoon. It was one of the new interns, a freshly graduated medical student, now starting his first days as an MD. He performed a full exam and then asked to take pictures. Finally, when he was done, as Betty expected, he said that he would report his findings to his attending physician, and they would all be by later.

Without answers Betty's anxiety continued to grow. Her mind would not rest. She had turned to Sandra, hoping that somehow she might help. But although Sandra seemed concerned about Richie's mysterious changes, she was unable to provide any information that might ease Betty's mind.

Despite all her worries and her inner turmoil, the remainder of the shift, at least outwardly, passed uneventfully. Late in the afternoon, as scheduled an escort came up from transport, pushing a wheelchair, to bring Richie down for his MRI. Richie's nurse had already saline locked the catheter and tucked the end of his central line under his nylon mesh vest so that he could travel without the IV pole tagging along.

Richie wore a top and bottom scrub set, with a tie gown over everything. He had a pair of hospital slippers and of course, his N95 mask. As he sat down in the wheelchair, Betty reached over and adjusted his head covering. "That looks better," she smiled and said, "see you later."

The aide flipped down the wheelchair footrests for support. Richie pulled down his mask briefly, smiled and gave a little wave as the aide turned him and pushed him toward the elevators.

As he arrived down in the MRI suite, which, as arranged, was empty that evening, the aide swiveled Richie around and locked the rear wheels. The aide reminded Richie that the very powerful magnet used by the MRI machine made it dangerous to have any metal nearby. He would have to walk from the radiology anteroom to the MRI machine, leaving the metal wheelchair behind. He would also be asked to leave any metal, jewelry and his cellphone behind when he went in for the imaging. After making sure Richie understood, he asked Richie to wait, while he checked in the MRI control room. A minute later, he came back out and told Richie that there was still a patient in the machine. He explained that once that patient was done, the radiology tech would come out and escort Richie in for his imaging. The aide would check back in about an hour when the exam should be finished.

Richard watched the aide leave. He had been thinking about this moment since yesterday afternoon. He'd been cooped up for weeks, and he was tired of that. He was antsy and fidgety and brimming with energy. He needed to get away, he needed to be moving. He was hungry all the time. He needed food, a nice juicy rare hamburger would be most welcome. He could feel his body changing. There was something inside him urging him on. It was impossible to resist.

He had a plan, it was not fully formed, but he had plotted out the basics. Richie imagined Betty finding the notebook he left under her mattress and how she would react. He couldn't think of another way to do it. He also knew that he would need to continue some of the medications for his transplant. He had located the outpatient pharmacy on the map of the hospital he took earlier that day. It was on the same lowest level as the MRI and close by. The outpatient pharmacy would be closed at this hour, but maybe, somehow, he could still get a supply of tacrolimus, Cellcept, and Bactrim for at least a week or so. Not wasting anymore time, he resolved to go ahead with his plan.

Richie looked around to be sure no one was watching. The coast was clear, he grabbed his cellphone and took off. He headed for the outpatient pharmacy, which, as he expected, was closed. It had a roll down gate and a keyed padlock hanging from the holes in the gate fitting. He banged on the gate and then tugged on the padlock. Nothing happened. Now what?

He tugged a bit harder, and then once more with all his strength. He heard a crack, and the padlock slipped down, exposing the shackle and its stripped notch. The lock then came off easily. Richie stared at the broken lock. He was puzzled. He couldn't understand what just happened, how was that even possible? But he needed to get going. He placed the lock aside and rolled up the gate. He searched the pharmacy and saw that the medications were arranged by category on labeled shelves. One shelf had transplant medications and he quickly found what he needed. He took a couple of bottles of tacrolimus and Cellcept, stuffing them into the pockets of his hospital wrap. He went to the antibiotic section and grabbed some bottles of Bactrim, he scanned the shelves, found some tubes of steroid cream and took two of those. That's all he needed, and he quickly headed out. He pulled the gate down, hung the useless padlock back into its fitting and stepped away. Just a few feet down the corridor he found the entrance to the stairwell that would lead up to the hospital lobby. It had been about 5 minutes since Richie left the wheelchair in the MRI suite.

Richie knew that no one would take notice of guy in scrubs walking around the hospital lobby. He quietly and without fanfare walked through the hospital exit. For the first time in many weeks, he was outside. Richie felt alive. He took a deep breath of the fresh air and smiled. Frankly, he was a bit surprised that he had made it out of the hospital without being caught. So far the plan was working, but he'd better get going. The weather was clear and balmy. It was, of course, dark at this late hour, but when Richie looked up at the streetlights, their bright light hurt, he had to turn away. A baseball cap would have been useful.

At first Richie was not sure which way to go, but he didn't hang around, he headed away from the hospital. He brought up Google maps on his phone, found the walking man icon and punched *home*. It quickly found the best route and told him that he would be there in 3 hours. The urge to move was strong. He set out at a comfortable jog, listening to the Google maps voice prompts. He closed his eyes for a moment. Was that the memory of his track coach urging him to move forward, or something else inside? As he worked to follow the prompts he was surprised at how strong he felt. He should have been deconditioned after being in bed for so long. But then again, he shouldn't have had his blood counts recovered so soon, or been able to break that lock. It didn't make sense. He shook his head, it was nothing to dwell on. He needed to get home, and while he jogged he created a mental list of things he would need.

Back in Richie's hospital room, Betty wondered why he wasn't back yet. It had been more than an hour and a half since Richie left for the MRI. Why was the scan taking so long? Maybe they found something in the imaging. Perhaps the radiologist asked for more scans to investigate something concerning. It was in Betty's nature to find a nefarious explanation for any unexpected event. Twenty more minutes passed before Betty walked over to the nurses' station to see if they could tell her what was happening.

The unit secretary called transport, and they connected her to the young man that had brought Richie down. He said that he had wheeled him to MRI a while ago, but he hadn't been called to bring him back. The secretary then called the MRI suite. It rang and rang. Finally, someone picked up.

The secretary explained that she was looking for a patient and got no answer from the inpatient MRI suite.

The operator told the secretary that she thought they were closed by now, but she would try to find out what happened. Letting it ring for a while, she also got no answer. Finally, the default connected her to the outpatient emergency radiology office. After ringing there for a while, once more someone finally picked up. Some back and forth continued. Eventually checking with the tech in the radiology office they located the order for Richard Samuelson's exam, but no imaging had been done. It was marked as a 'no show' and canceled.

Betty, already on edge, broke down completely. "Oh, my god," cried Betty. She was scared and angry. Where was he? She picked up her phone and punched the speed-dial for Richie. It rang and rang, and finally went to voicemail. Betty heard the standard invitation to leave a message and she hung up.

By now the word was spreading that Richie was missing. The unit secretary had called security and a code yellow, missing person, had been announced over the hospital PA. The secretary then notified the nursing supervisor. Betty texted Sandra, and Roland called Dr. Stanner.

Betty was frantic, pacing around the unit, with no idea what could have happened. She was terrified. Where was Richie? He could be anywhere, dead in some hospital stairwell with his body jamming the door shut. Had he become dazed and confused, wandering around outside in the dark, and run over by a drunk motorist. "Where the fuck are you Richie?"

Unable to think, she went back to their room and sat on her bed. Betty scanned the room, looking for a clue. She saw the Creature from the Black Lagoon poster and tore it down, maybe he had scrawled a note on the back. She sat back down on the bed, the torn poster in her lap, no hidden message and she cried. But as she rocked on the bed, she felt something hard under her. Betty stood up and pulled the sheets off. She found nothing. What felt lumpy? She reached down and swept her hand under the mattress. Her hand hit something, she grabbed it and pulled out his composition notebook. She sat on the bed and began turning the pages, there were several dozen filled with his writing. She saw pictures along with notes. The first pages were written early in his hospital stay. She skimmed over the notes from those early days. Some of it was about Nancy, and Betty flipped passed those. Many of the pages had dates at the top, and as she flipped through to the last couple of dozen pages, she came to the ones dated July 2 and July 3. Betty skipped several sections, but then something caught her eye. She started reading.

'Just today, Dr. Stanner talked about the chimerism test, and it resonated with me. I'm a hybrid. I feel that I am not alone in this body anymore, it's like I'm sharing it with something or somethings else. I need to be outside, I need to be moving, I've been caged in the hospital too long. I don't know if this makes any sense. I don't think it's just me feeling this, there's something else in here with me. The skin and tail are just the parts that you can see. It's insistent that I leave. I was pretty sure that if I said anything, you would've tried to talk me out of going, you might have alerted people, and perhaps I would have been restrained or there would be a guard at my door. I need time to work this out. I'll call you when I can. I love you, Mom. Please don't be angry with me or worry about me.'

There was a picture he drew, next to the writing. It seemed to be of him, with a long tail. The tail was curled up, with a devil's point at the end of it.

Betty tried to call Richie again, but she got the same result. Then she called Nancy, who answered on the second ring.

"Hi Betty, is everything OK?" she asked.

"Nancy, did you talk to Richie today?"

"Yes, we had a nice long talk, he seemed OK. Why are you asking me? What's happened?"

"Nancy, did you know? Please just tell me," Betty said.

"I'm not sure what you're asking me, Betty. Did I know what? What's happened?"

From the way Nancy was talking, Betty was pretty sure that Richie hadn't told her. "He's gone, Nancy!"

Nancy gasped, "what do you mean he's gone? Betty, what are you saying?"

"I mean he left the hospital. He's gone. He was supposed to be down in radiology getting an MRI and he took off. He left a note, a very strange note.

"Oh," Nancy breathed a sigh of relief. "When you said he was gone, I..."

"Listen, Nancy, he may try to contact you. It's very important that he comes back to the hospital, please tell him that, and please let me know if you see him or talk to him, OK?"

Betty didn't wait for an answer, she said, "thank you Nancy," and disconnected. She gathered some things together and found Richie's nurse, Annie. Betty quickly told Annie that she found a message from Richie and that he had left the hospital. Annie promised to inform Roland and Dr. Stanner, as well as the nursing supervisor, who would alert the hospital administrator on call. Betty told Annie that she was going home and hoped to find Richie there, and then she left. She was soon down in the parking lot, cranking the engine and heading home. She repeated to herself, over and over, a mantra, "please be safe, Richie, please be safe."

Back at the house, Richie knew that his mom had called about 30 minutes ago. It had been a little over two hours since Richard walked out the hospital exit doors. He had jogged the entire way home, and he was just coming up to his front door. Richie picked up the fake rock where an emergency key was hidden, and he was soon inside. He sat down in the kitchen, and looked around. He was home at last. A dozen memories flashed through his head, all those times, just he and Mom, sitting at this table.

He rested for a few minutes, but he knew he had to get going. He figured that his mom would have left the hospital. She'd be here soon. He was hot and sweaty, at least his head and brow were wet. He used a dish towel to dry his head and legs, but he didn't need to use it on his arms or chest, they were dry. He went up to his room to gather things he needed. He pulled out the medicine bottles he purloined from the pharmacy and swallowed two of the Cellcept tabs and two of the tacrolimus pills. He took off the tie gown wrap, scrubs and slippers and threw them in a pile in a corner of his room. He put on his jeans, a dark T-shirt, a pair of socks, and his track running shoes. He got his backpack and filled it with some extra shirts, underwear and socks. He stuffed the bottles of medicine in the zippered front pocket of the backpack. Richie also took a bottle of hand sanitizer, his toothbrush and toothpaste, a box of Band-Aids and triple antibiotic ointment, you never know. He packed a paperback book to read, a composition notebook and a pen to write with. From his utility drawer he pulled out an old Swiss Army knife, that he'd received for one of his birthdays. Next to the knife was a Zippo lighter, he thought he might need, and an old watch, one that he rarely wore anymore, it had luminescent hands and was water resistant down to 100 meters. He got his wallet, with his ID cards. Richie dug out an old green army blanket from the back of the closet. He rolled it up and strapped it to the bottom of his backpack. He took the navy-blue hoodie from his closet, his track baseball cap, which fit over his durag, his wrap-around polarized sunglasses, and a water flask, which fit in the side holster of his backpack. He quickly looked around for anything else.

Richie decided he had everything he needed from upstairs and went back down to the kitchen. He opened the cookie jar where his mom kept some emergency cash and took five twenties. From the pantry he took a half dozen quart size sandwich zip lock freezer bags, and a couple of gallon size bags. He found a couple of packages of dried Ramen noodle soups and he emptied a box of organic granola bars. In the refrigerator, he found a package of pre-cooked roasted turkey slices and one of sliced cheddar cheese, he packed those along with a half loaf of sliced whole wheat bread. There was also a take-out carton of half-eaten Chinese food that he grabbed. He filled the water flask from the filtered pitcher sitting in the fridge and put that back in its place. Richie repacked his briefs, socks and T-shirts in the larger bags, and some of the food went into the smaller bags. He threw in a couple of packages of plastic service ware that were always around from all the take-outs. Finally, he reserved one of the granola bars to stash in his jeans' pocket. He wore the hoodie, put on his sunglasses and track cap, and donned the backpack. He checked his watch and synched it with the clock on the kitchen wall.

Richie looked around once more and was ready to leave. He wasn't sure where he was going, but he had to get out of there quickly. He thought about Nancy. He started to reach for the door, then stopped and turned back. He took out his cellphone and left it on the kitchen table. He didn't want to be found, not yet. Then he stepped outside, pulled the door closed and disappeared into the night.

Nancy had been reading in bed when she got the call from Betty. She was relieved that he was alive, what she first thought when Betty said he was gone, that was awful. Why she chose to use those words, she couldn't say. For that instant, her world fell apart, those few seconds felt like an eternity in hell. But she needed to concentrate on the fact that he was missing, he took off and that was not like him. She worried about Richie. What was he doing? She was annoyed that Betty had accused her of colluding with him, but she decided that she needed to focus on Richie, not Betty and her problems. She was sure that Richie would try to contact her in some way. Nancy went over to her bedroom window that overlooked the driveway, it was lined with solar powered landscape lighting, leading up to her house. She had a crazy romantic idea, from old movies, that he might try to climb up to her window. She opened her window enough to poke her head out and looked down to see how he might do it. Satisfied there was a way, she lowered the window, but not all the way, she left an inch or two open at the bottom. She made sure to keep her bedside lamp, with the pink tasseled shade, lit. Nancy sat down at her bedroom vanity and checked the mirror to make sure she looked good for Richie. She smiled, turning side to side, still in her PJs, and decided that she looked pretty hot. She picked up her favorite flacon of perfume, inverted it twice and using the glass stopper, touched herself on several strategic parts. She was excited that he might meet her for a clandestine rendezvous in her bedroom. Her dad, just down the hallway, would be in bed, asleep by now and not likely to wake up until his alarm went off for work in the morning. Nancy climbed back into bed. She lay under a single cotton bed sheet. It was warm in her bedroom, the A/C couldn't keep up with the outside July air, as it poured through her open window. She closed her eyes. She imagined Richie lying next to her, unchaperoned. It brought a smile to her face and with that vision in her head, she drifted off to sleep.

Richie found a bench in a small park near his house, and sat next to a sign that read 'Closed after Dark.' Except for the possibility of a dog walker or two, he was not likely to run into anyone at this late hour. He used one of the plastic forks he packed to finish off what remained of the Chinese food he brought. He would have preferred it to be hot, but under the circumstances, he couldn't complain. It was the first solid food he had since the transplant preparation started two weeks ago. He tried to think about what he should do next. He was tired and confused. His mind was a jumble, it was difficult to concentrate. Richie began to wonder if he'd made a mistake leaving the hospital, but he'd felt desperate and trapped in that room, he could think of nothing but escape, and so he did. Still sitting on the bench, he leaned forward, his hands pressed to his temples, he shook his head and moaned, there were few good options left for him now. Richie was scared, but at least he was free from that hospital cage. He thought his mom would be home by now. She would have found the house empty and be worried about him. Richie had left a short note on the kitchen table, by his abandoned cell phone, it said that he was OK. He hoped she wouldn't worry. He would call her when he could. He couldn't help her any more than that, at least not now.

Resolved, Richie stood up, pulled the hood of his sweatshirt over his baseball cap, swung the backpack over his shoulders, dropped the empty take-out container in the trash and left the park headed to Nancy. He imagined that she would welcome him as he was and comfort him. There would be no judgement or expectation, he would be safe. And laying in her arms the constant din in his head might be quieted.

Betty finally arrived home, panicky, she fumbled with the key, but finally got the door open and walked in. The house was eerily quiet. She saw Richie's cell phone and the note on the kitchen table. She knew he wasn't there. She called out his name anyway. Mentally exhausted, she sat in one of the kitchen chairs. She laid her head down on her folded arms across the table and cried. She was lost and had nowhere to turn. After a while, the tears stopped. She stood up and took a few aimless steps around the house. She was not ready to read his note, Betty knew what it would say anyway. Without thinking, she grasped the newel post and climbed the stairs, headed up to Richie's room. She sat on his bed and looked around. Betty reached out and swept her hand across the bed, where he would lie. There was evidence of him everywhere. The posters on the wall, the mess on his desk, the books scattered about, his open closet, with some items on hangers and others laying disheveled on the floor. She saw the pile of hospital clothes in the corner where she envisioned him recently discarding them.

Just then Betty's phone rang. She anxiously reached for it, hoping it was Richie calling from a different phone. But when she looked at the screen, she saw it was Sandra. Betty hit the accept icon and brought the phone up, but didn't say anything.

"Are you there Betty? This is Dr. Gardner."

"Hello, Dr. Gardner."

"Word gets around," Sandra said, "I know that Richie left the hospital, is he there with you?"

"I came home, Dr. Gardner, and he's not here. He was here, but I don't know where he is now."

"Oh. I see, do you know what happened?"

"He left a note in the room, he was feeling anxious. He said that he felt like he was sharing his body with something. He had to leave." Betty was exhausted. It was all too much.

Sandra was silent for a while, she was trying to process what she had just heard.

"Betty, maybe Richie is right."

"What do you mean, Dr. Gardner?"

"I shouldn't say too much, but Dr. Belkin and I were thinking about the changes we saw in Richie, and OK, listen, we don't know, but maybe, somehow, the infusion cells were contaminated."

"I don't understand. What are you saying, Dr. Gardner?"

"Are you OK, Betty?"

"Yes. No. I just wish I could hear something from Richie."

"Did you hear about the pharmacy at the hospital?" asked Sandra.

"I didn't hear anything. What are you talking about?"

"Someone broke into the outpatient pharmacy tonight, and it happened right around the time that Richard was scheduled for his MRI. There's some video, and they see someone there, but there's no view of his face."

"Why are you telling me this?"

"The timing is interesting. All they found is that some transplant medications and Bactrim were missing. And when I say someone broke in, I mean they *broke* in, the padlock on the gate was mangled. Listen Betty, Dr. Belkin and I are working on this, we're going to figure it out and help Richie. This isn't his fault." Sandra disconnected before Betty could say anything else.

Betty sat there on Richie's bed, trying to make sense of what happened and what Sandra said. She was angry, worried and sympathetic all at once. Betty thought about the message in Richie's notebook. She tried to imagine what he'd been going through. The cancer, locked up in a hospital, being with Nancy, but then again not with her, the chemotherapy, the bone marrow transplant and all the crazy changes happening to his body. An overwhelming assault on his mind and body, no doubt enough to mess with anybody's head. "God," she thought, "what would I be like if all that happened to me. I would be a fucking mess, that's what."

What she didn't know, what she couldn't have understood was how those changes in his body from those infused cells were also working on his head.

46.

It was an hour or so after midnight and Richie came up to Nancy's house. The walkway was lit up like an airport runway. Richie avoided the lit path, electing instead to approach the side of the house by crossing through the shadows covering the lawn. He looked up as he got closer. The house was dark except for a corner window on the second floor, with a muted light. He had never been here, but he knew it was Nancy's room. Richie saw the open window, and the fluttering of a pink lacey curtain, as the bottom edge would briefly escape the room and then be drawn back in. Richie smiled. It looked like an invitation. He saw the ledge on the window under hers, and a drainpipe running vertically along the corner of the house. It didn't take much effort for him to climb up. He found the edge of a brick for a toe hold, grabbed the pipe with his right hand and reached up to her windowsill with the other. He raised his head up to the window opening. He saw Nancy, asleep in her bed. He watched her for a moment or so before lightly tapping on her window. She was beautiful. Nancy didn't wake. He considered dropping down and walking away. But his desire was too strong. He tapped again, a little bit harder this time. He saw her eyes open, and her face lit up as she saw Richie in the window. She jumped out of bed, and pulled the window open as much as it would go. Richie pulled off his backpack and handed it to her, before climbing through himself.

Nancy wrapped her arms around him, pulling him toward her, bringing her lips up to meet his. Richie returned the kiss, ardently, fervently. Their bodies pressed against each other, mouths open, tongues tasting each other, greedily, needfully, they clutched at each other.

Nancy touched his lips with her fingers. She whispered, "I'm so happy that you came to me, Richie. I've been so worried. Are you OK?"

"I am now," said Richie.

Nancy went over to be sure her bedroom door was locked, though she didn't really think her dad would be awake at this hour. "We're OK, here, as long as we're not too noisy." Nancy smiled, thinking about a noisy encounter. "Are you ready for me, Richie?"

He looked at her, he hoped she meant what he thought.

She reached up and removed his baseball cap, and the head covering, setting it aside. Then she walked behind Richie and helped him take off his hoodie, folding it and setting it on her vanity, while Richie eagerly tugged at his shirt, and tossed it aside. She then knelt in front of him, slowly unlacing his running shoes and pulling them off along with his socks. She set them aside, neatly by the bed. While she gazed up into his eyes, she undid his belt buckle, and pulled down his zipper, letting his jeans fall around his ankles. She stood up again, close enough to feel his breath on her face. He kicked his pants away and she reached out to take his hand in hers, "come here," she said as she led him to her bed. Lying together they kissed again, their mouths tasting each other.

"Hmm, that's nice," she said, her lips brushing his ear. He kissed her neck, tasting her. He pressed his face there, into the crook of her neck, her perfume was intoxicating. He watched, mesmerized by the gentle pulse under her jaw. He had wanted her for so long. And now together, finally, embraced in each other's arms, they lay like that for a while, Richie enjoyed the feel of her against him.

Nancy held him. She saw the changes in his eyes, and her hand strayed across his chest. His skin was different, smooth and dry as she touched him. He was much stronger. She could feel the changes. "What have they done to you Richie? Turn around, I want to see."

Richie hesitated for a moment, then turned over, his back to Nancy.

Her hands wandered across his back, and downward, toward his bottom and that thing resting there. Her fingers slid across his bottom. "You have such a cute butt, I've always liked this side of you," she smiled. Then her hand traveled a bit higher to the base of his spine. She held it, feeling it, examining his tail. "It does look like the pet turtle I used to have. What does it feel like?"

"Mostly, I don't notice it," said Richie, "except if I sit the wrong way or if you're touching it like that."

"Really?" Nancy fondled it lovingly, and she brought her lips there, kissing it softly.

Her touch was thrilling. It traveled through him, like a jolt of electricity, from his back to his front. He responded to her caress. He felt her heat. His heart raced, and his breathing became heavy. He thought only of her. He wanted her. Nothing else mattered. Irresistible urges flooded his head. They were impossible to ignore. He turned to face her again. "Nancy," was all he said, but her name was full of sex and wanting, he pushed himself against her once more.

Nancy felt it too. She needed him. How many times she imagined this moment with him. He pushed again and she responded.

"Richie, I want to do it with you tonight. I've been waiting for this to happen, with you."

Richie looked at her, he was in love, and he wanted this more than anything, his body was demanding it, but still he asked, "are you sure, Nancy. I want this too, but are you sure?"

Nancy sat up and pulled her top off, and then pushed her bottoms down, kicking them away, she pressed herself against him, as hard as she could, feeling him against her. She reached down, removed his briefs, and tossed them aside.

He felt her body against his, her softness, her scent, her hands seeking him. His hands wandered over her, his mouth met hers and any semblance of restraint was gone.

She felt his hardness pushing against her as she pressed herself to him. She wanted him. Her body responded to his. Soft sounds of pleasure welled up from somewhere deep inside.

Nancy gazed into his eyes. She was ready. She kissed him again, softly, expectantly. "It's time," she said. "There's a packet over on the nightstand, will you get it for me. I've already opened it, so we'll have to use it." She cooed at him, a wanton look in her eyes. Richie reached over, found the packet and handed it to her.

Nancy pulled out the condom. She smiled up at him and then looked down, "it doesn't look like you need any more encouragement." Her face was right there, he could feel her breath on him, it was hot and exciting. He lay on his back. She held him in one hand. She kissed him there and let a string of saliva fall from her lips onto him, sliding her hand up and down, circling gently, stroking him.

He felt the wetness of her fingers as she grasped him.

She marveled at how her touch could make him so hard. It thrilled her to feel him respond. Nancy squeezed the tip of the condom, and then bringing it down, she slowly unrolled it over his length. She inspected her work and said, "I think it's ready Richie, do you think it's ready?"

"Oh, yes, Nancy, please."

Nancy sat up and lifted one leg across his body as she straddled him, her knees tight against his hips. She leaned forward, pressing herself against him, her breasts brushing against his chest. She brought her mouth to his, biting his lower lip first and then kissing him, tasting him. She could feel him pushing into her, wanting her. Her hips edged upward. Nancy reached up to her mouth to wet her hand, she was ready, and she wanted him badly. She held him, lowering herself onto him, slowly. She grimaced at first, feeling him there, opening her up. The first time. She paused for a moment, took a few breaths, and then continued to ease down. All at once, he was inside. He was hard and excited, she slowly continued down, pushing herself onto him. Intense feelings traveled from her bottom all the way up and throughout her body. Finally, she sat all the way down. Their hips were joined. He was deep inside, completely engulfed. She brought her hand up to her mouth to stifle a cry. Her body filled with sensation, her head was ablaze. She had only imagined the feeling, but it was way more.

Richie was a storm of electric sensations as he felt himself inside her. "Oh, my God, Nancy, it's amazing."

"Shh," Nancy put her fingers across his lips, "we have to be quiet." Nancy felt him deep inside, her eyes closed, intent, as the feeling changed from the initial pain to something wonderful. For a moment or two, she stayed still, not wanting to move.

But Richie couldn't remain still, his body demanded that he push, his hips began to move, following the program long etched in his genes.

Nancy felt him inside, moving and she responded, she pushed herself down, urging him on. She matched his thrusts. It was new and exciting. Their bodies flooded with signals of pleasure. Richie grabbed her hips, trying to bring her even closer, and then, together, they turned over. She was underneath, and he was a piston, pushing into her as she responded. Her legs wrapped around him, her ankles crossed above his tail, her fingers dug in, wanting him, urging him on. She bit down on her lip, feeling him inside, trying not to cry out.

They were beyond control, their bodies tensed. He felt her tighten around him. They were breathing hard, gasping for air, their hearts pounding in their chests. Richie's body arched, every nerve in his body was on fire. There were no longer any thoughts, only pleasure flowed through him. Thrusting, pushing himself inside her, again and again and then it all exploded. He emptied himself inside, spasms of pleasure passed up and down his body.

She felt his throbbing and his pleasure as her body followed, seized with tiny convulsions rippling across her, millions of nerves ignited, heat shooting upward and throughout her body.

Nancy held on tightly, her arms wrapped around him, wanting him to stay right there, not to move. She kissed him once more, tenderly, lovingly.

"Oh, my God, Richie."

"I know!"

She felt him softening, "Richie, be careful when it comes out."

He knew what she meant and held on so that nothing spilled. Then he slid the condom off, and they both examined the reservoir filled with his juices. "Oh, my, Richie, that seems like a lot." He tied it off and threw it in the trash by her bed. Richie lay on his back, his breathing slowed. Nancy draped herself across him, lying on her side, one leg resting between his. She looked at him, relishing the feel of his body against hers. She pressed her lips against his face, her hand softly caressing him, across his chest, on his face.

"That was wonderful, Richie. I have wanted that for so long, dreamed about it, imagined it. It still feels good, even now." Nancy ran her hand down her body, across her belly and down below, touching herself, feeling the heat and the wetness. And then she slid her hand across to him, it was soft and sticky as she held him. She looked up at him, still pressed along his side. He saw her look transform from a loving angel to a wanton devil. "When can we do it again, Richie?" She squirmed against him, pressing on him, "I want to do it, again!"

He looked at her, smiling, "wow," he thought, "she wants more!" He had forgotten about everything else in his life. There was just his girl, Nancy, with him, how amazing she was and how lucky he felt that she liked him. He kissed her, and held her, "soon," he said.

"That's good, but I'm not sure how long I can wait," she smiled, "I might have to start without you," she giggled and snuggled more.

"Richie, can I tell you something?"

"What is it?"

"Well, you know the window was open when you came to the house, right?"

"The one I climbed through, with the pink curtains fluttering in the breeze."

"Yes, well I knew you'd be coming, because your mom called and told me that you left the hospital. You know, she's worried about you. She thought you might be here. And she asked me to call her if you showed up. She wanted me to try to convince you to go back to the hospital, she thought you needed to be back there."

Richie held her and took some time before he responded. He kind of already knew everything she said.

"I know I have to leave before the morning gets here. Why I left the hospital is complicated. I'm not even sure I can explain it. It was a feeling I had, an urge really, and I just needed to be out of there. I also know that I probably should go back there, but not yet, I need some time away.

You can call my mom after I leave. Tell her that I'm OK and that I made you wait until I left. You can tell her you tried to talk me into going back, but I was just too stubborn, OK? Blame me, tell her you tried."

"OK, Richie, I will. Will you call me, I need to know how you are?"

"I went home first, and I left my phone there, I know mom has a tracker app. I'll try to get a burner phone during the day, and I'll call you. You won't recognize the number when I call."

"OK, Richie, what will you do? Where will you go?"

"I don't know yet, but I'll figure it out. Nancy, I can feel my body changing. It's like I'm sharing it with something. That probably sounds crazy."

"You're not crazy, Richie. I love you, and I know you love me too, so you have a responsibility to take care of yourself, for me, Richie. You'll do that for me, right?"

He looked at her. He felt their connection, and their love. Richie knew he had to keep her safe and he realized that meant keeping himself safe. Whatever other tragedy she had in her life, he would not let her go through anything like that again, not because of him.

"You really care about me?" he asked.

"Of course, Richie, I care about you, I love you and," she smiled, "we've shared a bed."

He turned to her, and kissed her again, their mouths open, pressing against each other, tasting each other.

"Ooh, Richie," she cooed, in her sultry voice, "I can feel you against me. Is it *soon*, now?"

As exciting and new as it had been the first time, it was even better now. She was ready, and they knew how to please each other. There was no pain this time, only the pleasure they shared. They took their time, exploring each other, pleasing each other, slowly building up to the climax they shared. And then there were two tied up condoms in her trash basket by the bed. "I guess, I'll need more of those," she said, with a grin as she lay against him, enjoying the warmth of fresh sex coursing through her.

"You're amazing," he said. "I just want to stay in bed with you and do this over and over again, but I need to leave."

"Just a few more minutes, Richie, hold me, please. I want to feel you next to me."

They lay there together, for a while, enjoying the closeness of their bodies. But it was getting late, the sun would soon rise, and Richie knew he had to go. Reluctantly he got up. Nancy put her PJ's back on and helped Richie with his things. He wore his hoodie, she adjusted his durag and then his baseball cap and finally his sunglasses. Nancy thought he looked kind of scary. She probably would have crossed the street if she came across a character like him in the middle of the night. But it also gave her a thrill to think that she was his girl. She reached up and they kissed once again. Richie turned and opened the window. He threw his backpack down and started to lower himself out the window. She kissed him once more before he tumbled to the ground.

"Wait," she called out. Nancy turned back and gathered the trash bag lining her wastebasket, tied it off, and went back to the window. She extended her arm, her hand opened, and the bag containing the evidence of their lovemaking dropped to the ground. "I'm sure you'll find a way to take care of that."

Richard gathered everything, pulled his backpack on and left in the very last minutes before dawn.

Nancy watched until she couldn't see him anymore, then she closed the window, turned off her bedside light and curled back into bed. Her last thoughts before falling asleep were of the night they had together.

Someone else was watching as Richard slipped away. As he went out of view, the curtain in Walter's bedroom fell back into place. "Oh, Nancy," he said to himself, "I hope you're being careful with that boy."

Richard left with a smile, and a memory of sharing the night with Nancy. He wasn't sure where he was headed or what he would do. He only knew that he had to find someplace where he could stay for a few days, without being found. But first, he was very hungry. Traveling unfamiliar roads, he came to a wooded area. Satisfied with the covering, he left the road and walked a few hundred yards into a covert, where he might be able to hide, have a bite to eat and think. When he turned back and could no longer see the road, he stopped, pulled off his backpack, unstrapped his blanket and spread it out, under a tree, and sat down. Richie rummaged through his backpack and took out a couple of slices of bread, the turkey and cheese slices and built a sandwich, it disappeared with four mouthfuls. Sated for the moment, he pulled his cap and head covering off. He rubbed his head. He tried to think. Nothing came to him. Exhausted, he lay down on the blanket under the tree, safely distant from the busy road, and fell asleep.

47.

Early Tuesday morning, Sandra was busy online trying to get as much information as she could about PGL. She learned that in addition to processing stem cell products, PGL had a separate division that conducted medical research using animal models. She was able to find bios on the heads of the many laboratories at PGL. On the home page of the PGL website, there was a tab for investors, and as Sandra perused that, she came across an announcement for several newly hired Ph.D. lab directors, and what important expertise they brought to the company. Because of their previous job applications, she was able to use social media, to find their posted CV's. She opened, read and closed many of those, mostly boring, self-aggrandizing propaganda. But one of them caught her eye. It listed references for several interesting peer reviewed papers by two of the same newly hired scientists that were featured under the investors' tab, namely Drs. Hans Benzi and Jordan Carlson. As a fellow at Memorial Medical Center, she had access to medical journals and so it was not hard to download PDF versions of their articles. When she finished reading those papers, she was stunned. She copied and pasted those articles, and sent them on to Paul, Roland and Miriam.

Betty's phone rang, she heard Nancy's programmed ring tone and answered it right away. "Have you seen Richie?" she asked.

"Yes, Betty, he was here," answered Nancy, "and he seemed OK."

Betty paused, processing Nancy's response. She took a breath, relieved that Richie was OK. "But I understand from your answer, that he's not there now."

"I'm sorry, Betty. Richard asked me to wait until he left to call you. He was afraid that you would try to talk him into going back to the hospital. I think that he knows he needs to go back, but he said he needs more time."

"I see," said Betty. She was not happy with that answer, but she didn't want to say anything to antagonize Nancy. Richie loved her and trusted her. It wouldn't be a good idea to do something that might drive a wedge between them. Betty needed to keep their lines of communication open.

"But he seemed OK, to you?"

"He did," said Nancy, "he seems heathy and strong, much stronger than when I saw him last. But, you know, the skin on his chest and his arms is still changing. When he came over, he had been walking and jogging, he was kind of hot and sweaty, at least his head and legs were, but not his chest or arms, they were dry as bones. And his tail is bigger. You know, he said he felt like he was sharing his body with something. I'm worried about him."

"Me too," said Betty. She thought about Nancy describing Richie's chest, how it felt and how long his tail was. What had they been up to?

"He wrote something like that in a note," said Betty, "*sharing his body*. What do you think he meant?"

"I don't know, it sounded kind of creepy, like some alien movie. You know like he's the host body."

It caught Betty's attention, as she said it that way, the transplant doctors were always talking about the stem cell donor and the host. Richie was the host. And what was it that Sandra had said, something about the donor marrow being contaminated. How did that all fit? She wondered.

"Nancy, do you know where he is now?"

"He didn't tell me. I don't think he knew what he would do or where he was going. He said he would get a burner phone and call later."

"Nancy, I'm glad that Richie has you as a friend."

"He's more than a friend," said Nancy.

"I know. Would you please give him a message from me?"

"Sure, Betty, but I'm sure he'll call you."

"Tell him that I love him. Tell him that I will do whatever he needs me to do. Tell him that he can come home, and that he can stay here as long as he wants, it will be his decision to go back to the hospital. Will you do that?"

"I'll tell him."

"Thank you and thank you for being there for him. I want to ask you something else, Nancy. You don't have to answer, but if you do, whatever you say will stay with me. OK?"

"OK."

"Nancy, does your father know that Richie came to see you?"

Betty waited, Nancy seemed to hesitate before answering. She imagined that Nancy was trying to formulate the right response. Finally, she answered, "no, Betty, at least I don't think so."

"Thanks for being honest with me. Walter's a good dad. He may be more understanding than you think. But he won't find out anything from me, it will be up to you. Will you text me when you hear from Richie?"

"I will."

"Thanks, Nancy, bye," and Betty disconnected. She thought about Nancy and her son together. Boys will leave their moms someday. She didn't know if that was happening already, she hoped not.

Betty was scared and desperate. She needed to help Richie, somehow. Something clicked, she remembered the reporter's business card that Carol gave her. She rummaged through her wallet and found it. "Hannah Darrow, AP News." Betty tapped the card with the cell number and email on it, trying to decide. She wasn't sure this was a good idea, but in the end she decided that she might need some big guns on her side to fight a pharmaceutical company. She was pretty sure that AP News filled the bill. "Well, Hannah Darrow, I think I have a newsworthy follow up for you to investigate," she thought. Betty picked up the phone and called her.

It was a very interesting and lengthy call. They were on the phone for nearly an hour. Betty told Hannah what had happened to Richie since she wrote that interest piece about the prom. There was the bad news about his leukemia mutation, the decision to take him to transplant, the search for a donor, and then the bone marrow transplant. Richie's body had changed, he thinks he's sharing it with something, and she mentioned the possible contamination at the Pharma Gene Lab. Oh, yes, and he's taken off and now he's missing, AWOL. Betty thought it was quite a story, and Hannah was intrigued. Betty was ready to sink the hook, "If you come over to talk, I have some pictures that I think will convince you that I'm not crazy."

"Betty, can you send me one of those pictures. This sounds like it could make a very good story, but I need to talk to my boss, and it would help if I had something to show him."

Betty sent the one with Richie's tail and her finger next to it for size comparison.

The conversation stopped for the time it took for the picture to cross the void and show up on Hannah's phone.

"I got it," she said. "Hold on."

Betty waited.

"It's not the best picture, it's a little hard to make out any details."

"There's more to see, if you come," said Betty, "and it's real. Something nefarious is happening, and it needs a good investigator to figure it out. Listen, even if you find out that I'm crazy, it'll still be a good story."

"Are you?" asked Hannah.

"What, crazy? No, I'm not. You can get back to me at this number. Let me know." Betty disconnected.

48.

When Richie woke up, he was disoriented. At first, he couldn't remember where he was or how he got there. He'd been in a very deep sleep, and it took several minutes to fully awaken. His body was repairing itself, and it seemed to do it best while he slept, and though he lay still, his body was working hard. There was a lot to repair, refurbish and reconstruct. New cells were forming rapidly, millions upon millions of iterations. Inside his cells, the Watson, Crick, Franklin and Wilkins DNA double helix would unwind and split like an opening zipper. The edges of each of the two zipper halves dangled, apart from its mate. And then each edge would be repaired separately, each tooth of the zipper, would mate with a new base pair, creating two new complete DNA helixes. There was a cost, of course, there always was, it demanded energy, lots of energy and elements, iron, essential vitamins, minerals, and water. He had immense needs. He was bigger and much stronger, but he needed to feed the humming machine inside of him. His metabolic demands were immense, and he searched for ways to satisfy it.

The sun appeared high in the sky, he looked at his watch and confirmed that it was late morning. He put on his sweatshirt, his cap and durag, with the hood pulled up and the wraparound sunglasses to protect his sensitive eyes. He rolled up his blanket, strapped it to his backpack and slung that over his shoulders.

Suddenly, something nearby scampered across the ground, the leaves rustled as it passed by. It was white and furry, and it looked like a meal with four legs and a tail. As he tracked it in his head the target's dash slowed, nearly grinding to a stop, like a movie playing in slow-motion. An outside observer would have seen a rabbit running along and then seemingly out of nowhere, a dark blue blur would have corralled it, lifted it up and made it vanish.

Richie cradled the rabbit in his arms, stroked its head and back a couple of times, then abruptly twisted its head, snapping the neck. It lay limp in his grasp. He put the rabbit down, gathered some stones, and arranged them in a small circle. He filled the circle with leaves and twigs and started a fire with the Zippo lighter he retrieved from his backpack. When he was satisfied it was going well, he added some of the larger branches. He sat down with the rabbit and using the Swiss Army knife, did the best he could to remove its skin and then slit the belly to gut the animal. It was something he learned from one of the many books he read. He found another bigger branch to create a skewer and propped it over the fire. Richie sat down, leaning against a large oak tree watching his meal cook, he turned it from time to time. The outside of the carcass began to sizzle and bubble. From time to time, the dripping grease would make the fire flare up. He added more branches to keep the blaze going. As he watched, smells of the cooking animal drifted toward him, and his mouth watered. He wished that he had packed some salt and pepper, but this would do. Richie pulled the rabbit from the flame and carefully ripped off some of the hot outer layers that were already done, before returning the rest to the flames. It wasn't home cooking, not surprising, but even without the seasoning, it tasted good enough, and helped quiet the grumbling sounds his belly had been making as he sought to meet his body's demands. He was soon finished, and he felt better. He threw dirt on the fire and scattered the ashes, making sure there were no dangerous hot embers. He tossed the bones and the rest of the carcass around. There would be morsels for scavengers to enjoy. Richie packed up everything. He dressed again, careful to wear those sunglasses, which protected his increasingly sensitive eyes. He pushed his arms through the backpack straps and headed through the woods toward the road. Once there, he chose to turn to the right, hoping he was headed into town.

From somewhere inside, he felt the need to follow the path eastward. After walking for many hours, he began to smell the fresh salty air of the nearby harbor. He'd been drawn to the sea. Whatever that was inside him was pulling him. It seemed to demand that he head toward the water. It became breezier and cooler as he got closer. He began to hear the sounds of rocking boats, and the sea bells chiming. The distinctive crack of the boating flags as they snapped in the wind let him know that he was near. Soon he heard the shouts of crews yelling commands. An idea began to take shape. Perhaps one of the fishing vessels could use an extra deckhand, it might be a good way to disappear for the few days he needed to be alone.

Richie walked along the dock in the small harbor village. There were at least a few dozen boats moored in the boat slips. As he strolled by, if he came across anyone aboard a boat, he would stop and chat them up. He had spent some time the previous summer on a fishing boat, so he had a bit of experience, which he mentioned to anyone who would listen. After stopping at a half dozen boats, asking if they could use help, one man finally seemed interested. It appeared that they were preparing to ship out soon. The skipper was on board, and he told Richie that one of their regular crew was unreliable, he was often passed out, from some late-night binge and he hadn't shown up again. The skipper really needed another deckhand. It didn't require much experience, just a willingness to help pull as the fish lines were hauled in. After a few minutes of conversation, the captain had decided. He spelled out a few rules and what Richie would be paid, and then, "OK, Richie, we're going to leave in the next hour or so and we'll be out at sea about a week, are you ready to do that?"

Richie smiled, "Aye, aye, Captain."

"Listen, there's a marine supply store, just across the way. We'll provide most of what you need, but you should get a good pair of work gloves, and a minimum 50 SPF long sleeved shirt to wear as protection against the sun. Be back in 15 minutes. The captain reached into his pocket, retrieved his wallet, and handed him $50. "You seem trustworthy, I'll have to retrim my radar if I'm wrong about you. Hurry up."

Richie pulled out his wallet and to reassure the captain, he left his backpack there on the dock before running over to get what he needed at the waterfront supply store. Richie picked out a 60 SPF fluorescent yellow long-sleeved rash guard top, with an image of an orca on the back. He asked the clerk's help to find a good pair of work gloves for handling the lines. The total was $65, so he added one of the twenties from his wallet and kept the change. He was back at the boat, ready to report for duty 20 minutes later. Richie climbed on board the *Sea Hunt*, put on his new shirt and stowed the rest of his stuff in a corner down below. Somehow, Richie felt that he needed to be here, on this boat, at this time. He was soon back on deck to see what his assignment was. He met the two other crew, who humpfed a bit, but seemed glad that there was extra help.

49.

The skipper started up the 1,000 horse power diesel engine on the 65-foot trawler and ordered them to cast off. Soon, they were headed out toward the horizon. The seas were calm, and the sun shone brightly in a cloudless sky. Richie followed the lead of the other crew members, Newt and Saul. They were readying the longline and its hundreds of hooks, each one linked to the main line by snoods. Each hook needed to be baited in preparation for its deployment. Richie watched and tried to copy what Saul and Newt were doing. Though it looked simple, it wasn't. They were smooth and fast, he was clumsy and slow, but he figured every bit he did, helped ease their chores, and he knew he'd get better. He liked the mindless work that kept his hands busy, it kept him from thinking about his personal challenges. As he worked the line, Richie tried to chat up Newt and Saul. He wondered how they came to be fishermen. He learned that they mostly caught pelagic fish and Richie remembered from biology class that those would be far from shore. Saul said it would be at least three hours before they came to the first good spot. The skipper would make the final location choice as they got closer. The captain had sonar and fish finding programs to locate the best places to set their lines. They were out to catch tuna and swordfish and so they headed up toward Nova Scotia and the Grand Banks.

The three of them sat on the deck baiting the line. The work helped pass the time. Richie had been so focused on their task that he was surprised when the skipper announced that they had arrived at their first site. They scrambled to get ready. The longline had more than 2 miles of baited hooks. Attached at the start, the radio buoy would mark the end of that long line. They played it out, hand over hand, as it was guided into the ocean by Newt, Saul and now Richie. The longline passed like a fireman's bucket brigade, snaking over the gunwale and into the icy waters below. It took more than an hour for it to be set. The line would lay below and drift for hours while the tuna nibbled at the bait and hopefully became hooked. The longline was kept a short way below the surface by floaters connected with float lines to the main line and spaced out along its length.

After hours of waiting and feeling the line being tugged on by whatever was out at sea, the skipper signaled that it was time. They should begin hauling the line in. This was physically the hardest part of the process. As the longline came in, the hooked fish were brought onto the deck matting. Richie remembered from his previous summer how important it was to minimize the time from when the tuna first landed on the deck to the time it was packed away in the hold below and covered with a mix of cold sea water and ice. A memory from that summer seemed to guide him as he worked. It was beginning to feel familiar. A long pole with a hook end helped release the fish from the line. Quickly, they had to spike its head, instantly killing the fish. The tuna was then bled, gilled, gutted and cleaned. Two or three fish were placed together in a large bag, awash with seawater, the bag was closed and then laid in the hold. After each group of bags were stored, ice chips were shoveled over and around them.

They continued for hours and hours: land, unhook, spike, bleed, gill, gut, clean then store and ice them in the hold below. They worked until they reached the end of the line, and every caught fish was stored below. It was exhausting work and it continued well into the night. The boat's spotlights aimed at the deck came on at dusk, and remained lit until all the fish had been stored below. Finally, the radio buoy was brought back on board, signaling the end of the haul. The longline was washed off, carefully wound and stored for use at dawn the next day. After some 16 hours of hard work, it was time to sit, eat sandwiches from the galley, hydrate and relax, enjoying the satisfaction of having hauled in an excellent catch of tuna. Captain Hansen gave them all a job well done, and a thumbs up to Richie, who more than met the low threshold for success that the captain had in mind. They sat around for a while. Richie listened to fisherman tales. He mind relaxed, the stories were comforting. He closed his eyes and the scary hospital was far away. As he lay there, Newt and Saul went down below deck to get some sleep.

The boat sat somewhere in the deep sea, almost a hundred miles from land and from any manmade light. As Richie lay on his back, looking up at the night sky, it was blacker than he had ever seen it, and yet it was ablaze with countless stars stretching from horizon to horizon. The Milky Way appeared in the sky as a brush stroke of white paint across a black canvas. It was magnificent and he imagined that this was what early people saw before there were factories belching their waste into the atmosphere, and before cities were covered with their obscuring lights. In the dark of night, he no longer needed sunglasses, his eyes felt cool and comfortable. He could have watched the sky for hours, but it had been a very long day, he was exhausted, and he would need to be up before dawn to do it all over again. He went down below deck to his bunk. A memory tugged at him and he pulled his transplant meds from his backpack. It was a glaring reminder of his reality. But still, he put his head down and was soon asleep.

Only a few hours later, it seemed, just before dawn, the captain had brought the boat to a new location. By the time the sun broke across the horizon, the boat was anchored and ready to repeat the process. Every muscle ached from yesterday's intense workout, but he didn't mind. He worked as hard as he could. The second day he was a more productive member of the crew as he worked the line again. By nightfall, the captain was happy with the day's catch, and he let the crew know that if they kept up the pace, they would be due for a nice payday at the end.

In addition to the sonar, the captain had access to radar, and satellite broadcasts providing government sponsored weather reports. Captain Hansen could see a large threatening weather system, but it was far to the east and headed away. For now, it was nothing to worry about, but he checked its progress frequently. The third day began with a brilliant red dawn, and another new site. Richie had become more proficient. He could almost keep pace with Saul and Newt.

Back at home, more than a hundred miles from Richie, Betty called Dr. Gardner, "Can you tell me more about how Richie's stem cell infusion might have been contaminated?"

"Betty, first off, we've been through enough, please call me Sandra. I've become convinced that Richie's stem cell product must have been contaminated, and if that happened, it most likely would've occurred at PGL. So, I went online, digging for anything I could find about that lab. It turns out that they've recently hired two scientists who have published articles about longevity genes in various animals, including the tortoise and the larger whales. It seems more than a bit curious that Richie's donor cells were processed in a facility where they are also carrying out experimental work with whale and tortoise genes and now Richie has something that looks like a turtle's tail and the skin on his arms and chest, has morphed into something that looks like it came from a whale."

"What are you saying, Sandra?" asked Betty, "that Richie is now infected with turtle and whale genes?"

Sandra hesitated. It was a direct, to the point question. Was she ready to say out loud the crazy ideas that had been percolating in the recesses of her mind. Finally, "yes, well infected is not the right word, but as weird as that sounds, it's the only thing that makes sense."

"What the fuck!" said Betty. "Is that possible? What will that do to Richie?"

"If you asked me that two weeks ago, I would've said that's impossible, but now, I'm not so sure and I don't know what it means for Richie."

"Sandra, I've been talking to a reporter from the AP news, Hannah Darrow. She was one of the people who reported on Richie and how his class photoshopped him into their prom. She called Carol, asking for follow up, you know human interest shit. But given everything that's happened to Richie, I got in touch with her, and I've told her some of my thoughts and fears. I think we may need someone like her on our side if we have to fight a powerful pharmaceutical company. I described Richie's changes. I even sent her a picture of his backside. I suspect that she thinks I'm crazy, or just desperate because Richie's disappeared. Would you talk to her?"

Sandra thought about what it might look like in a news story for her to be quoted as saying there are whale and turtle genes in one of her patients, "I don't know, Betty."

"I believe that if Hannah thought this was real, she'd be able to convince her boss to let her investigate and maybe help figure this out. What if I told her that you would be willing to talk, you know, off the record, deep background sort of thing, without using your name? I think she might want to go over there, to the lab. She could poke around and hopefully find out stuff that could help Richie."

Sandra wanted to help Richie and expose whatever it was that was going on at PGL. After a few moments of thought she said, "OK, I'll talk to her, on the condition that I could remain anonymous. I'm not sure it would be good for my fellowship program if my involvement got out. I can see getting an unpleasant visit from the hospital lawyers."

"So, it's OK for me to call Hannah, let her know your conditions and give her your contact information?"

"Go ahead," said Sandra. "And please let me know when you hear from Richard again. He needs to be back in the hospital."

"Thanks," and Betty disconnected. She immediately called Hannah Darrow to tell her about Richie's doctor, and that his doctor could confirm what she had told her earlier. Betty gave Hannah all the contact information she needed and added that it would have to be confidential.

50.

It was late in the afternoon on the *Sea Hunt*, and they were busy hauling in and processing the day's catch. The seas began to turn choppy, white caps appeared on increasingly larger swells. A dark line in the sky appeared far out to the east. Captain Hansen didn't like the way the sky looked, and he went back to check his radar and the weather reports. The storm had grown in size, it was about 100 miles east of them, but it was no longer heading away, it was spinning in place. The captain left the cabin and told his crew what he knew. He asked them to try to pick up the pace. An hour went by, and the skies continued to grow darker. Richie could feel an easterly wind blow across his face. He knew there was trouble coming. He looked around the boat, which suddenly seemed too small and started to worry about how safe it would be in a storm. The boat began to rock. The captain came out again and now he told the crew that the storm had changed course and was coming around toward them, it looked like a big one. There was no time to haul in the longline, he ordered them to cut it and secure the deck as quickly as possible. He hoped to be ready to pull anchor and get underway in the next 15 minutes, putting as much distance as they could between the storm and them.

Richie followed the lead of Saul and Newt, securing what they could. The equipment was stowed. The hatches were battened down. What was left of the lines and gear was secured. The anchor came up and soon the boat was coming about turning away from the storm and gathering steam. The boat rose and fell as it cut across the menacing waves that were steadily increasing in strength. The gusting winds hammered them, forcing them to lean forward to make any headway. They used the boat lines, holding on for support as they tried to navigate across the increasingly slick deck. A few drops of rain soon became a torrential downpour, demonstrating the fury of mother nature and how rapidly she could turn threatening. The skies darkened ominously, and lightning cracked across the heavens. Richie and Saul had gotten their life jackets on and cinched the fastenings tightly and securely, but Newt was having trouble with his. He slipped on the deck, trying to grab onto anything he could to secure himself, but everything was wet, and as he tried to grasp the lines, his fingers lost their grip. He slammed against the forward mast, and became entangled in the boat rigging. He struggled to get free. But just as he seemed to have twisted away, another wave crashed over the sides and onto the deck. The boat listed violently, thousands of gallons of seawater picked Newt up and carried him uncontrolled across the deck. He hit his head on the portside gunwale and flipped head over heels disappearing over the side and into the churning sea. Richie and Saul rushed to the side. In the ever-deepening darkness, they could barely make out a waving arm. His hand appeared and disappeared as the waves rose and fell. Saul grabbed a life ring and threw it toward where he last saw Newt. He wasn't sure if it landed anywhere near him or if Newt might have been able to grab hold of it. Saul leaned against the gunwale, holding on, trying to scan the waters, hoping to spot Newt.

Richie ran to alert the captain who immediately spun the ship wheel, bringing the boat about, heading toward where Newt had last been seen. Captain Hansen switched on the ship's powerful searchlight, pivoted on a gimbal mount. He swept the beam across the water lighting the area that Saul pointed to.

While Saul and the captain were desperately trying to spot Newt, Richie stepped back, out of their line of sight. His new friend was in trouble, and somehow he knew he could help. It screamed at him. He quickly pulled off his life vest, his raingear, his socks and shoes, and then his pants. He started to remove his SPF shirt with the orca on the back but decided it would be better to leave it on. He was now only clad in his sun shirt and briefs. He took a few deep breaths and before either the captain or Saul could stop him, he leapt over the side into the dark seething waters below. Saul yelled but it was too late, Richie was already overboard and soon he too disappeared beneath the waves. The skipper and Saul watched, stunned. Now Richie was gone too.

"The fool!" said Captain Hansen.

Richie swam downward, below where he last saw Newt's waving arm. The water felt comfortable, and he could see clearly as plunged further below. He knew that he was swimming toward Newt, he could sense his movements below. But as he dove deeper, whatever it was that he was feeling, the thing that was guiding him abruptly ceased. That was not good, he knew that he didn't have much time to find Newt. He continued deeper, heading downward toward where he had last sensed him. A drive within him led him further into the depths. Then, just below, Richie noticed a string of rising bubbles, he followed those downward toward their source. He pulled with his arms, like a breaststroke underwater, and his legs pumped up and down together in a wave, a butterfly kick, a swimming technique, drawn from whale genetics. He continued deeper. The bubbles seemed more numerous as he descended. He was closer.

Richie felt completely at home in the dark icy waters. He willed his heart to beat slower, decreasing his oxygen demands. He had no idea how he was doing this. There was no urge to breathe. He had all the oxygen he needed. It had been nearly five minutes, searching, and then, just below, he saw an arm. It was not moving. It was raised toward him like a student trying to get his teacher's attention, attached to a body that continued its slow descent. Unseeing eyes looked up towards him, the hair on his head waved in the deep ocean currents. Richie redoubled his efforts, swimming toward the arm, quickly closing the distance. Finally, Richie was there. He grabbed Newt by his wrist. He first slowed his descent, and then turned upward toward the surface. He held Newt's wrist with his left hand and stroked the water with his right. He worked his legs, in a frog kick, to help bring him and Newt back toward the boat.

More than five minutes later, still comfortable under the waves, he was close to breaching the surface. As he looked up, he spotted the underside of the hull bobbing in the water above, and headed for it.

Captain Hansen and Saul had been searching the dark waters for any sign of life. They swept the powerful searchlight across the water. Seven minutes had passed since Richie had jumped into the water and they saw nothing but stormy seas. The captain had sent out a Mayday distress call, and his automatic emergency system kept repeating the call, along with their location coordinates. By now they only hoped that they might somehow at least be able to recover their bodies.

Ten minutes had passed, and Saul thought he heard something. He couldn't be sure. At first it was just a noise in the storm. Then, again, he heard it, more clearly. "Help," he heard. It had a gurgly quality, a voice and then water bubbling. He turned the light toward the source and saw someone in the water. Saul called to the captain, and he threw another life ring in the voice's direction. Saul saw someone fighting the currents, headed toward the boat. He dropped a rope ladder down the side of the boat to the water, and still wearing his life vest, he carefully climbed down the ladder to the water's edge. Saul clung to the ladder with one arm hooked around the vertical rope and his feet perched on the lowest rung. Waves were crashing over his body, the ladder swung out and back as the boat rocked in the storm. Saul desperately held onto the ladder as he reached out with his other arm. It was Richie paddling toward him, trying to grab hold. Saul could hardly believe that Richie was still alive, he was certainly happy about that, but his heart was also heavy with the loss of his friend, Newt.

Richie came closer and Saul was finally able to reach him with his outstretched arm. Saul was ready to pull him from the water. Suddenly, Saul, barely able to believe that Richie was still alive, saw that Richard held Newt with his other arm, still down beneath the waves. Incredible, his mind scrambled, he tried to process what he was seeing. But there was no time to figure out how any of this could be, there were now two souls to rescue. Saul, along with Richie tried to pull Newt from the water. Newt was cold and blue. He wasn't breathing and his body was limp. He looked like a dead man. And yet sailors knew that a cold lifeless body might look dead, but it might not be, he could still be saved. A brain could survive without oxygen, without a heartbeat even after many minutes in the extreme cold of the ocean, its metabolic needs reduced, it might still recover.

Saul was doing what he could, but it was clear that there was no way to bring Newt onboard without help. He yelled up to Captain Hensen to throw a line down. The captain quickly fashioned a bowline knot. The loop in the knot looked like a noose, but the captain fastened it so that it was large enough to hold a man around his chest. He threw the line over the side down toward Saul who still had one arm hooked through the ladder. As the boat rocked in the sea, Saul reached out, franticly trying to catch the tossed line.

Once Saul finally caught the line, he and Richie struggled to fasten the bowline securely around Newt's chest and under his arms. Saul then pulled the knot taut behind Newt's shoulders. With the line now tethered to a winch, they were able to raise Newt up and onto the deck. Saul then helped Richie climb the rope ladder, following him from below, supporting him, and ready to catch him if he slipped.

Once on board, they turned Newt to his side and worked to expel the water that filled his lungs. It seemed like gallons of water spilled from his mouth. When the gushing sea water finally ebbed, they turned him flat on his back, still cold, blue and lifeless. Saul and Captain Hensen quickly carried Newt inside the cabin, stripped off his clothes and dried him as best they could. They rubbed him vigorously using whatever towels they could find. He had no pulse, no breath. The captain gave two breaths and then began to perform chest compressions. Richie sat to the side, watching, still recovering from his underwater ordeal. Saul shouted above the shrieks of the storm for Richie to get the AED from the captain's wheelhouse. With Richie gone, Saul and Captain Hensen continued CPR, cycles of thirty compressions and two breaths. The men alternated, trying to preserve their strength and stay on Newt, all while the boat rocked violently in the storm. Richie was soon back with the AED, but the cabin was too wet to safely use the machine. CPR continued. They switched places, now Saul was pushing on Newt's chest, and the captain gave rescue breaths. Captain Hensen yelled for Richie to turn the heat up all the way. Newt had to be warmer, they couldn't hope to bring him back to life until his body temperature neared normal.

As they worked on Newt, the boat rocked in the storm. It was a herculean effort to keep from being tossed around the cabin. They had to brace themselves against whatever they could find and continue CPR if Newt were to have a chance. They were working on fumes, and they needed Richie's help.

Richie was still recouping from his dive, he had used all of his oxygen reserves, he was short of breath. But he knew what he had to do, he gathered his strength, and made his way down below deck to change into dry clothes and gather as many dry towels and blankets as he could. Within minutes, Richie was back in the cabin, with all the towels and blankets they needed. And now with dry clothes, he could safely help. He had a change for Saul too. They wiped the cabin and Newt as dry as possible while they continued their rescue efforts. Once it was dry enough, they could use the AED. Saul flipped the switch, and followed the AED's instructions telling him where to paste the pads on Newt's chest. Saul shouted over the thunderous storm for the captain to stop compressions and lean away. They watched the monitor as the AED analyzed Newt's heart looking for a shockable rhythm. It showed a flat line. No electrical activity. The AED could not help. Back to compressions and rescue breaths. Each chest compression squeezed Newt's heart and forced some blood to circulate. Their CPR was having an effect, Newt began to show a bit of color. It was better than nothing, but Newt needed a real heartbeat.

The rescue effort was exhausting, but they wouldn't give up. After several more cycles of compressions and breaths, they paused again, hoping for a change. They paused for a few seconds, allowing the AED to analyze. Finally, it detected a signal, the line on the monitor was squiggly now, its robotic voice, spoke, "V-fib, prepare to shock!" The machine was charged to deliver 200 joules of energy. Saul yelled "clear," everyone's hands raised up and away, and he triggered the shock. Newt's body jumped with the electric impulse. CPR began again. After two more cycles the compressions were paused again. They watched the screen. No change. Once more the machine detected V-fib, and robotically announced, "prepare to shock!" Richie shouted "clear," all hands lifted as they leaned back and away. Richie triggered the second shock. Newt's body again jumped as the electric charge passed through him. They waited, a second or two passed, but he was still in V-fib. There was no pulse. Back to compressions, pounding Newt's chest and filling his lungs with their breaths. Two more cycles of CPR finished now with Richie pushing, keeping the pace. The compressions were paused. Once again, the machine detected V-fib, and the robotic voice announced, "prepare to shock!" They needed more juice from the AED so they increased the energy level to 360 joules. Captain Hensen shouted, "clear," everyone sat up, they raised their hands off Newt as they leaned back and away. Captain Henson initiated the third shock. Newt's body seemed to jump even higher as the bigger surge of energy passed through him. A second or two passed, they waited, not daring to breathe, staring at the monitor. But this time, the AED sounded a ping. Eyes glued to the screen, watching the tracing, one normal wave, a short pause, then another, then a string of normal peaks and troughs. Newt had a normal rhythm!

Saul again laid his fingers on Newt's neck. The captain and Richie watched Saul, as he smiled and nodded, "he has a pulse." Newt started coughing just a bit at first, then harder, they turned him to his side as he continued to cough. More sea water poured from his mouth. After another minute or so, the coughing stopped, and Newt lay back. Saul gently coaxed him back to his side. Newt was breathing. His color pinked. Captain Hensen covered him in more blankets, keeping him warm and dry. Newt opened his eyes briefly, but they quickly closed again. He was asleep. His breathing seemed rough but steady. The boat had quieted. The brunt of the storm had passed. The captain, Saul and Richie just looked at each other, a quiet victory over death. They savored a moment together that not too long ago seemed impossible. Captain Hansen announced that they'd be returning home immediately. He raised the Coast Guard on the radio, reporting the emergency, a near drowning, and that he needed an ambulance standing by for one of the crew as soon as they docked in port. Captain Hansen turned the boat about and sped home.

After some time had passed, Richie heard the captain call them into the wheelhouse. "I don't fully understand what just happened," he said, looking squarely at Richie, "but this will forever be a terrifying memory with a good outcome. Not the nightmare ending that I had feared." He passed out three paper cups, and they each received a generous pour from the single malt, that he pulled from the cabinet. Captain Hensen toasted, "to life and its mysteries." The Scotch was strong, and Richie made a face as it went down. The captain was watching Richie and he seemed to want to hear something from him. He smiled broadly, "that'll put some hair on your chest." Captain Hansen laughed and downed the rest of the drink.

Richie felt the warm liquid flow down through his chest. It quickly went to his head. A little light headed, he looked around the wheelhouse and noticed Saul watching him. He wasn't sure why. His first thought was that Saul had noticed something different about him.

"I seem to want to ask you some stuff, Richie," Saul paused, looking directly at him, "but then, I don't know if I want to hear the answers."

"It's complicated," said Richie, not sure exactly what to say.

Richie was looking to change the subject when he suddenly thought of his mom and how worried she was. The Scotch was making it difficult to focus, but he turned to ask the captain, "is there a way for me to make a phone call?"

"Sure, I can do that for you son," said the captain. He handed him a notebook with a pen, "write the phone number down." Richie jotted the number down and handed the notebook back. The captain got the ship to shore, and soon Betty's phone was ringing. He handed the phone to Richie.

Betty had been frantic and ready to answer any phone call, any number could be Richie, or it could be from a hospital or a morgue, delivering bad news. Now in the middle of the night her phone rang, she didn't recognize the number, but when she answered, she immediately recognized the voice, "Oh my god Richie, are you OK? Where are you?"

"I'm OK, Mom, really. I've got quite a story to tell you, hold on a second." Richie asked Captain Hansen which port they would be coming in to and when they'd arrive. Then back to Betty, "Mom, can you meet me in three hours?" and he told her where he'd be. "I'll tell you, everything when I get there, OK."

"Sure Richie," she said, "I'm so happy you're OK, I've been worried sick about you."

"I'm sorry, Mom, but I had to leave. I'm sorry that I put you through that. Would you please let Nancy know that I'm OK, I had to borrow a phone, so you can't call me back on this number. But I'll see you in three hours. I love you, Mom, bye."

51.

Betty was able to hold it together during the call, but as soon as she disconnected the tears flowed. She'd been tense, on edge. Betty hadn't seen Richie since he left for that MRI so many days ago. And there'd been no contact at all for the last three days. Betty had imagined the worst. The relief of hearing his voice and knowing he was okay, was overwhelming. Those weren't the tears of sadness or the tears of joy, it was the release of emotions that had been churning inside her, threatening her sanity that caused the flow.

It was almost 4 in the morning. She wasn't going to call Nancy at that hour, but she texted her, letting her know that Richie was OK. Betty cleaned up a bit, washed her face, and quickly got ready to pick up her boy. She peeked in Richie's room. Betty had left it exactly as she found it, seemingly ages ago. Now, that she knew he was OK, she quickly made up his bed, fluffed up his pillows and picked up the laundry that had been scattered around the room. She opened his window to let some of the night air freshen his room. Betty turned his night light on, and walked out, with a smile. She carried his dirty clothes to the hamper and then went downstairs. Using Google maps, Betty found the port where Richie told her they'd be, it was 45 minutes away. Betty didn't expect much traffic at this hour. Meeting Richie at a port? She couldn't imagine what his story was going to be, nothing seemed to make sense, but he was alive. She picked up the cell phone that Richie left on the kitchen table, and out she went.

Betty arrived about 20 minutes before she expected Richie. She parked in an angled parking space, facing the harbor, where she'd be able to see any approaching boat. She waited anxiously in the car. Betty turned the rearview mirror, to see if she looked decent. While she sat, an ambulance pulled in, there was no siren, but the lights were flashing. It had Memorial Medical Center, arced across its side. The ambulance parked not far from where she sat. The lights were turned off, and the engine was cut. A moment later, two EMT's left the van, and walked over to sit on a nearby bench, facing the sea. They could be taking a break from a recent run, but Betty didn't think so. She had a feeling they were waiting for someone from that damn boat. Somebody needed an ambulance, a sinking feeling returned in the pit of her stomach. The minutes passed slowly, the analog clock on her old Subaru clicked, marking each second. She tapped her thumbs on the steering wheel, muttering to herself, come on Richie, where the fuck are you? Are these guys waiting for you?

Frustrated and anxious, but feeling a little safer with the EMT's nearby, she got out of the car. She paced back and forth, passing by the small shops in the little mall by the harbor, all tightly closed at this hour. After a little while, she saw the EMT's stand up and walk back to the ambulance. The engine started and the flashing lights turned on again. They sat there waiting. Betty once again looked out over the harbor and this time she saw lights. As it neared, the boat slowed, the bow fell, and the bow wave softened. It made its way slowly toward the slips. Betty could see two men on the deck scurrying about, preparing to dock. She could see through the windows of the wheelhouse, a man, who she presumed was the captain, guiding the boat into its slip. One man jumped off and onto the dock. Another hand, still on board, tossed a line to him. The engines were cut, and the harbor was suddenly quiet. The flashing lights of the ambulance played eerily on the men producing a stroboscopic effect as they worked to secure the boat. Betty heard the shouted commands as the man on the dock, tugged and pulled, finally cinching the line to a cleat.

The EMTs came out of the still running vehicle, walked to the back and pulled out a gurney. They guided it to the boat, locking the wheels when they were close. The captain and another man on board, carried a third person, someone who lay still in their arms. The EMTs and the man on the dock, helped take him, as he was lowered down. The limp body was carefully laid onto the gurney, one EMT applied an oxygen mask to his face and the other, wrapped him in blankets. The head of the gurney was raised, the sides were brought up, the wheels were unlocked, and they pushed the gurney across the lot to the back of the ambulance and then guided it inside and locked it in place. Both EMTs hopped in and began working on the patient.

Betty walked apprehensively closer, trying to see if it was Richie. After a few minutes, one EMT jumped out of the back. Betty got a glimpse inside as the doors closed. The driver ran around to the front and hopped into the cab of the ambulance. He shifted into gear, the vehicle backed away, then turned, the gears shifted again, and the ambulance sped off. She hadn't been able to see very much inside the ambulance, but it did seem that the EMT who stayed there was tending to someone who was alive.

As she watched the ambulance leave, she noticed three men from the boat walking toward her. The one with the backpack suddenly broke away from the others and ran directly toward her. As he passed under the harbor lights, she saw his hoodie and then his face, it was Richie. "Oh," she yelled, not so many words, but laden with emotion. She ran toward him, and they embraced, rocking together, she held him tightly, and then, she leaned back a bit, holding his face between her hands, inspecting him, examining him for damage, and then kissed both his cheeks and hugged him again, tears streaming down her face.

"Oh, my God, Richie are you really OK? I sat here for a while and watched the ambulance waiting for somebody. I was so frightened."

One of the other two men, approached Betty, he was the one she saw through the wheelhouse window. He struck out his hand, offering to shake hers. "Hello, ma'am, I'm Captain Hansen, it's my pleasure to meet you."

Betty took his offered hand, and they shook. Betty held her son, one arm draped around his shoulders.

"That man, that you saw being taken away in the ambulance," the captain said, "he goes by Newt, his real name is Graham, and he's alive only because of what your son did. Richie is a true hero. And I don't use that word lightly."

Betty looked from the captain to her son, not sure what was going on.

"Richie will tell you the story, he may be a bit modest in its telling, but that would be inaccurate. What happened this morning at sea will be reported and there will be a full accounting made to the Coast Guard. You might look for it in the papers. I can tell you, ma'am, that my memory of this day, something I will carry with me for the rest of my life, is dramatically better than I feared it might have been, because of your son."

Captain Hansen turned to Richie, "I hope that everything goes well with you, and please, if there is anything I can do for you, call me. I mean that, anything." The captain handed him his business card and an envelope. "The money is your share of the catch. We had a pretty good haul for the few days we were out at sea. There may be more when I know the final sales figure."

Saul came over to Richie and embraced him too. "Thank you, Richie," was all he said, a single tear fell down his cheek.

They turned to walk away. “Captain,” Richie called out, and they stopped, looking back, “I’ll text you my number, please let me know how Newt is.” The captain nodded and they continued on their way.

Betty and Richie got into the car and sat side by side for a while. Betty turned to him several times, looking at her son carefully, she saw someone different. He had changed since the last time they were together. His eyes were even lighter, almost devoid of color, he seemed bigger, stronger, whatever was happening from the transplant, but there was more, something in his demeanor, the way he held himself, a new maturity that he seemed to carry.

“What was that all about?” Betty asked.

“Mom, while we were out there, there was a storm, and Newt fell into the water, and I helped get him back on board.”

“I see,” said Betty, “that sounds like it could have been dangerous.” Somehow, she didn’t think that she was getting the whole story. She felt like yelling at him. She was angry that he put her through such horror. But she was mostly happy that he was alive and here with her. And something still could happen to her son. She never wanted their last words to be those of anger.

“Well, that’s what you have to do, you know at sea,” he said, “we have to help each other. They would have done it for me.”

Betty started the car, “are you hungry? We could go to one of the all-night diners.”

Richie’s eyes lit up, that was the old Richie, “sure Mom, I could eat a horse.”

They pulled into the diner parking lot. Once inside, they were directed to sit anywhere. The diner was starting to fill, it was still dark outside, though the first light of dawn was beginning to show. They found a booth and sat down. The waitress came over, and Betty asked for a coffee, with milk. Richie asked for a hot chocolate, with whipped cream and lots of water.

They opened the menu, but Richie knew he wanted a big fat juicy, rare cheeseburger with fries. Betty was a bit less ambitious at this hour. When the waitress came back with their beverages, Richie was ready with his order. Betty only asked for a couple of slices of whole wheat toast with orange marmalade. The waitress left to put in the orders, and Betty sipped her coffee as she watched Richie. The physical changes from his transplant were continuing and she was scared. And still nobody knew what was wrong.

"Richie, what happened that made you leave the hospital?"

Richie sat unanswering for a few moments. He seemed to be organizing his thoughts. "It's hard to put into words, Mom. I was feeling anxious and boxed in. I couldn't sit still. I had an urge to be moving. There was, what do they call it, a wanderlust in me. And I felt stronger, I was pretty sure that I didn't need to be there anymore. I wasn't worried about my leukemia, I was pretty sure it was gone, but I did worry about the changes happening to my body, and it didn't seem like the doctors were. I guess I was in search of answers. It was weird, like I was sharing my body with something."

"What does that mean Richie?"

"It's like there's someone else inside me, kind of like Richie, but not me."

"Richie, do you know what you did the night that you left the hospital?"

"It's kind of a fog, I can sort of remember walking around and then I was in the lobby, and I walked out."

"You know that you broke into the outpatient pharmacy, and you took some medicines."

"I kind of remember."

"The pharmacy has a gate with a padlock and somehow you broke the lock, no one can figure out how you did that. The only items that appeared to be taken were the medicines you needed for your post-transplant care. The hospital is pretty sure that you did it, though I don't think that they can prove it. There's no clear image of you in their video. But other than destroying the padlock, you didn't cause any damage and you didn't take any controlled substances. Of course, they could also be worried about what their liability might be for the strange effects you're having from the transplant. Better not have an angry family. Anyway, given all of that, the hospital doesn't seem interested in pressing charges against you. Do you remember any of that?"

"Not really, I have a memory of being on a mission. I had orders to follow, but it's fuzzy."

"Richie, you probably need to go back to the hospital, there are things happening to you, changes and you just had a bone marrow transplant, you can't just walk away. There's still lots that can go wrong."

"I really don't think I need to be in the hospital, Mom."

"Dr. Gardner has been trying to figure out what's wrong, she has some ideas, and she's worried about you, too. She also thinks you need to be back there." Betty understood that it was important to get Richie back in the hospital. But she had to be careful not to push too hard. And she wasn't sure how to navigate the tricky balance of concern and understanding.

"Really, gee Mom. I can't go back there now. Wait, doesn't she have a clinic? I would go to her clinic. I just can't be caged up again."

Betty looked at him, "okay, Richie, I'll talk to her in a few hours during the day. Maybe we can work something out."

The waitress came over with Betty's toast and Richie's meal. Richie attacked the hamburger with all the fixings and his hot chocolate with whipped cream. Betty was more demure, she spread the marmalade on the toast and took a few bites. She wasn't really interested in food.

"Richie, can I see the business card the captain gave you?" Richie was busy devouring the meal, but he reached into his pocket and handed the card over.

"I'd like to talk more to Captain Hansen, is it OK with you if I call him?"

"Sure Mom, that's fine. You know I'm feeling tired, it wasn't easy to sleep on the boat, and I worked really hard. I hope we can go home soon."

"Yes, honey, I'll get the check and we can leave."

Richard seemed very tired on the way home. He didn't say anything during the ride. But Betty's head was busy, she reviewed everything she learned in the last few days. First off, Sandra suspected that somehow Richie's stem cells became contaminated while they were being processed at PGL, the same company where two scientists are leading experiments in their lab involving genes from different animals, including whales and tortoises. And Richie now has physical manifestations of those animals, and somehow, he wound up at sea, and Richie did something that made an impression on a veteran captain and a crewman. How could all those things be connected? Or were they somehow just weird coincidences? What were the odds of that?

She needed someone to poke around inside PGL and find out what the fuck happened there. She hoped that Hannah would be the one to do that. Betty needed to make sure that Hannah had enough information to convince her boss that there was a real story. Well, Richie was back now, and Hannah would be able to see the changes for herself. She also remembered that Richie had blood samples taken on the morning he left the hospital. She needed to find those results. Somehow, she thought the captain might be helpful, she wasn't sure how. She needed to talk to him again.

52.

As soon as they arrived home, Richie announced that he could barely stay awake, his body was drained from the fishing and from whatever happened just a few hours ago in the storm. He was ready to go up to his room and get some much needed sleep.

Before heading upstairs, he rummaged through his backpack. He found his morning transplant pills and took those, as he had done diligently every day since being on his own. He had some laundry tucked away in there too, he handed those over to his mom. He dug out the turkey and cheese, which needed to be tossed. He came across the envelope the captain gave him and opened it. Inside were five crisp one hundred dollar bills. That was more than he was expecting. Richard remembered that he'd taken a hundred dollars from Mom's emergency stash. He handed Betty the envelope, "one of these is yours. I borrowed some money from you."

Betty looked curiously at the bills. It brought images of Richie working on a fishing trawler far out in the ocean, of a storm plummeting the boat, of her son in danger as he helped save Newt. What was going on inside his head that pushed him out of the hospital and made him step on board a boat leaving the harbor? It was all too much for her to wrap her head around. She took the money and put it in the cookie jar to restore the missing dollars in emergency stash.

Before Richie went upstairs, he asked to get his phone back, he kissed his mom and climbed the stairs, closed the door to his room. He was quickly asleep.

While Richie slept, Hannah called. They talked for a while. Hannah said that she spoke with Dr. Gardner who confirmed everything that Betty had told her. Hannah had shown the picture to her boss, and also to several colleagues, including some of their science and health reporters who had been helpful in the past. No one could make much of the fuzzy, grainy image, and there were some doubts about its authenticity and what they were supposed to be seeing. Nevertheless, there was some intrigue and Hannah's boss said that he would consider sending her to PGL, to investigate further, but only if she was able to see Richie herself and verify what they might be seeing in the picture. Images could be created by AI, and he wasn't about to waste money on some wild scam.

Betty told Hannah that she would figure out a way for her to see Richie.

Betty next called Nancy. "Richie's home now."

"Oh my God, is OK? Where's he been, I wanna talk to him."

"Nancy, he's fine. But he's asleep right now. I'm sure he'll want to talk to you and tell you everything. I just wanted you to know he's OK."

"Richie's really OK? Why didn't he call me? I've been terrified for the last few days. If he's really OK, I'm going to kill him."

"Tell you the truth Nancy, I wanted to kill him too. I didn't hear from him either, until just a little while ago. Listen he couldn't call anyone from where he was and I know he wants to tell you everything. I promise to get him to call you as soon as he wakes up."

Nancy was quiet for a few moments. Betty heard her heavy breathing on the phone. "I don't understand, Betty." She paused again. "I'm just so glad he's alive. Betty, please tell Richie that I won't kill him if he calls as soon as he's awake. I'll be waiting. Bye."

Betty knew that she had to call his doctor, and she was on her speed-dial too. "Sandra, Richie is home, it's hard to believe, but somehow, he wound up on a fishing boat, he was part of a crew, and they were out at sea for three days. He came back today. I met him at the harbor early this morning. He seems OK, but he's exhausted and right now he's upstairs sleeping."

"Have you noticed any more changes?" asked Sandra.

"The only thing I could see were his eyes and the color seems even more washed out. Something strange happened on the boat, Sandra, but I haven't been able to learn any of the details. The captain came over to me and said that Richie was a hero. But later when I asked Richie what he was talking about, he basically said it wasn't anything."

"I'm not sure how that's related," said Sandra, "but strange things have happened to Richie. Betty, he needs to come back to the hospital. He can't be just wandering around like this so soon after a bone marrow transplant."

"I know, but I don't know if I can get him to do that. But he said he would come to your clinic, he trusts you."

"Listen, I'm not scheduled to see patients today, but I can let the outpatient clinic manager know that Richie's coming and that I'll see him. Betty. I need to convince him to let us admit him to the unit."

"I'll talk to him when he wakes up, and I'll bring him in to the clinic," said Betty, "where is it, and what time should I be there?"

Sandra gave Betty all the information she needed, and then she rang off.

Betty still needed to give Hannah enough ammunition to convince her boss to send her to PGL. She kept thinking about what the captain said. '*He's a true hero.*' Something happened out there on the seas. She didn't know how, but maybe the captain had something to say that would help. She had his business card on the kitchen table, and she dialed the number. It rang for a while and then went to voicemail. Betty left a message after the tone, saying it was Richie's mother and she was sorry to bother him, if he could spare a few moments to talk to her. She thanked him for taking care of Richie, and then disconnected.

Betty was exhausted and wasn't sure what to do next. Then her phone rang, she saw it was the same number that she had just called, and she answered.

"Hello, Betty, I'm sorry I didn't answer, I get so many calls, I have to let most of them go. But your name will show up now and I will always answer. How is Richie?"

"He seems alright, he was pretty tired. He's sleeping now."

"That's good, I'm sure he needs it after all he's been through. He's a really good kid. How can I help you?"

"Well, I was just trying to wrap my head around the things you said about Richie back at the port. You called him a hero. He's my Richie and of course he's my hero, but, that description from someone outside is unexpected. When I asked Richie about it, he said that Newt fell in the sea, and he helped get him back on board. He didn't make much of it."

"Well, ma'am, he is a hero, and that narrative is accurate but hardly descriptive of what happened. And if you didn't have him right there at home safe in bed, I would be a bit reluctant to tell you the details, but I reckon that you should know what your son did, and it was remarkable. You might want to be sitting down, perhaps with a drink in hand."

Betty was bewildered, she could not imagine what the captain was going to say, but she could probably use a drink now anyway, even this early in the morning. "Hold on a minute," she said and walked over to the cabinet and got the bottle of bourbon and one of her juice glasses. She poured herself two fingers worth and sat down on her couch. "I'm ready," she said and swallowed her first sip.

Betty listened as the captain told a truly unbelievable story about how her son dove into a raging ocean, stayed underwater for more than 10 minutes, found that man in the pitch black water and saved his life. It was a completely unbelievable story, except the captain swore by it, and it was her Richie, part whale, part tortoise. What the fuck was going on inside her son?

Betty had finished two glasses of bourbon listening to the story. "I don't know what to say, Captain, and I don't know if I should go upstairs right now and knock the living shit out of him or pin a medal on his chest."

"Well, I think I know what you mean Betty. I tell you that I got home, and I hugged my two children and my wife, and they all thought I'd lost my mind."

"I have a favor to ask you Captain."

"Sure Betty, whatever I can do, just name it."

"Well, Richie had been in the hospital for a while, I won't trouble you with the whole story, he seems to be better now, but some things happened while he was there. Anyway, there's a reporter that's been interested in his story, trying to figure out what happened and she's trying to help us, her name is Hannah Darrow. If it's OK with you, I would like to give her your name. I'm asking if you would please talk to her when she calls, and it would help if you could tell her that story. If you want, you could ask her not to use your name. Would that be OK?"

"I hope Richie is better, I hadn't known he was in the hospital, I guess... well I didn't know. But if you think it will help Richie, I'll be happy to talk to her and tell the story."

"Thank you very much Captain, and thanks for suggesting the bourbon, it was quite a story and the drink definitely helped."

"Take care Betty, and I hope to hear from you and Richie again. Bye now." The captain disconnected.

Betty put the phone down and took another swallow of the bourbon. That was a fucking crazy story. Somehow, this was all linked, it had to be.

Betty's head was spinning from everything that had happened. At least Richie was home and safe, for now. She refused to think about how much danger he'd been in when he jumped into the water. God, fucking teenage boys! Betty decided she needed a power nap. The bourbon was having an effect. Two hours would help enormously. She set the alarm on her phone and went upstairs to catch a few z's. Her head barely had time to hit the pillow before she was deeply asleep.

Betty woke up about five minutes before the time she'd set. She blinked her eyes a few times and stretched. She reached over, turned the alarm off and got up and went to the bathroom. The power nap worked, she felt refreshed and ready to go. Betty walked across the hall to check on Richard, she knocked on his door, once and then louder, with no response she cautiously opened his door. Richie was wrapped in his bedsheets like a caterpillar in a cocoon, dead to the world. She walked in, trying to make noise, to no avail. She had to lean over, reach out and shake him by the shoulder and call out his name before she got any response. Finally, he moaned and groaned and his eyes began to blink. "Oh, what time is it?" He tried to turn over again, but Betty wouldn't let him.

"You have to get up Richie, we have an appointment. I've talked to Dr. Gardner, and she will see you in her clinic, we'll need to leave soon. I know that you want to see Nancy. Maybe you can call her and we can all go out there together."

Finally, Richie reluctantly sat up. "What?" He rubbed his eyes, trying to shake off the sleep and looked up at his mom. "OK, OK. Give me a few minutes, I'll call Nancy."

Nancy, Betty and Richard pulled into the parking lot of the Memorial Medical Center. It took about an hour with a bit more traffic this time of day. They headed up to the pediatric hematology/oncology clinic on the fifth floor.

53.

Richie was now wearing sunglasses all the time, even inside the building, to protect his ever more sensitive eyes. They were waiting for only a few minutes in the exam room when there was a knock on the door and Sandra came in. "Well, I see that there's a bit of a crowd here," as she looked around.

Sandra was looking at Richie. "You look remarkably well, Richie, I was afraid of what I might see. I'd like to hear more about your last three days, but I want to examine you first. Can you please take off your sunglasses?"

Sandra came over, and looked closely at his eyes, they were almost pink. Nearly all the pigment was gone. It recalled her medical school clinics caring for people with albinism. His pupils were pinpoints. "Does the light bother you?"

"Yes," he said, "it's much better with the shades. Otherwise I feel great."

"What happened Richie? You just took off, only a few days after the infusion, that wasn't good. I've been very worried."

"I'm sorry, Dr. Gardner, but I just couldn't stay anymore. It was almost like it wanted me to hide."

Sandra was curious about how he phrased that, "what do you mean *it* wanted you to hide?"

"I don't know really," said Richie, "like I said, I've been feeling like I'm sharing my body with something, and *it* wants things."

"I see," said Sandra, though she really didn't. "I'd like to continue the exam with everyone outside, and then I'll go over the lab reports we have from the day you left. I've ordered some new testing for today. I understand that you've been taking the tacrolimus, Cellcept, and Bactrim, is that true?"

"Yes, I've been pretty good about that."

"That's good, considering the effort you made to get them. You pretty much destroyed the padlock on the pharmacy gate. What did you use on it?"

"Nothing, I just tugged on it a bit, and it opened. It must not have been really locked properly. I don't remember much about that."

Sandra looked at him, she had seen the damage to the lock, it had been ripped open. "You're telling me, that you didn't use any tools, you just tugged on it?"

"That's all."

Sandra didn't say anything, she remembered how much trouble Paul had trying to straighten Richard's arm when he resisted. She added it to her list of his changes. "OK, I'd like everyone to step out, and I will too. There's a gown under the exam table, please take everything off and I'll be back in a minute."

They all stepped out, giving Richie a chance to change. Betty briefly relayed the story she heard from the captain about what Richie had done. Dr. Gardner listened, it didn't seem possible, but she began to wonder, what's possible for this boy? The whole story was crazy. And what did happen in the lab at PGL? Thoughts went through her head, but first she had to help Richie. She went back in to examine him.

"Richie, this is going to be a complete exam, head to toe. I would like you to take your sunglasses off again, for a few minutes, while I use the ophthalmoscope, then you can put them back on." Sandra tried to check his pupillary response, but they started out so small that it was hard to discern any changes.

She watched him track her finger across his field of vision. She then came in close with the ophthalmoscope to examine the back of his eyes. The light was very bright, his pupils were very small and it was hard for Richie to keep from looking away, but he did his best. When she was finished, he put the sunglasses back on. Sandra searched for any enlarged lymph nodes, she listened to his heart and lungs and pushed on his abdomen. She ran her hands over his chest and arms, feeling his skin. There was clear progression of the changes. His skin was completely smooth, not a hair or pore to be found. While she did that, Richie offered that when he ran, or worked hard, he sweated from his head and legs, but his chest and arms were dry. Sandra nodded, acknowledging his comment. She examined the rest of the body, leaving the growth at the base of his spine for last. Finally, examining the tail, it was bigger than before, and was clearly reptilian in appearance.

"I'm told that you can move it, Richie, will you show me?"

And he did, he had become fairly adept at it. He wagged it right and left.

"Can you move it up and down?" she asked, still processing what it meant that he had a reptilian tail at all. It still made no sense.

"No, just sideways."

"I see," said Sandra, "you know the drill, is there anything else you want to tell me while we're alone?"

"I'm worried about the changes. It feels like there's something else in me that has a will of its own. And it's getting stronger, louder. I guess that sounds kind of crazy. I had an urge, that I followed, that brought me to the harbor, I hadn't known I was headed there until I was close enough to smell the sea. And when I jumped off the ship, I knew I'd be fine. I could see perfectly underwater, like I was wearing goggles, but I wasn't. I guess that I was underwater a long time, but I never felt that I needed to take a breath. And the man that fell over,

Newt, I knew exactly where to find him in the ocean. I know it all sounds very strange."

Sandra was listening, and she thought it was crazy too, but she didn't think it wasn't real. "I'm going to leave for a minute while you get dressed, then we'll all come back in."

While Richie dressed, as arranged in Betty's phone call, Hannah arrived at the clinic. She was hoping to gain more information that she could use to help convince her boss that there was a story. Hannah knew there was, she could smell it.

They were all gathered around, and Sandra made sure that it was OK with Richie and Betty that she could talk in front of Nancy and Hannah. They nodded.

"First off, from his exam, mostly it's good, but there is progression of the unusual findings we saw before. His eyes have lost more pigment. His skin is continuing to change, it feels even more like a marine mammal than before. You may know that whales and dolphins do not have skin pores and they don't sweat, just like Richie. His tail is bigger and longer. Richard's metamorphosis is accelerating."

"Metamorphosis, that sounds like he's a tadpole or a caterpillar," said Nancy.

"Well, maybe it does sound like that, changes directed by gene programming," said Sandra. "We need to understand why they're happening, and I don't think we have much time.

One of the tests we ran from Richie's last day here is something called a protein electrophoresis profile, it measures the different proteins circulating in the blood, and of course, there are many. The results are presented as a graph, with peaks or spikes along its horizontal axis. Each spike represents a different protein in his blood, and its position along the X axis identifies it." She pulled up the study on the C.O.W. and showed them. She pointed to two of the larger spikes, explaining that one represented albumin and the other showed the globulins, two normal human blood protein groups. "There are no spikes consistent with known pathology, like we might see in some cancers. But there are a few other interesting peaks along the graph," she indicated with her finger, "and based upon their positions along the graph, these are proteins that we don't normally see, at least not in humans. We also have a preliminary result from the genetic microarray test, and it identifies several genes that are *not* part of the human genome. We will eventually know which genes they are, but for now we just know that they shouldn't be there. It seems evident that Richard's stem cell product was contaminated. We see the signatures of animal genes inside his cells. Those genes are directing the production of unique proteins. It's likely that those novel proteins are responsible for the changes we see around his body. As far as I or anyone else we've been able to talk to knows, this has never happened before."

Betty had steeled herself for some news like this. Sandra watched her carefully trying to gauge her reaction. Betty wasn't falling apart. In fact, she appeared to harden and pretty soon it was clear that she was angry. "It's that fucking lab. What can we do?" asked Betty.

"We don't really know yet. One option we're considering is that Richie may need to undergo a second bone marrow transplant."

"Oh, no," said Richie, "I can't do that again, we need to find another option."

Betty looked at Richie, she wasn't sure that she could sit by watching him go through another transplant.

"It seems to me that someone needs to go to PGL," said Betty. "Hannah needs more evidence to convince her boss that there's a story here. That seems to be where the money is, as Willy Sutton is believed to have said. So," Betty looked toward Richie, "I hope that Richie will let her take some pictures, including his tail. Hannah will need copies of the lab reports and testimony from you, Sandra, as well as from the captain to convince her boss. Sandra, I'm hoping that you will consider going with Hannah to help with her investigation. Only you have the medical expertise to walk through a lab and see what shouldn't be there. This won't work without you."

"Betty," said Sandra, "you may be right and it's something I've considered." Sandra seemed to be thinking for a few moments. "I do want to go. I want to see Richie get better. I need to see where the stem cells were processed and how this could've happened.

I'm still getting oriented in my lab, and I haven't started any bench work yet, so it shouldn't be too hard to get a couple of days off, to do some important clinical work."

"Thank you, Sandra," said Betty, "I hoped that you'd agree."

"I want to go too," said Nancy, "I want to see the place that fucked up Richie's transplant. I'll get Dad to pay for my ticket."

"Well, first we have to get Hannah's boss to agree," said Betty. "Richie, will you let Hannah take some pictures?"

"Sure, maybe Nancy can help," said Richie. Betty and Sandra stepped out and left them to get the photos Hannah needed. Sandra went over to the workstation to order the labs she wanted, including a CBC with differential and another chimerism study. Normally, a decreasing chimerism result would imply that the patient's leukemia was returning, but for Richie, in this strange circumstance, it could mean that it was detecting more foreign DNA and not the return of his cancer. None of this made much sense, but Sandra was determined to get to the bottom of it.

Richie's exam room door opened, and they came out. "I've got some really good pics," said Hannah. "Nancy helped so I have a size reference for his tail. I've also got nice shots of his chest and those eyes. Once I'm finished talking to the captain, I should be set to present this all to the old man. It'll be an opportunity he can't refuse."

Betty gave Hannah the contact information she needed, and Hannah stepped aside to make the call.

"Richie," said Sandra, "we'll figure this out, I promise. The assistant is printing the labels now and she'll be right over to get the blood samples I ordered. She can do a peripheral stick, so we won't need to access your central line, will that be OK with you?"

Richie agreed.

As she finished, the assistant came over with her tray. She had the tubes, labels, tourniquet and needle to get the samples. She went into the room with Richie and closed the door.

Hannah was still on the phone with the captain. Nancy, Sandra and Betty were busy chatting. Ten minutes later the MA came out and said she couldn't get the samples Sandra had ordered.

"It's hard to find a vein in his arm, and the three times I tried, from his antecube, the needles bent, they wouldn't puncture his skin."

That was weird. Sandra went over to try. She tightened the tourniquet, asked Richie to make a fist and pump it, flicking the site in the crook of his arm a few times, hoping to encourage a vein to show itself, but she saw nothing. Richie's skin was smooth, thick and leathery. There was nothing to access. Finally, Sandra turned his hand over. The skin changes stopped at his wrist, and the back of his hand looked like a place she might be able to draw blood from. Sandra tightened the tourniquet low on his forearm and some beautiful veins popped up. Soon all the samples were collected.

Hannah was back, after speaking with the captain. "He tells quite a story, sprinkled with some very salty language. Listen guys this started out as just a follow up human interest story, but it's turning out to be much more than that, literally! My visit to PGL will happen, I guarantee it. And this will be a big story, I can smell it!

I'm going to powwow with my boss. I'll text him the pictures and lab reports. I've no doubt that he'll be interested. I want to leave tomorrow, fly into SAN, the San Diego International Airport, rent a car and drive out to PGL. I'll text everyone my itinerary, and we'll smoke out those bastards! By the time I'm done, there will be tons of personal injury lawyers salivating." Hannah took off, she had to talk to her boss and get ready for the trip out west.

"I'm not going to try to talk you into coming into the hospital right now, but please stay, at least until the CBC's back," asked Sandra, "I sent it stat. I've also got to talk to my lab director to let her know I need a couple of days off."

Nancy walked off into a corner to call her dad. Betty could hear one side of the conversation, and it sounded like some serious negotiating going on. Betty was betting on Nancy.

Richie and Betty went to the hospital cafeteria to get something to eat while they waited for the test results. Betty wasn't very hungry, but she ordered coffee and a blueberry scone. Richard, on the other hand, always seemed to be famished. He wanted red meat and found what he was looking for. They sat down at one of the open tables, by the window. Betty nursed her coffee while Richie's meal was disappearing. They sat and talked. They hadn't done too much of that since the transplant started. He sat with his back to the window, facing away from the sunlight. The hood of his sweatshirt was pulled up and he wore his wraparound sunglasses to protect his sensitive eyes. People seated in the cafeteria peeked at him nervously. His appearance was apparently intimidating.

"Richie, when you first said that you felt that you were sharing your body with something else, it didn't make much sense to me. I thought it was some sort of trick your mind was playing on you, maybe all those cancer drugs, you know, chemo brain. But I think maybe I get it now. I feel bad that I dismissed what you said, Richie. I should've paid more attention."

"Gee, Mom, it's OK, I hardly believed what I was saying. Who would've thought that something like that could happen."

"I know, it's incredible," said Betty, "but still, I should have listened to you and realized there was something wrong."

Both Richie and Betty looked down when they heard pings on their phones. They saw a text from Hannah. She'd convinced her boss that there was a story, and he agreed to send her to investigate. In the text, Hannah gave all the details for tomorrow's flight to SAN.

Soon after, they received a text from Nancy, who also copied Sandra and Hannah, "I'm going. I have my dad's permission and he'll pay for the ticket. I can meet you all at the hospital or wherever in the morning."

"I certainly hope that there won't be any trouble for them at PGL," said Betty. "We should get back to the clinic, hopefully your results are back. We'll talk to Sandra and find out what she's planning."

"The results are remarkably good, his white blood cell count of 7.1 and his platelet count of 175,000 are unbelievable and completely normal, but the hematocrit is 65%, it should only be about 35 to 40%. It appears that all the blood lines have recovered, in fact his red blood cell count is *higher* than normal." She said that could happen if Richie wasn't drinking enough and his blood was concentrated, or if his oxygen was low or he had been exposed to carbon monoxide on the boat.

Betty, thinking outside the box, quickly Googled hemoglobin results for whales, and sure enough, they had hematocrits normally in the mid to high 60 per cent range. They could stay submerged longer, not because their lungs were bigger or they could hold their breath longer, but because their entire body was an oxygen storage vessel. Using their incredible supply of hemoglobin and myoglobin they could store enough oxygen in their body to remain underwater for as long as two hours.

Betty also learned from Google that some marine mammals had vibrissal crypts scattered throughout their skin. The crypts functioned as electroreceptors. They could detect weak bioelectric fields, like those generated by the muscle activity of their prey. That helped them track their food, even in the inky black seas.

Sandra was beginning to get how much Richie's genome had been manipulated. It made the story of his dramatic sea rescue not so far-fetched.

"That's remarkable," said Sandra. "So, Richie has the skin and hemoglobin of a whale, along with the tale of a tortoise. He's definitely a chimera."

Sandra used Hannah's information to book her flight to San Diego. They'd meet in the hospital lobby very early tomorrow morning and then head out to the airport.

Hannah had contacted PGL and spoke to a woman from public relations to explain that she was a reporter for AP News and would be out there looking for information as part of a follow-up piece on one of the transplant recipients whose cells were processed there. The lady at PGL was very cordial and said she looked forward to meeting the group in the morning. She would send detailed directions from the airport and arrange a personalized tour of the facility.

Richie was finishing in the clinic, his catheter was flushed and capped off to keep it patent. He had his transplant medications refilled and they headed back home. Betty and Richie chatted in the car, buoyed by a sense of hope that finally, they might be able to explain this crazy shit.

But as they arrived back home and pulled into their driveway, Richie began to complain about a tightness in his chest. It felt harder to take a breath. He got out of the car and walked around a bit. Standing up and moving around seemed to help.

"Maybe I should call Sandra," said Betty.

Richie took a few deep breaths, he shook his mom off. "I feel better now, walking around. It's OK."

Richie was glad to be back home. He grabbed the newel post and climbed the stairs, headed to his room. That was his sanctuary, his little world. He was prince of the 12 by 14 foot room he called his palace. Richie sat in his comfy rocker chair, his legs propped up on the desk, he put on his headphones and enjoyed the latest pop and hip-hop music. Soon he was lost in the music. He didn't have to think about anything else when he was transported to that world. Of course, his headphones were linked to his cell, and he heard it ring with Nancy's tone. He answered it by tapping the earpiece, "Hi, Nancy."

"Hey, Richie," said Nancy.

"So you're going to PGL tomorrow."

"Yeah, I want to see those fuckers that did this to you, they need their asses handed to them. And I can do it, believe me."

"That's my girl," said Richie, "you don't ever want to get on your bad side."

"You got that right. They'll rue the day that they messed with my guy!"

Richie giggled. He could imagine the trouble Nancy could dish out. "I wish you could be wearing a videocam so I could watch you kicking butt."

"I do plan to have my phone and record what I can."

"Nancy, I was kidding about the videocam. Please don't get into trouble."

"It'll be fine. Don't worry, no one will know."

"OK, just be very careful. I miss being with you, Nancy. I can't wait until we can be together, alone, again. That night was amazing. I think about it all the time. I can reimagine everything, it's like you're right here, I can feel you next to me."

"I think about it too. Being with you, like that, it was perfect. Tomorrow night I'll leave the night light on and keep my window open."

"I can hardly wait, Nancy. I love you..."

"Me, too," said Nancy, she kissed the phone and disconnected.

Richie was all hot and bothered just talking with her. That night in her bedroom played over and over in his head. He needed a shower. It might help until he could be with her tomorrow. A few minutes later, he was standing in the hot shower, soaping up and letting the steamy water splash all over. But soon the usual hot water began to feel uncomfortable, and he turned the shower knob toward colder. Cooler was good, but it felt even better as he continued moving the handle further toward cold. And then it was all the way, as cold as it could get. The shower washed over his chest and arms, the water bounced off, ricocheting from his body. It felt natural, he recalled the feeling he had, far from land, diving to find Newt. He hadn't said it before, but it'd been exciting. He felt at home in the icy waters of the Atlantic. He stood in the shower for as long as he could, until he heard knocking on the bathroom door. He couldn't tell what his mom was saying, but he expected that they weren't endearments. He turned the water off and dried himself. Richie felt better. He came out of the bathroom, smiling, with a towel draped around his waist, "it's all yours." Betty watched him saunter across the hallway, go into his room and close the door. She had a glimpse of his chest, as he walked by. It hardly looked human. He had definitely bulked up. His skin was smooth and gray, water beaded up on his chest, and dripped down to his towel. He was gone for a couple of minutes, and then the door opened, and he came out, wearing his PJ's.

"Headed down for some milk and cookies, then I'll be off to bed. I'm kind of tired."

54.

The three ladies landed at SAN, with only backpacks carrying some essentials. They planned to fly back on the Red Eye later that night. It was late morning, local time, and it was not too busy at the Dollar car rental, where they picked up the Jeep Wrangler that Hannah had reserved, using her AP business credit card. They started on the San Diego Freeway, then exited onto State Route 94, about 45 miles all told to Potrero, not far from the Mexican border. There on a windswept plain, half buried in ground, sat the Pharma Gene Laboratory. It was isolated, yet less than an hour from the airport. The proximity to the airport simplified shipping and receiving products. The lab was a virtual fortress, protected with electrified barbed wire fencing around its perimeter. There was a guardhouse at the gate, still about a half mile from the buildings. The guard stepped out, carrying his clipboard with the list of the day's expected visitors. There were about a half dozen names on his sheet. He quickly found Hannah Darrow on the list and waved the car through. Land was relatively cheap out here. The facility was composed of twin one-story buildings, covering more than an acre. The exposed roofs were laden with solar panels, using the abundant sunshine of southern California and ensuring their independence from the grid.

They were met at the front entrance by their host, Charlie. After introducing herself and welcoming them to PGL, a '*Lab with a View to the Future,'* she led them down a narrow concrete stairway, to the lobby below. Once there, she took them to the business counter where a camera snapped their pictures and a temporary ID was created for them to wear during their tour of the facility. She had a few rules to go over. They weren't allowed to make recordings or take pictures, and they had to stay with her at all times during the tour. Some areas would be off limits and she would let them know where those were. They had to leave their backpacks and purses in a locker just off the lobby, near the bathrooms.

The three ladies went over to stow their carry-ons in the lockers. While they were there, Hannah checked the micro camera in the broach she wore to be sure it was functioning, it would record pictures and sounds when activated by the touch surface on her linked wristwatch.

The tour started at the loading docks where the products arrived. The cells would typically have been flown in on a commercial carrier and then brought from the airport to the lab in one of their vans with the PGL logo. The product would be scanned in, and the electronic log would be downloaded and examined for any deviations from protocol. The temperature inside the box was recorded every ten seconds during its trip and that became part of its electronic document. It was then left in the cold room until the lab technicians were available to begin processing.

Charlie used her ID badge to open the electronic lock on the cold room door. She led them through the small room off to one side. There were several shelves, and a worktable in the tiny room. Charlie pointed out the three containers sitting there, each holding a precious cell product. She explained that one of them would be processed later that day, and the two others were already prepared, waiting to be shipped out. After a brief look-see, they left the cold room and headed over to the main processing area. As the tour continued, Charlie described what they were seeing. The enormous room was lined with high flow HEPA filter hoods, each of which had a lab tech busily at work in front of a stainless-steel table. The work surface sat within a transparent plastic enclosure. The front of the enclosure was fitted with a window on a track that could slide up and down. The hood included a HEPA unit connected to a duct that led the air through several layers of filters, trapping all particles larger than 0.3 microns. It would remove 99.97% of dust, pollen, mold and bacteria. That kept the space under the hood clean. The exhaust was guided to a specialized handler below ground so that no particles escaped the facility.

They stopped to watch the workers. As typical, working under a clean hood, their arms passed through the front window of the hood, using attached protective sleeves ending in gloves. The system meant that they were technically outside the hood, while their hands and arms worked inside. As they watched the accordioned black sleeves in the hood move it looked like robot arms as they transferred the cell solution from a hanging IV bag into the specialized container needed for the next processing step. The container, with the stem cell product safely inside, would then be removed from under the hood and carried over to an automated processing unit. From there, the procedure was finished by computer controlled robots, no human was needed during that portion of the operation.

Sandra was looking for vulnerable steps in the processing during which contamination might have occurred. As she tried to picture the cells on their journey through the lab, it seemed to her that whatever happened to Richie's cells must have occurred during one of the steps that required human hands.

As they moved along the tour, Sandra probed, "Charlie, this all seems so complicated and yet it appears to move smoothly. I wonder if there are ever any problems here."

"Oh, no," she answered, "this unit is run meticulously. Every step of the way has been planned, monitored and double checked for errors. We're very proud of our work."

"I see." Sandra watched Charlie as she asked, "but humans do make mistakes, don't they? So, nothing, no unusual events could have occurred, say in the last few weeks of June?"

Charlie paused before answering. She fidgeted a bit, seemingly uncomfortable with the question. Finally, she said, "no, I'm sure that there haven't been any problems during that time, or since I've been working here."

Charlie turned away quickly, but Sandra thought she saw her lips twitch as she pursed them. She had a few more questions. "I understand that there is also animal research at PGL. I wonder how that may be connected to the stem cell processing unit."

Charlie seemed even more uncomfortable. "The research division is completely autonomous from the processing division. They are absolute silos. No one from the research building would have access to this area."

Sandra thought that Charlie tried to appear very sure about her answer. But she wasn't convinced. Something wasn't right, Sandra could feel it. But she decided that pushing Charlie any further would not get any more information.

Several minutes later, as they were being led to another set of workstations, a worker carrying one of the specialized containers scurried down the aisle. He seemed to be headed right toward them, apparently in a rush to get across to the other side of the lab. The ladies tried to stand aside to give him room, but he still managed to collide with Hannah who teetered from the contact. Losing her balance, she was about to crash onto the hard floor when the tech reached out, grabbed hold of her, and helped guide her to a soft landing. He turned to rest the box on the counter, apologizing profusely and reached down to help her back on her feet. Another quick apology and he was off to the cold room side of the work area with his precious cargo. The technicians seemed to be working under enormous pressure. It was fertile ground for mistakes. Hannah brushed herself off, staring at the jerk who just toppled her. She assured Sandra, Nancy and Charlie that she was fine, and the tour continued.

They were told about the proprietary processing, but none of those details were shared. Once the automated segment was completed, the container was returned to the hood, where one of the lab technicians transferred the suspension into a new sterile single use transfusion bag. It would then be repacked and returned to the cold room where it would sit waiting to be shipped to the appropriate treatment center.

The tour of the facility lasted about 90 minutes. Sandra noticed that there was some time when the transfusion bag, with the stem cells inside, was sitting in the locked cold room, unattended, and not yet sealed in the shipping container. It was another vulnerable link in the process.

They ended the tour in the area around the reception lobby, near where the bathrooms and lockers were located. Hannah peppered Charlie with several questions while she led her away from the lockers.

Nancy stayed behind while Hannah was jawing Charlie. Nancy was an experienced high school locker user. She knew that if they were not secured, stuff would go walking. She noticed that several of the lockers had no padlocks. Most were set aside for staff. While Hannah kept Charlie busy, Nancy peeked into a few of the ones that weren't padlocked. Inside one of them she saw a hanging white lab coat alongside an ID badge fixed to a lanyard suspended from a hook inside. She closed the door quickly. She checked around as she did that, but she didn't think anyone saw her. Nancy went to the locker she used at the start of the tour and retrieved her own backpack.

Soon, they were sitting in their rented Jeep, with the A/C on full blast, still in the parking lot of PGL, talking about what they'd seen. Hannah thought the processing lab was just what it appeared to be. She had a series of pictures that she could look through later, but til now she didn't think they'd uncovered much.

Sandra spoke up, "I didn't see too much either. But I think that there are some security soft spots in the lab. I noticed a few places where the product was vulnerable and something could have happened."

It was sharp eyed Nancy, who hated using lockers at school, that added, "you know it was kind of weird, in a place that's supposed to be so careful, many of the lockers were not secured. I opened a couple of them and peaked inside. The third one I looked in had an ID badge, just hanging from a hook inside."

But in the end what had they learned? It didn't seem like much.

Hannah also complained about the jerk that had knocked into her. "At least he was polite enough to stop and help me up." She rubbed her hand on her hip, looking down at it. "I bet there's going to be a bruise."

Hannah cranked up the Jeep, backed out of the space, and then turned toward the gate.

Nancy was quick to speak up, she was urgent and commanding, "wait, just turn here and drive around to the back of this building. Don't leave!"

"What," said Hannah.

"Just do it," said Nancy.

Hannah pulled around to the other side of the building and parked in a shaded area that left them out of sight. "What's going on?" Hannah was perplexed and a bit annoyed that Nancy had diverted them, they had a plane to catch.

"Don't you think that was kind of weird, Hannah," said Nancy. "Some guy bumps into you and then stops and reaches out to help you up. He put his hands on you, didn't he?"

Hannah looked at Nancy, she was trying to remember. She put her hand back on her hip, where she remembered being touched. Suddenly she stepped out of the car. There were a few pockets to check, and sure enough, one of them at her hip contained a note. It simply said, "Call me," and there was a phone number.

Hannah looked at the note and read it again. "Fuck me!"

She passed the note around, and Nancy said, "call it, go ahead."

Hannah called the number, and someone in a quiet, hushed voice answered. "I only have a minute, but I heard one of you ask about a connection with the animal lab and mentioned the end of June. Charlie told you there was no connection, but one of the animal lab docs, Dr. Benzi, was asking some funny questions about how we do things, just a few days before that. He said that he needed it for some upcoming lab inspection. It sounded fishy to me. One morning at the end of last month, when I reached in my locker to get my lab coat and ID badge, it was hooked on the wrong side. I always have my badge hanging from the hook on the right side, but that morning it was hanging on the left. I didn't think much more about it. But later that day, some security types were poking around the lab, asking if anything was missing. I kept quiet. If I were you, I'd call Bill, he works in Dr. Benzi's animal lab, he's a straight up guy. I'll give you his number." And he did.

55.

Betty was awakened by her phone. She looked at the clock, it was too early for calls. She rubbed her eyes, trying to shake off the sleep. She picked up the insistent phone and was immediately on alert when she saw that it was Richie, "what's going..."

Richie interrupted her, barely getting the words out, "Mom, it's hard to breathe, please come."

Betty rushed over from her room across the hallway. She saw Richie, he was a dusky blue, agitated and struggling to breathe.

"It hurts." His voice was raspy, and barely louder than a whisper, "it feels like someone's sitting on my chest. I tried to sit up, but I can't. I called out to Siri to get you. I'm scared."

Betty tried to help him sit up, she propped some pillows behind his back so that he was elevated at least a bit. "Take it easy, Richie, just take little breaths, it will be OK, I'm here for you." She picked up Richard's phone and dialed 911. When the police operator answered, Betty quickly told her, "It's a medical emergency, my son who has cancer is having trouble breathing, he's blue and he needs an ambulance," Betty gave her address.

The operator tried to ask some more questions. Betty quickly became frustrated and angry. "Please," she shouted, "he's turning blue, he needs help, he needs oxygen, please send an ambulance right now. Oh, my God, please."

"OK, ma'am, stay on the line, I'm sending an ambulance right now, it'll soon be on the way. What's your son's name and how old is he?" Betty answered her questions.

"Can he still talk to you? Is he awake?"

"Please hurry, he's getting weaker, his color is darker. He can't talk."

"OK, ma'am, try to keep him calm and still, he shouldn't try to speak, the EMT's are on the way."

It seemed forever, but it was about 4 minutes. She heard the siren. They weren't far. She spoke to Richie, "I'll be right back honey, I have to go downstairs to open the door, and flag them down. They're coming. Please, just take small breaths."

Betty left him propped up, on his bed, and ran down the steps, she opened the door and saw the ambulance, down the road. She waved to get their attention and guide them to the right house. They screeched to a stop at the house, and two EMTs popped out. She yelled at them, "It's my son, he can't breathe, he's upstairs. He needs help." Betty left the door open and ran inside and up the stairs to Richie. He was very dusky, his nostrils flared as he tried to get enough air. His chest was barely moving, he tried to talk, but no words came out.

The EMT's climbed the steps carrying their emergency medical boxes. Betty heard them and yelled, "he's in here." Betty held Richie. She was sobbing, tears rolling down her face, "Please help him, please help Richie."

Mark came in first and immediately saw that Richie was in trouble. He took his stethoscope from around his neck, listening to his heart and his lungs. He felt Richie's pulse, it was weak and thready. He placed a pulse oximeter on his finger.

Mark turned to Betty, "did I hear that your son has cancer?"

"He's being treated for leukemia," said Betty, he had a bone marrow transplant."

"I see," said Mark, "is he DNR?"

"What?"

"Is he DNR, ma'am, do you want us to treat him, or just make him comfortable?"

"What the fuck!" she almost screamed, "he is not DNR, do everything, he needs help, now! Please help him."

"OK, we're going to put an oxygen mask on him, but he needs to be intubated, right now, he's not making adequate respiratory efforts, and he's not getting enough oxygen, just putting a mask on him won't help much. We are going to have to breathe for him. Do you understand?"

"Yes, you need to put in a breathing tube, can you do that here, now?"

"Yes ma'am, we're going to bring some equipment up to do that. I'm going to start with a face mask, and I'll need to start an IV, so he can get some medicine to relax him for the intubation and in case we need to give him anything else. I'm going to talk to my partner."

"Ok, I understand," said Betty, "but you won't be able to start an IV in his arm but he does have a central line."

"Thank you, ma'am," said Mark, "we have it."

Mark and Jim worked quickly to set up for the intubation. They couldn't be worrying about the panicky mother. Their focus was now on getting the patient an airway and oxygen.

An oxygen mask was placed over Richie's mouth and nose, and the flow rate was turned all the way up to 15 L/min. They prepared what they would need. They would first try an 8.0 size endotracheal tube, but they were prepared with one a half size larger and a half size smaller if that one didn't fit. They set up a roll of tape and a 20 ml syringe to inflate the ETT cuff. They prepared the laryngoscope attaching a Macintosh size 3 blade. An end-tidal CO_2 detector was ready. The detector would tell them if the tube was inserted correctly in his trachea.

Richie was fading quickly. They needed to intubate him right then. There was no time to hunt for IV access. They'd do it without sedation.

They worked closely as a team. Jim lubed up the end of the no. 8.0 ETT, and attached the 20 mL syringe to the cuff, making sure it was deflated. The stylet inserted in the tube was bent slightly into a curve that matched the anatomy of Richie's trachea. Jim picked up the laryngoscope and swung the blade out from the handle, making sure that the integrated light in the blade worked and was secure. He held the scope in his left hand, ready to slide the tube in with his right. He stood at the head of Richie's bed, looking down at his patient. Mark gently lifted Richie's chin to allow better access. Jim slipped the laryngoscope blade into his mouth from his own right side and used it to sweep Richie's tongue to the left and out of the way. He advanced the blade downward to just above the vocal cords. Jim pulled up and away on the handle of the laryngoscope, which helped him visualize the airway. Mark pushed down slightly on the cricoid process in his neck, making it easier to see the target. With that Jim announced that he could see the vocal cords. He held the ET tube with his right hand, and turned the bevel face slightly to his right. With a steady hand he skillfully guided the tube down his throat, watching the tip advance down the center of Richie's trachea, and disappear between the two sides of the laryngeal cords. He advanced it just a bit more.

"I'm in."

He removed the stylet and attached the end tidal CO_2 device. He inflated the cuff of the tube to help secure it in his airway and then removed the syringe. Using the connector he attached the ambu bag. The color of the device changed from purple to yellow, as the stale air from Richie's lungs exited through the detector. Mark listened to each side of Richard's chest while Jim gave a few puffs with the bag. Mark gave thumbs up, he heard breath sounds equally on each side, agreeing with the end tidal CO_2 device that the placement of the ET tube was good. It was then taped in place. The ambu bag connector was hooked to the O_2 tank, and very quickly Richie's color improved from that dusky blue to a more appropriate pink. They continued manually squeezing the ambu bag to breathe for Richie. Eventually, once they were inside the ambulance, they planned to replace the ambu bag with an automatic mechanical ventilator.

Betty, who was holding Richie's hand the whole time, breathed a sigh of relief as she saw his color improve. "Thank you so much. I'm sorry if I was bitchy before."

Mark waved her off, "already forgotten ma'am," he said. "Let's get him in the wagon and roll."

"He's got to go to Memorial Medical Center," said Betty.

"Well, that's not the closest hospital," said Mark.

"That's where they know him," said Betty, "that's where his doctors are, they've got all his records, and there is nowhere else even remotely near that is set to care for kids with cancer, he has to go to Memorial."

Mark and Jim looked at each other, "Ok, we go to Memorial."

"I will be two minutes while you get him into the ambulance, I need to put some clothes on, and grab a toothbrush."

Jim went down to the ambulance to get the stretcher, while Mark stayed with Richie. Together they eased him on to the stretcher, managed the staircase, and continued the breaths, something they had done a thousand times before. By the time he was secured on the gurney in the truck, Betty was down, locking up the house and ready to go. Jim stayed in the back with Richie, and Betty climbed in to join them. The truck sat at the curb for a few minutes, while Jim tried to hook Richie up to the ventilator in the ambulance, but it wasn't working. The machine would cut out because it sensed the pressure needed to fill his lungs was too high. The thick skin covering Richie's chest was strangling him.

"We'll have to manually ventilate him, with the ambu bag. Ma'am, you watch how I'm doing this, because we may need to switch off at some point. Slow, long squeezes on the bag, about ten times per minute. Normally we look for the chest to rise with each squeeze, but we're not going to see that, his chest wall is too stiff. We'll know he's OK if his sats stay good and his color remains pink." Jim looked at Richard, "give me a thumbs up if you understand." And Richard did.

"OK, let's go." And they took off, lights flashing and the siren screaming, they needed to get to the hospital quickly. Anything could happen on the way over. The tube could dislodge, and Richie would be up shit's creek, or anyway, up shit's highway.

56.

Sandra, Nancy and Hannah were still sitting on the other side of PGL, hoping no one would notice them parked in the shade behind the building. "What do we do?" asked Nancy.

"We call Bill," said Hannah. "I think Sandra should do it. They can speak medical to each other."

It rang while she held on, Sandra had him on speaker so they could all hear Bill when he answered.

"Hello," Bill answered.

"This is Dr. Gardner."

"I just got a call from the tech on the cell processing side," said Bill. "He said you guys were asking a lot of curious questions. And he told me, what he knew about Dr. Benzi and his ID badge."

"I'm here with a friend and a reporter. I'm the doctor for an adolescent boy who had a transplant using stem cells that were processed in this lab. He's had some very strange changes since the transplant, and we're hoping you can explain what's going on."

Bill didn't say anything for a while. Finally, "what kind of changes?"

Sandra hesitated, not sure what to say. Direct is best, she figured, "he has the tail of a fucking turtle!"

"Oh, shit," he said and nothing more for a few seconds. "Where are you?"

"We are in the parking lot, on the backside of the processing building, hidden in the shade, sitting in a red Jeep Wrangler."

"OK, I'm in the other building, come around to the door in the back, I'll meet you there."

As they approached, Bill appeared in the doorway, he poked his head out, looked around and then let them in.

"We're alone, right now, I don't expect Dr. Benzi until later this afternoon. Tell me again about the patient, he's just a boy?"

"He's 17, and he received cells that were processed here." Sandra asked Hannah to show the pictures she had.

Hannah turned her camera so Bill could see the screen and showed him how to scan through the images. Bill saw the tail, the eye color, and Richie's chest. He sighed. His worst fears confirmed.

"Come into the animal room, I want to show you some things."

He led them inside. They could see rows and rows of cages on shelves, each cage labeled, and each had a mouse inside. As he pulled the cages down, some looked sick, lying on the bottom of their cage, not moving, panting heavily. But these mice all looked like regular sick lab animals, with normal mouse skin and normal mouse tails. Hannah and Nancy looked at each other, it was upsetting to see the caged animals that were being experimented on, but they were not sure what this had to do with Richie.

Bill led them further down the rows of cages. A squeaking sound grew louder as they followed Bill. Nancy asked about the sound, "what's that?"

Bill brought one of the noisy cages down onto a table they used to inject the mice. Inside, they saw a mouse, busy on the exercise wheel, running, not fazed by the cage's movement.

"It looks like Richie, running on the track," said Nancy.

Bill brought up his flashlight and shone it on the mouse, it immediately left the wheel, scurried to a corner of the cage, and started digging furiously at the side, trying his best to escape. Bill turned off the light, and the mouse stopped digging. He took the top off, reached in, and brought the mouse up, turning him, so they could see its backside. Sure enough, he had a tail that was a miniature version of the one on Richie's back.

"Certain animals seem to hardly ever develop cancer," Bill began. "There are many researchers trying to understand why, and there are multiple theories about what genes might be responsible. Among those animals, the giant tortoise that inhabited the Galapagos Island was one, and the large bowhead whale is another. Both are resistant to developing cancer. In theory, bigger animals that lived longer were more likely to develop cancer, because they have lots of cells dividing for a long time. Although researchers had looked at individual genes that might be responsible for their remarkable resistance, so far, they found no single gene that could explain the phenomenon. The doctors here, Benzi and Carlson, believe that looking at individual genes isn't the answer. Their idea is that it's a specific combination of genes that protects those animals. So, they've been testing various permutations of gene combinations." Bill explained that "each of these surviving mice had received a unique set of genes from a bowhead whale and a tortoise and that after a few days, when the new genes were functioning, they were injected with a lethal dose of leukemia cells."

Bill continued, "almost every other mouse died within a week of the injection. But now, after years of study, we've found two mice that resisted the lethal injection. Dr. Carlson was very excited, and he set up a new trial to verify the effect of this particular gene combination. All the mice in the control group died, but the others that received the same combination of genes from a bowhead whale and a tortoise, lived. It was remarkable. And all those mice had these same strange external traits.

Dr. Carlson was riveted, and he outlined new experiments to determine which of those genes were important, and which ones might be unnecessary. He began to work on a paper to publish his findings. He knew that there were years of work ahead before this could be tried in humans.

I wasn't sure, but when I spoke with Dr. Benzi, he seemed to ignore protocol. He muttered some things like, this can't wait, and walked off like a man possessed. I didn't know what he was planning."

Sandra filled in what she had deduced. "So, it seems, that Dr. Benzi came to the cell processing side of PGL, he asked some questions, nosed around and likely saw the same weaknesses in security that I did. One night, I imagine, he brought some container, holding a syringe full of this gene combination, 'borrowed' an ID badge from one of the lockers, sneaked into the cold room and injected the contents into a bag of stem cells waiting to be shipped to some unsuspecting donor. He didn't pay too much attention to exactly how the badge he picked up was stored, and so it went back into the locker on the wrong hook. What the fuck he was thinking when he did that, I haven't a clue. Clearly, he is mad, and he will pay for this. But now one of my patients, a kid, looks like one of your fucking mouse experiments!"

"Yes, you're probably right," said Bill, "I need to show you something." He appeared to be very disturbed, and he picked up a set of log records. "The first two mice that received this gene combination, lived for six more weeks. They had the same external manifestations that you saw on these mice. But those two eventually died of asphyxia, they were suffocated by the changes in their bodies. When they underwent a postmortem exam, there was no leukemia, so their disease was cured, but the treatment killed them."

Nancy, gasped, and started to cry, "no, that can't be." she said, "You're fucking monsters!" She started to beat her fists on Bill.

Bill didn't stop her, he stood there while she pounded on him. Hannah went over to take Nancy in her arms and try to comfort her.

Finally, Bill said that there was more. And he went on to explain.

While they were standing there trying to absorb what they had just heard, Nancy and Sandra received a text, telling them that Richard had been admitted to the PICU, he required intubation.

Sandra immediately called Paul to see what she could find out, but Paul didn't know much yet, he was just getting ready to head over to the intensive care unit to find out what happened. Sandra went on to explain what they discovered at PGL. She told him that they were shown caged lab mice that shared the same changes as Richie. From what she learned at PGL, there may be a way to help Richie. She told Paul that when she gets back to the hospital she can explain in more detail. For starters, he will require another stem cell infusion, preferably from the same donor. Sandra recommended that they try to contact the IBMTR as soon as possible with an emergency request to harvest Richie's donor for a second stem cell collection. And they should prepare Richie for tumor lysis syndrome.

Paul told her he would see what he could do. They would talk again after he saw Richie. He rang off.

Paul soon found Dr. Street at the workstation in the PICU. She quickly reviewed Richie's presentation to the ER. He was in acute respiratory failure, but the strange thing was that there was nothing wrong with his lungs. He was being strangled by the changes in his chest wall.

Dr. Street recounted the events, starting with Betty's 911 call, the EMTs finding him dark and dusky, intubating him at home and not being able to use the ambulance ventilator.

"Paul, I tried several different modes of ventilation before settling on high-frequency ventilation," said Dr. Street.

Paul, of course, knew how this setting of ventilation worked. But he had only seen it in the very premature babies. It was needed for them because of their extremely fragile, immature lungs. Paul could imagine the extreme level of pressure conventional ventilation would require to move Richie's strange chest and how that would eventually damage his lungs. He immediately understood how Dr. Street's brilliant idea would get around the problem. High-frequency ventilation would deliver very frequent, small, gentle puffs of air down his trachea. It would create tiny eddies of air in Richie's alveoli. Thousands of tiny mini-tornadoes spinning in every air sac of his lungs, allowing the exchange of oxygen with carbon dioxide, without expanding his lungs.

Dr. Street went on, "but Paul, this isn't sustainable. Eventually something needs to be done about his chest."

"I understand," answered Paul. "When I talked to Sandra, she told me that she's learned information that may be used to help Richie, but she didn't have time to explain the whole thing. She just told me that he needed to be prepped for a new transplant and an upcoming tumor lysis crisis."

"That sounds like another mess on top of his impending respiratory failure. I've already restricted his fluids to help his lungs. Preparing him for tumor lysis would seem to require that he's well hydrated, and that's what I've been working to avoid."

"OK, Dr. Street, just start the allopurinol and remove any potassium from his fluid," said Paul, "we'll worry about the hydration later. Do what you have to do to keep his breathing safe."

"Paul, we have to move fast with whatever Sandra has in mind. And I sure hope it's going to work, cause Richie is in deep shit right now."

"I know," said Paul. "I know."

57.

Landing back home, Sandra left the airport and headed directly to Memorial Medical Center's PICU. She was upset seeing Richie with a tube down his throat, hooked to a monitor, clinging to life. The continued progression of his physical changes was a reminder of what she had seen in the animal room at PGL and a warning about those animals' ultimate demise.

On admission to the PICU, Richie was initially sedated with midazolam and a continuous fentanyl drip. The sedation allowed Richie to tolerate the tube he required for his respiratory support. Once stabilized, the midazolam was switched to a propofol drip. The drip could be adjusted to reach the proper level of sedation, or even turn it down briefly if they needed to speak with him. It was a tricky balancing act, trying to keep him comfortable and informed.

Sandra steeled herself for the unenviable task of speaking with Richie and his mom. It wasn't easy. Being a physician wasn't just a job for Sandra, it's who she was. She made deep personal connections with her patients. Sandra had made a choice to help children with cancer, most of whom did well. There was nothing more satisfying than that. But there were still some children whose disease was very aggressive and unresponsive to treatment. And watching those children and their families was so very difficult. Sometimes the best she could do was to ease their suffering. Every child that died, took its toll on Sandra. She thought about them now, but she wasn't ready to add Richie to that list. Sandra sat down by Richie's bed, looked into his eyes and held his hand. She reassured him that there was a plan, they had new information. Their plan would work. He just needed to hang in there a while longer.

As Sandra turned to leave she wiped a tear that had fallen down her cheek. She took a deep breath, all she could think was, "this has to fucking work."

Sandra stood in front of an anxious group of docs that was waiting to hear the plan to save Richie. She carefully explained what she learned from Bill, the tech who managed the laboratory animal room at PGL. Sandra said that Bill was stunned to find that his worst fears about Dr. Benzi were true. But he also said that there was reason to hope that the damage could be rectified. Sandra went on to detail what she found at PGL. It was Richie's only hope, and though in theory it should work, no one had ever done it under these circumstances. It was an unknown.

"We've contacted the IBMTR," said Paul, "and we're waiting for a response to our request to get in touch with Richard's stem cell donor about another harvest. I've also been in touch with an agent at Takara Bio. The director of our pharmacy and one of our medical center VPs are working with the company to expedite the shipment of the needed product. It should be here tomorrow or the next day at the latest."

"What about the other drug, Paul. We need that too!"

"Well, the sirolimus is commercially available," Paul said, "and it'll be here tomorrow. I've also talked with Dr. Street in the PICU. She's making changes in anticipation of another tumor lysis syndrome, but she can't safely increase his fluids right now. So, we've got to work with that restriction. If it comes to it, Dr. Street said they could consider hemodialysis to remove excess potassium."

Everything now depended on the availability of a new shipment of stem cells, which would not go through PGL for any reason.

Hannah had been on a conference call with her boss, and the risk management lawyers at the Associated Press. She gave a detailed report on everything she'd discovered during her trip to PGL. She presented interviews, pictures and voice recordings. She even sent a picture of the original handwritten message passed to her by one of the lab techs. Everyone at AP knew it was one hell of a story, but they had to be careful about how it was handled. Hannah had begun writing a draft of her article. She had prepared two versions, one with a happy ending, and one with the other kind.

When Nancy arrived at the PICU, Betty stepped out so that she could be alone with Richie.

Richie lay there, terrified. It had been better since the tube went in, but now he was dependent on that damn machine. He could hear the machine whirring. He was constantly aware of the air swirling around in his lungs. He felt his chest tightening. It was closing in on him. Richie knew that the breathing tube would not help much longer.

But she was here. He felt her by his bed. The sound of Nancy's voice comforted him. It was sweetness in the face of looming disaster. But he worried about her. His pain would end if he died, but not hers. He hoped his mom would be there for her.

"Hi, Richie, it's Nancy," she held his hand, "I know you can hear me. I love you so much. I need you to get better and come back to me. I have plans for you, Richie. So, you better come back." Nancy sat near him, whispering so that only he could hear. "See, I'm wearing the bracelet you gave me. You can hear it jingle." She wiped a tear. "When I wear your bracelet, you're near my heart. I close my eyes and I can feel you in my arms, just like that night we shared." She opened his hand and kissed each finger. Then she stood up and leaned over him. She kissed him near his mouth, on either side of that damn tube. She dabbed another tear that fell on his cheek.

If Richie could have smiled, he would have. He tried to think of how wonderful it would be to be with his girl again, but the propofol caught up with him, and he was out.

Richie remained intubated, using the high frequency oscillatory ventilation mode requiring relatively low levels of supplemental oxygen. The machine had been running continuously for more than 36 hours, and Dr. Street knew they were running out of time. Her last trick was to add nitric oxide to the inhaled oxygen. The NO would help relax the smooth muscles in his bronchioles. That would be a temporary stopgap. Something had to be done about his chest wall. They had maybe a day or so to act. If nothing changed, it would become difficult to ever wean him from the machine.

They had yet to hear back from the IBMTR. They didn't know if anyone had reached Richie's donor. Paul called again. If they couldn't get in touch with the original donor, or if he weren't willing to undergo a second cycle of harvesting, they would have to find a new HLA matched donor. That would take time, and there wasn't much of that left.

The medications he needed arrived at the medical center. But they needed a new supply of stem cells to replace the ones that would be destroyed during the rescue.

Paul was frustrated, it took every bit of control to keep from losing it while he continued to try to locate the right person at the IBMTR. The request was now two days old, and the situation was desperate.

Nearly ready to give up, he was finally connected to a helpful representative. Paul worked to keep his voice even-tempered as he again expressed the urgency of the request. Paul read the case number, the date of the harvest and the confidential identity data required to locate Richie's donor. A few minutes passed while the agent brought up the appropriate page in the IBMTR electronic record.

"Yes, I have the record, here and your emergency inquiry," he spoke English perfectly, but with an Eastern European accent that Paul had trouble placing. "Hold on, I'm reading through the notes. We're still trying to locate the donor, it says that we've tried several times, phone calls and a certified letter went out as well.

Wait a minute, I'm still reading. It says that we had an excellent yield from his first harvest, in fact we had collected twice as many CD34+ stem cells as you'd requested. So, half the harvest was frozen and is stored here at our collection facility. There's some paperwork that needs to be done, which you can fax over, including the medical reason for the request, but we can ship that out to PGL tomorrow."

Paul could hardly believe the good news. "Oh, thank God, that's wonderful, so amazing. That certainly gives our patient a chance. I'll give you the fax number for sending the forms that I need. It should only about an hour or so after I get it. But it's very important that you do not send the stem cells to PGL. I'll give you a different address to send the product to. It's very important that the cells are shipped to the Memorial Medical Center Blood Bank, not PGL. I'll fax all that information to you. Can you please repeat that back to me."

The representative repeated the instructions, to close the loop.

"That's it, thank you again." said Paul and he disconnected. He could hardly believe it. He couldn't wait to tell everyone. They could start the rescue, as soon they knew the cells were on the way.

Paul came back to the fellow's room, where the doctors had been trying to plan how they might proceed under various scenarios. The mood was grim. Everyone involved was there, Drs. Lester, Reed, Gardner and Stanner. They looked up expectantly when they saw Paul. He tried to wear his poker face, but he couldn't help the grin that popped through.

Sandra saw the smile, and guessed, "I see that look, Paul, they found the donor and he's agreed, right?"

"Even better," said Paul, "they had collected enough cells for two transplants during the first harvest, and half of the harvest is just sitting there, frozen in storage. They can ship that bag to us as soon as we fill out the paperwork."

"No fucking way!" said Sandra. "Oh, my god, we've all been sitting here, about to turn blue, we're breathing again, cause the fucking cells are there and we've got a mission to run!"

If they had champagne bottles, they would've shaken them and sprayed each other with the foamy bubbly eruptions. They shared a few moments of giddy relief, with high fives and embraces. Dr. Stanner, let it go on for a few minutes before calling everyone back to order, "let's get to work," he said, "we've no time to waste."

Paul went to work completing the forms that the IBMTR needed. He hesitated a moment, there was a box to check for the reason for the request. There were choices: graft failure, disease relapse, graft vs. host disease, CMV infection. None of the choices seemed to fit the actual reason. He smiled a bit, "I guess they hadn't considered whale and turtle gene contamination as a possible explanation." Finally, he checked, "other, see attached" and wrote a brief explanation.

Sandra was ready to talk to Betty and Richie about what the doctors learned and their plan. She asked Dr. Street to lower Richie's sedation, so he could understand the information and be able to make an informed decision.

Sandra started with a brief historical background. "Typically, larger animals, that lived longer and were composed of trillions of cells, were more likely to get cancer. There were more opportunities for a lethal mutation to occur. But a few animals defied this typical pattern, among them were the giant tortoise and the bowhead whale. Many researchers surmised that there was something different about their DNA. They must have evolved protective genes. There have been legitimate studies to find out which of those genes might be the key to their good fortune.

At PGL, there's a lab, which is set up to be independent of the cell processing division. It's engaged in that kind of cancer resistance gene research. The lab was appropriately carrying out experiments using animal models to test their theories. They narrowed their focus to a small group of genes that showed promise."

Sandra went on to describe the research at PGL and what some of the mice they'd seen looked like. She also told them about Dr. Benzi and what he'd done to the stem cells that wound up in Richie's infusion. His cells were deliberately re-engineered.

Dr. Gardner went on, "Hannah Darrow will soon have a byline on a story about a major investigation into the PGL lab. AP News has sent an early version of the article to the Federal Drug Enforcement Agency. I expect that DEA agents will soon be swarming all over that lab. But it turns out that previous misfortune has led to some hope. Sandra explained that because of horrific tragedies in previous attempts at gene therapy, scientists had developed a series of fail-safe emergency gene inserts, sort of like the self-destruct button on an errant rocket tumbling out of control. If any infused cells unexpectedly turned out to be dangerous the inserted gene would be activated and they would initiate apoptosis, cell self-destruction. Sandra added that a collection of blood stem cells, from Richie's donor, would soon be on the way. This transplant would be different. He wouldn't need preparative chemotherapy because his leukemia's gone. The programmed destruction, apoptosis, would leave an empty bone marrow space. The new donor cells will be able to move onto a relatively healthy bone marrow foundation, implant and develop. He will still need medications to minimize GvHD which will be created as the donor cells adjust to their new home."

Sandra had finished telling them all she knew. But she added, "we're in completely uncharted territory, no one really knows what will happen. We can, if you choose not to do this, just watch and wait, but I don't believe that is a viable alternative for Richie." Sandra paused and took a breath, "I know that's a lot to process."

Betty looked at Richie, their eyes met in silent communication, he nodded to her, and squeezed his mom's hand.

"We've been through a lot in these weeks at the medical center," said Betty, "and we've gotten to know the doctors and nurses here, who've all been wonderful. Watch and wait, given how we've seen these changes unfolding, does not seem like an option. The transformation's happening faster and it's become clear that Dr. Street won't be able to keep up with that much longer. We're grateful for your dedication, and persistence. You've gone well above and beyond what anyone could expect. So, do what you can, we're ready. But please make sure that Richie doesn't suffer." Betty looked at Sandra, "don't let that happen, OK?"

"OK, I promise." Sandra listened to Betty's appeal. None of this was easy for Sandra, and she could only imagine how much worse it was for Richie and his mom. On top of it all, she couldn't help feeling some guilt as part of the team that had given Richie those fucking cells. It was an effort to present the reassuring face that she knew Betty needed to see. She wasn't sure any of this would work, but she'd make damn sure that whatever happened, at least Betty would not see Richie suffering.

"We're ready to start as soon we know that the rescue stem cells are en route," said Sandra. She left to find Dr. Street to review the plan's details. They had one chance to get this right, and there was no precedent to guide them.

Dr. Street had a cot in her office that she rarely used, but tonight, she wouldn't leave the building, something could go south quickly and without warning. She needed to be available immediately and so her cot would be occupied tonight.

When she reviewed everything with Arnie, the night nurse, she saw his look of concern. "What are you worried about?"

"It's Richard's central line catheter. It's a subclavian and it runs through his stiffening chest skin. The blood flow had been good, but not so much anymore. The tube is being pinched as his chest wall tightens. His pump is sensing higher resistance. It alarms, and then shuts off. I've had to restart the pump several times. So far it restarts, but I don't think it'll work much longer."

Dr. Street saw the looming problem. "I see. He's going to need a new line inserted in his groin, below the chest, where the skin is normal. I don't want to do that yet, but please make sure that there's a kit available at his bedside if it needs to be done emergently. How's his level of sedation?"

"It's good right now," answered Arnie, "he's asleep most of the time, but you can wake him if you need to ask a yes/no question. He can blink once or twice. If you need more than that, we have an alphabet board."

"Good," said Dr. Street, "I'm going into my office to lie down but call me immediately if there are any concerns at all, OK Arnie? If you are wondering whether to wake me about something, just wake me."

It was shortly after 3 AM, when the text went out confirming that the stem cell product had shipped. It was on its way to the medical center and expected to arrive in 12 hours. That was the news they'd been waiting for. They could now start Richie's rescue.

Arnie called Dr. Street at 5:30 AM, to let her know that the central chest line was extremely finicky. He'd started a peripheral IV in the greater saphenous vein medially above his left ankle. That was working OK, for now. It could carry the sedation medications, but not much more.

Dr. Street came out five minutes later and told Arnie to prepare for the placement of a central femoral line. They had an ultrasound imager, to help visualize the anatomy in his leg, and help find the best access path for the canulation.

Dr. Street sat down with Betty, and explained the problem, and what needed to be done. But Betty had been watching Arnie restart the pump multiple times, she already understood the problem and knew something needed to be done. So, when Dr. Street asked her about the new line, Betty had already decided to agree to the procedure.

Dr. Street asked her to wait outside the room until the new line was secured.

Betty was exhausted, the pressures of the last several days had taken a severe toll. She needed to leave the unit, even if it was only for a short break. She used the opportunity to head down to the cafeteria for coffee and nourishment.

Dr. Street put on a sterile dressing gown, gloves and a mask. Arnie brought over the ultrasound machine. Using the transducer probe and watching the generated images, she felt confident that she knew the best approach. Arnie had the femoral line kit set up and ready to go. She made sure that Richie was well sedated. Dr. Street prepped the site on his right leg using three betadine swabs. The area was covered with a fenestrated sterile dressing, its opening over the access point. She infiltrated lidocaine into the subcutaneous tissue, numbing the region before making the first scalpel incision in his groin. Using the Seldinger technique, she punctured the deeper tissues with the introducer needle. With the help of ultrasound imaging, she was able to find the deep large femoral vein. Once inside the vessel, she advanced the guide wire forward tracking upward toward his heart. The introducer needle was removed and the larger catheter was inserted over the guide wire. Once that catheter was in place, the guide wire was no longer needed. It was removed and discarded. Continuing with the aid of ultrasound, she threaded the catheter up and into the inferior vena cava, just short of the small heart chamber, his right atrium. The line was then secured. Dr. Street tested that it could draw and flush readily. It was ready to be used.

Arnie transferred the IV fluid, D5W with 25 mEq/L $NaHCO_3$, from the finicky central line above, to the newly placed inguinal line, and they were in business for whatever was to come. Arnie flushed the chest line with heparin and capped it off, hoping that if the day's treatment plan worked, the line would be useful again.

Sandra called Dr. Street to get an update on Richie and learn when she could start the rescue. Dr. Street reported that his new line was functioning. They were ready for the next step.

"That's great," said Sandra, "I'll be up soon, with Stacy, and we'll have everything we need to start.

Down in the hospital cafeteria Betty saw Nancy and Hannah at a table, deep in discussion. Betty walked over carrying her breakfast tray and sat down with them.

"You guys are up early," said Betty.

"I heard from Sandra," said Hannah, "that the donor stem cells are on the way, and they're going to start the reversal drugs very early this morning. I called Nancy, and we came over together. I want to cover the rest of this story. I hope to get some good pictures too. I understand that there should be some dramatic changes once the suicide genes are activated."

"I saw that the exposé with your byline made the front page in several of the big national papers," said Betty.

Lab Covertly Employs Experimental Animal
Genes on Teen With Leukemia
by Hannah Darrow

"That was very impressive, you certainly nailed it. I hope PGL gets what they deserve. I'd like to see that God damn CEO forced to come to the hospital and see what his company did to my son, and humbly apologize to him."

They finished in silence, each alone with their private thoughts. Then they headed to the bank of elevators and back up to the PICU, to be there, supporting Richie as he faced an uncharted therapeutic intervention. Nancy held Betty's hand as they left the elevator together. Through all of this, they'd connected. They shared a harrowing journey watching the boy they both loved as he endured a horrific scourge and now teetered between life and death. They had managed their feelings and fears, they had given him all the love and support they could. But it was done at a very high cost.

58.

The team was outside Richie's room, reviewing what was expected over the next several hours. They developed planned responses to each of the potential contingencies they envisioned. But they also knew that they had to be ready for the unexpected. Stacy was there, beside a cart stacked with a pair of labeled IV bags. The doctors were present, Stanner, Street, Belkin, Gardner, Reed and Lester. Sandra tried to look confidant, but inside she was a bundle of nerves. She closed her eyes and prayed for this to work. She was going into battle against an unknown enemy, with no certainty of success.

Leslie was taking over for Arnie after his busy shift. Richie was hooked to the monitor. They heard the steady blip, blip of his heartbeat as it played in the background. The crash cart was set inside his room, and the fully charged automated external cardiac defibrillator sat just outside in the hallway. Richie had an IV in his left foot, but the larger, newly placed line emerging from his groin was now his primary vascular access. It was a single lumen catheter, hooked to a "Y" extension, allowing two IV pumps to deliver different fluids or medications at the same time. The fluids would start out on separate journeys as they left the pumps but would then join at the "Y" extension, before flowing into Richie's large femoral vein. He had just completed the 30-minute infusion of Rasburicase, 6 mg IV, to treat the expected rise in uric acid. Sandra's nerves were on edge. She had never wanted something so uncertain, so badly.

Everything was ready to activate the safety suicide genes, which they hoped would initiate a cascade of events. All cells were filled with tiny cellular organelles called lysosomes. These tiny membrane bound sacs were scattered throughout every donor cell. The sacs were packed with enzymes, just waiting for someone to push the destruct button, the signal to release their contents and destroy the cell they occupied. They were true sleeper cells.

Stacy had two IV bags ready and labeled, each filled with one of the drugs that would signal the start of the cellular dissolution. One bag contained 32 mg of the drug, AP 1903, and the other bag had 900 micrograms of an analog of sirolimus called ABT-578. They would be infused simultaneously over 30 minutes. Using two drugs, each activating a different pathway, was like lighting two fuses to be sure the dynamite exploded. It should ensure the destruction of every single one of those damned transformed cells that were now strangling Richie. Stacy worked with Leslie, to hang the bags from the IV poles. With the go ahead from Sandra both pumps began propelling their drugs down the tubes, and into Richard's blood stream. Thirty minutes later the bags were empty, the drugs had been infused and they were now circulating throughout his body, hopefully delivering their signals to the intended targets.

Sandra was anxious. Her hands were clenched tightly as she paced back and forth. It had to work. That's all she could think. It had to work. They planned to send stat blood samples every 30 minutes, to be alerted for dangerous elevations in potassium, uric acid and phosphorous. So far, the cardiac monitor showed a steady rhythm, those pesky T waves maintained their normal appearance. Outwardly, nothing seemed to have changed.

An hour went by, then two, but still they saw nothing.

The steady oscillation of the ventilator continued. The vital sign monitor displayed stable telemetry. Richie, who was sedated, lay on the hospital bed, quiet and asleep. Urine dripped into the collection bag, and the IV pump chugged on. His maintenance IV fluids flowed through his femoral line.

Doubts began to grow. Sandra was worried that their plan wasn't working. Maybe the drugs were ineffective. Maybe they were given bad information. Maybe there were no suicide genes in the viral vectors that Dr. Benzi injected into Richie's donor stem cell bag.

Nancy watched too, waiting for something to happen. She was the first to notice a change. "Look, something's different." She pointed.

The others looked to see what caught Nancy's attention. At first, no one else noticed anything different.

Nancy's voice rose, she couldn't understand why she was the only one to notice, "it looks like he's been sitting on the beach all day. Don't you see? His chest and arms are bright red, like he's on fire."

Sandra walked over to him, and laid her hand on his chest. She quickly pulled away, "it's hot! He's burning up." She touched his forehead and his legs, they were cool. "We need to cool the skin on his chest and arms. Let's get an ice chest in here, now, fill it with cool saline water and soak some bed sheets in it. We need to cover his chest and arms with chilled sheets. Now!"

The staff scrambled to get it done. One ran down to the lab where they had ice chests for transport. In the meantime, they filled a sink with saline and ice and threw bed sheets in to soak up the cold liquid. Soon the cool sheets were wrung out and laid over Richie's red hot skin. As the sheets absorbed the heat, they warmed and had to be replaced with new ice and saline soaked sheets. Richie began to moan. He seemed agitated and fidgety. He began to scratch at his chest and arms, lightly at first, but then more strenuously.

Sandra ordered 50 mg of IV Benadryl to help with the itching, but Richie still scratched. Chunks of skin were now coming off wherever his nails raked across his body. The tissue revealed underneath was raw, red and oozing blood. The meds were working for sure. But now she began to worry that Richie was losing too much skin, too fast.

Dr. Street picked up her phone and called the hospital operator, on the PICU stat line, "this is Dr. Street, please page whoever's on call for the Burn Unit and have them call me back at this number, it's urgent, thank you." Sandra suggested adding a dose of solumedrol to help mitigate the inflammation. Meanwhile, Dr. Street increased the sedation and ordered morphine. Richie raised his arm one more time and then mercifully the sedation and morphine kicked in. He was asleep.

Another nurse was called over to help Leslie manage his "burns." Fresh cold saline sheets were replacing the warmed ones. Together they logrolled Richie, by his near side, tipping him up, like the lid on a storage chest, so they could place cold dressings underneath to cool his back. As they smoothed out the linens he'd been lying on, and readied to ease him back down, Leslie's arm grazed against Richie's tail.

She was a veteran nurse, and had seen nearly everything you might imagine, but Leslie shrieked, it was brief, and she was immediately sorry. But she had been unnerved and lost it for a moment. She hadn't been prepared to see his tail drop off as she brushed against it. Leslie was able to quickly compose herself, and using her thumb and forefinger, with her gloved hand at arm's length, she moved the tail out of the way.

Roland, also watching the proceedings, came over to help, and also with gloved hands, picked up the tail, placed it in a freezer bag, labeled it with one of Richie's ID stickers and for now, placed it in the PICU freezer. It would eventually be sent to the pathology department for examination. It could later be used as a specimen to extract DNA and gain valuable insight about what happened to Richie.

Meanwhile, Hannah was snapping away, taking pictures of everything she could and jotting down notes. She was making a record. Nancy and Betty watched, horrified. As the scene played out, it became grislier and more frightening. They tried to comfort each other but it was difficult watching pieces of his skin fall off. They had to turn away.

Sandra was thinking about how to manage what was happening, she couldn't let the cure be worse than the disease. Suddenly she realized that there would be no massive tumor lysis. The internal cells that would lyse and dump their contents inside his body were almost exclusively the stem cells and the white blood cells. Since more than 99% of his leukemia had been eliminated the risk of tumor lysis affecting his blood salt levels was very low. What she hadn't counted on was that most of the tissues affected by the aberrant genes were now peeling off Richie. As the skin and tail fell off, it carried the bulk of that toxic content away. The anticipated massive tumor lysis syndrome was not going to happen.

The big concern now was the loss of Richie's protective skin. Those open sores were a portal for bacterial infection, and that was especially dangerous now that his immune system was virtually absent. He would also be subject to significant fluid loss and dehydration as his skin sloughed off. It would be painful. He would need intravenous morphine to manage the nociceptive signals. And it would be even worse later, if he survives this, when he would have to undergo the inevitable debriding and dressing changes.

Richie needed first-class burn care. Oncology was pushed into the background, at least for now. And he desperately needed the new donor stem cells. They couldn't come fast enough. It would be at least another seven to ten days after the infusion before the new cells he needed for healing and fighting infections would be available. There was a long way to go.

Nancy, standing with Betty, away from the apparent chaos, was drawn to look back. And in the midst of the unfolding calamity, Nancy noticed something else, "look!" she exclaimed, pointing to Richie again.

Everyone turned, and once again it took a moment before the others saw what she had. But then Sandra saw it, too. "Richie's breathing. See, his chest is moving up and down, he's breathing!" It was what they had been trying to achieve, shedding the strangulating transformed cells, allowing him to expand his chest again, so that he could breathe. And now he was.

Dr. Street walked over and watched for a minute. She pulled the stethoscope from around her neck. She found a small island of intact skin on his chest, where she could carefully hold the bell of the scope and lay its diaphragm against him. She listened. It was not the turbulent sound of air from the oscillating ventilator, but rather the normal sound of laminar airflow, entering and leaving his lungs as his chest expanded and relaxed. Dr. Street found several other patches of skin on his chest that she could safely listen from. As she moved the chest piece of her stethoscope around, she heard the encouraging sounds of normal air flow.

She leaned over, and spoke softly to Richie, "it's Dr. Street. You're breathing now, Richie." She smiled. He was still in lots of trouble, but those strangling cells were being destroyed and that gave him a chance. "Richie, I'm going to try to get you off this ventilator.

I'll leave the tube in for a while longer, but I'm going to disconnect the machine, the tube will just be connected to oxygen. You'll be doing all the work. I'm going to ask the nurse to dial down the sedation. The morphine will still be there to help control pain. If it goes well, we can remove the endotracheal tube, if not, we can restart the ventilator. You'll be safe either way. Squeeze my hand if you understand?" She put her hand in his. And after a moment, she felt his grip tighten. "OK, here we go." Dr. Street disconnected the ventilator and connected the newly opened end of the ET tube to a humified oxygen source. It was now up to Richie to move the air. And he did. The oxygen saturation sensor continued with good readings, it stayed at 98% and his end tidal CO_2 monitor displayed acceptably low stable readings.

"Richie, it's looking good," said Dr. Street, "I'm going to give you an hour, breathing on your own, and if you're still keeping up with your respiratory demands, I'll take the tube out, OK?"

He squeezed her hand.

Betty and Nancy approached, wearing masks, and Dr. Street nodded that it was OK. She stepped aside to give them privacy.

Betty held his hand and smiled, doing her best to keep from crying. "Hi, Richie, we've been here all the time, me and Nancy. We've been at your side, and there are lots of others all over, rooting for you. There are texts and letters from everywhere, wishing you the best. You've got lots of fans. There was even a story about you in the news, and we have tons of mail for you to read when you're feeling better."

"It's me." Nancy moved closer so he could see her too. "I've been praying for you to get better, Richie. And now you're breathing without that fucking machine. You're amazing. Keep it up and they'll soon be taking that damn tube out. Dr. Gardner says your leukemia's gone. Hey, guess what? Your fancy turtle tail fell off, but they saved it in the freezer, I've got a picture of it. I don't think I'll miss your tail, Richie. I just want you back, so we can be together."

Just then, Dr. Street's phone rang. "Hello, PICU, this is Dr. Street."

"Hi, Rachel, it's Jack Pyre, from the Burn Unit, I understand you called."

"Hi Jack, I've got a kid here in the unit, who came in with respiratory distress, intubated and now he's got desquamating skin all over his chest and arms."

"Sounds like he was in a bad fire, but you know I don't take care of children," said Dr. Pyre.

"First off, he's going to be 18 in two months, and he wasn't in a fire, and he has no lung disease, Richie, that's his name, was intubated, before his skin started peeling off."

"I don't think I'm following you. Does he have Steven Johnson's syndrome? Why would he be intubated if he doesn't have lung disease? It's not making any sense," said Dr. Pyre.

"Sorry, Jack, I understand why it sounds confusing," said Dr. Street, "but it's not Steven Johnson's syndrome, it's not a reaction to a drug, and he wasn't in a fire, and he did require intubation without any lung disease. It's complicated, but it'll be easier to explain when you're here. I do need your burn care expertise to help treat this young man for large swathes of desquamating skin. Right now, he's getting pain control, fluids and we're using cold saline soaked sheets as temporary dressings."

Dr. Street added, "before you come over here, you may want to Google a story by Hannah Darrow about Pharma Gene Laboratories, it may help answer a lot of your questions."

"OK, Rachel, if nothing else, I'm intrigued, it sounds like an Agatha Christie mystery novel. I'll be over soon. Keep doing what you've started. I'll ask my nurse practitioner from the Burn Unit to come up as well. You can call me on this number if something changes and you need to talk to me sooner." Dr. Pyre disconnected.

Sandra came over to talk to Dr. Street. "What do you think? Is he going to make it?"

"Let's go to my office," she said.

Once inside they sat down, "I don't know," said Rachel, "his skin loss is huge. His chest and back comprise 18% of his body surface area, add another 9% for his two arms, so at a minimum, 27% of his body is covered with severely damaged, peeling skin. That's a lot. If he's lucky, it's only the superficial epidermal layer and then he may have a shot. He seems to be breathing better, and that's obviously good, but he needs an immune system to heal his skin and fight infections. So, what can you tell me?"

"His donor marrow stem cells are on the way," said Sandra "they should be here this afternoon. But I think we should wait at least 18 hours after the drugs we just gave, so he has enough time to clear them from his system before we infuse the new stem cells early tomorrow morning. I could be here at six. I only need the frozen unit from the blood bank and a body temperature water bath, and of course, I'll need central line access. It'll be at least a week before he has any new white blood cells."

"Sounds like we'll need to be super vigilant this week," said Dr. Street, "if the skin damage is superficial and we can extubate him successfully, he might have a chance."

Dr. Street walked over to Richie, glanced at the vital sign monitor and once again used her stethoscope to listen to his chest.

"You've been breathing on your own for more than an hour. It's looking good. Are you ready for me to take the tube out?"

He squeezed her hand.

"I need to raise the head of your bed a bit more, so you're sitting higher."

Leslie held his feet, while Richie bent his knees and pushing with his legs and using his strong arms, he was able to scoot further up in the bed. Once there, Leslie raised the head of the bed so that Richie was sitting nearly upright.

"I'm going to ask you to keep taking deep breaths," explained Dr. Street, "and then on my signal, you will breathe out as forcefully as you can. I will take the tube out while you're exhaling. Are you ready?"

Leslie used a suction device to remove any secretions that might interfere with his breathing once the tube was out.

Richie nodded.

"OK, here we go," said Dr. Street, "take several more deep breaths."

He did, and Dr. Street lifted the tape and used the syringe to deflate the cuff that had helped keep the tube secure.

"OK, now breath out as hard as you can," said Dr. Street.

As he exhaled, Dr. Street, in one continuous fluid motion, smoothly pulled the ET tube out. As soon as the tube was removed Leslie replaced it with a humidified oxygen face mask.

"Breathe and cough, Richard, it's good to cough now, it helps keep your lungs expanded and it recruits more alveoli to absorb the oxygen."

Richie coughed several times, it hurt and felt good at the same time. Then he settled down, just sitting there, thinking about one breath coming in and one going out. It helped to concentrate on just that. In and out, one at a time. One at a time, just breathe. His chest hurt where the skin was damaged, but he felt free, no longer restricted from taking a normal breath, that simple act of breathing, now restored, was wonderful.

Betty and Nancy watched, they held their breaths while his tube came out, and now they were breathing with him, taking big breaths as he was, encouraging him. They smiled and cried, tears of joy ran down their faces, as they watched Richie, moment by moment, breath by breath, continue to grow stronger, no longer dependent on that fucking machine for his life.

Richie saw them watching and smiled, he gave a thumbs up, but he wasn't quite ready to use his voice, not just yet. For now, just breathing was all he could manage. Richie knew that he had been very near death. And from watching his doctors, he had surmised that they had never been sure that he would be able to pull through. Richie was counting his blessings, his leukemia was gone. And all those fucking contaminated donor cells were gone. Whatever he felt he was sharing his body with, was gone. It was just him inside, all alone as he should be. His mom and Nancy were nearby and he was not ready to lie down.

59.

Sonya Tarret, NP, arrived first from the Burn Unit. She carried all the supplies that the nurses would need. Dr. Pyre was not far behind and when he arrived, he greeted Dr. Street, and introduced himself to Sandra. Sandra gave a quick presentation of Richie's history and why he required specialty burn care. Sandra also mentioned the AP story by Hannah Darrow.

"I read it. It's hard to believe that something so wicked could be done to anyone, let alone a kid," said Dr. Pyre, "I'm here to help, what can I do?"

Sandra continued, "as you'll see, it looks like an extensive burn, but since it wasn't caused by a fire. I'm hoping that there's no underlying damage, and no injury to his lungs. I'd like to know the extent and degree of the damage, and how best to manage it. And by the way, he'll have no white blood cells for a week, so there's that."

"OK, I should be able to help you. Sonya brought some of the materials you will need for his care and she can show the nurses how to apply the dressings. Let's go over and see Richie."

Sandra led him over, and introduced Dr. Pyre to Richie and Betty.

"I've been told about your injury Richie, and I want to say how sorry I am. I'm the burn doctor, and I'm here to help your doctors get you better. First, I'll need to examine you. Do you have any questions before I begin?"

By now, Richie was ready to try out his voice. When he spoke it was raspy, he hardly recognized the sound of his own voice. And as expected, it felt quite sore. "Good afternoon, Dr. Pyre," he said. "I'm ready. The medicine is helping, but it still hurts."

"I understand how painful an injury like this can be. I'm going to be as gentle as I can during the exam. I'll ask that mom step outside before I start," Dr. Pyre said.

"I'll be right outside the room, Richie," and Betty stepped out.

Dr. Pyre put on a mask, a gown and gloves. He examined him thoroughly, gently touching and pushing around the areas of damaged skin. Once in a while, he would ask Richie how it felt where he touched, if it was painful, if he had any feeling at all. It took about 20 minutes for him to complete the exam. When Dr. Pyre finished, he asked if he had any questions.

"Maybe I will," said Richie, "but can my mom come in now?"

Dr. Pyre opened the curtain and asked Betty to come in. "From my exam I'm classifying Richard's injury as an extensive first degree burn. To be honest, I'm not sure I understand how this damage occurred, but how it happened isn't so important. What's important is the extent of damage.

I find that it's only the most superficial layer, the epidermis, that's injured, the deeper layer, the dermis was spared. Since the dermis was not affected, it should heal without scarring or permanent damage. The fact that Richie is feeling pain in the damaged areas may not sound good, but it's actually a positive prognostic indicator. It means that his nerves are still working and that is what I would expect in a first degree burn. I've seen this kind of damage often. He should do well. Do you have any questions?"

Betty asked, "what happens now? I've seen stories about burns and all the treatment that needs to be done. From what I've seen, it seems horrible."

"Well, there will be a lot of work to help Richie. The skin will need to be debrided. The damaged skin is necrotic, it's dead tissue and it needs to be removed in order to allow healing. The underlying layers needs to be protected with special bandages. That will minimize the risk of dehydration and infection. He will definitely need strong pain medication while the debridement is being done. The doctors will be able to control the worst of the pain, but there will still be some. He will need antibiotics to protect him until the tissues heal. And that is especially true while his white blood cell count is so low."

Betty shook her head, and looked at Richie.

"It's going to be OK, Mom. The doctors will help, and I will get better. Remember, the leukemia is gone and so are those nasty turtle and whale genes." He smiled and reached out to his mom.

Dr. Pyre, waited a moment more, and then said, "I'll speak with Richie's doctors now."

Dr. Pyre spoke with Rachel and Sandra. He said he agreed with the dressing changes that Sonya recommended. She had brought an initial supply of the active synthetic hydrogels, which would cover the affected areas, providing the needed heat absorption and wound protection. He added the need to apply bacitracin under the dressings to reduce the risk of infection. Parenteral antibiotics should only be added if Richard becomes febrile or shows other signs of infection. After he explained everything, he left his card with his personal cell phone number and then went over to speak with Nurse Tarrat.

After Dr. Pyre left, Sonya carried the supplies over to Richie's bed. She showed Leslie how to apply a generous layering of Bacitracin over all the open areas. Once that was complete, she unwrapped the active hydrogel dressing and helped Leslie place it properly over Richie's wounds. Sonya suggested that they shouldn't be stingy with Richie's morphine, especially during debridement. She reviewed that the necrotic tissue will stick to the bandages and so when the old dressings are pulled off, the attached dead tissue will come with them. That will be painful, but essential for the healing process. She left printed instructions with illustrations of the technique, including how often to do the dressing changes and her contact information. She promised to be back to monitor Richie's treatment.

Several sets of blood tests had been done over the day, and though his white blood cell count was dropping, the results were otherwise rather benign. His potassium, uric acid levels and other electrolytes remained normal. His chest central line, no longer pinched by the alien skin, was now working again. If that continued, by the next morning, the inguinal line would no longer be needed. And without a tube in either his groin or his mouth, he might be only a few days away from being able to stand and walk. Moving around would facilitate the healing. Tomorrow would also bring the infusion of pristine, unmanipulated donor blood stem cells, and then, hopefully, he would truly be on his way to recovery.

"I've gotten a lot of pictures today," Hannah told Betty, "I think I'm done for the day. But I'll be back tomorrow morning for the stem cell infusion if that's OK?"

"Sure, that's fine, you've been a great help," answered Betty, "we want to make sure that your boss is happy."

Betty went in to sit with Richie. He was completely wrapped with bandages over his arms and chest. But at last he was sitting up, breathing and quite talkative. Betty had been terrified that she might lose her son, but now she began to relax, just a bit. The tension in her shoulders eased. She could finally imagine an end to the horrors that his disease brought. The knot in her stomach loosened, and she could even manage a smile. "Hey, you know you look like one of those monster creatures on your posters."

Richie smiled, Betty hadn't seen that in a while.

"It's good to see you smiling Richie, and looking more comfortable," said Betty, "how do you really feel?"

"You know it still hurts," he answered, "and when I talk it feels funny, but the morphine helps, and shit Mom, you can't imagine what it feels like to not be able to breathe. That was so freakin scary, but I don't feel that way anymore, it's such a relief to be off that machine."

"I can't even begin to imagine what it's been like for you. That memory will be with me the rest of my life." Betty began to sob, "Richie, you can't ever do that to me again, I don't think I would survive another horror like that."

Richie reached out to comfort his mom. "I promise not to."

Betty smiled. "OK, let's turn out the lights and close our eyes."

60.

The next morning, after his first good sleep in weeks, he woke up hearing Sandra setting up for the stem cell infusion. "Good morning, Richie."

"Hi, Dr. Gardner, so this is Infusion II, the sequel? I hope it's better than the first, I didn't like that version very much."

"I don't think anyone did. We've bypassed PGL, and these cells should work as they were intended.

Before you get any of the stem cells, I'll ask Dr. Street to remove the inguinal line. After it's out, she'll place a dressing over the exit site and a 5-pound sandbag over that. That'll sit for about 30 minutes to make sure that the wound doesn't open. We'll do that before the cell infusion. If we pulled the line out later and you bled, we would be losing some of those precious newly infused stem cells. I'll be back in about an hour to check, and if it's all good, we can proceed with the next step."

Dr. Street removed the dressing over the inguinal line site, snipped a couple of sutures and slowly but steadily pulled the line out. She quickly held a gauze with hand pressure over the site. After a few minutes, and no bleeding, Dr. Street folded a larger sterile gauze over the first one, secured it with some hospital tape and then positioned a sandbag over everything. "I'll be back to check that in 30 minutes."

A half hour later, Dr. Street was back as promised. The site of the line removal looked good. She removed the gauze and tape, and applied Dermabond to glue the edges together. A few seconds later the glue was dry and the wound was additionally secured with several sutures. Dr. Street let Sandra know that it was safe to infuse the stem cells.

As preparation, Richie received extra fluids so that he was well hydrated, and Zofran to preclude any nausea. As standard procedure, before storing, the donor cells had been frozen in a solution with an agent called DMSO, dimethyl sulfoxide, which allowed the cells to remain functional even after being frozen and thawed. They were kept safe that way during their journey to the medical center.

"Richie, you may notice a garlicky taste or smell as the cells are infused," said Sandra. "That's the DMSO mixed in the solution with your cells. Sitting next to you is a body temperature water bath. The cell product came up from the blood bank, still frozen in its cooler. It must be thawed, of course. I'll take it out and gently swirl the sealed infusion bag in the water bath which will thaw the product fairly rapidly. As soon as it's a liquid suspension, the nurse will connect it to your central line. It'll take about 5 to 10 minutes to infuse. As the solution of cells circulates inside you, I'll be able to smell the garlic like odor of the DMSO on your breath. That will confirm that the cells are circulating as they should. After a few hours, the stem cells will settle in your bone marrow. Over time, those cells will produce all the blood cells you'll ever need, sort of like planting perennial seeds in a garden." Sandra looked at Richie, "are you ready?"

Richie gave a thumbs up. Richie was more than ready to put this nightmare behind him. He thought about the first transplant, and how many things had gone wrong. Yes, he was ready. Richie was hoping that transplant number two would be the boring sequel.

Sandra checked the label on the stem cell product, visually and with the scanner against his wrist ID. It was also confirmed by Leslie. When everyone agreed that it was the right product and the right patient, Sandra took the frozen product, placed it inside another sterile bag, and began to swirl the package in the body temperature water bath. She double bagged it so that even if there was a leak, they wouldn't lose any of those precious cells. Every few minutes she would remove the bag and feel it, squeezing the edges, checking to see if it had melted completely. Finally, when she pressed around the bag and there were no more frozen chunks, she asked the nurse to spike the bag and begin the infusion. This part of the transplant was rather anticlimactic.

Dr. Gardner stood, making sure that everything was running as expected, After just a few minutes, she smiled, "I smell the garlic scent, Richie. Those cells are on target."

Richie gave the thumbs up. After everything that happened with the first transplant, he was confident that he could manage whatever cropped up this time. He was a veteran. The infusion finished in just over 10 minutes, Sandra ran a bit more saline into the bag, inverted it a couple of times and then ran the wash through Richie's line, being sure to capture every last cell. Once completed, the bag was taken down, packaged, labeled, and sent back to the blood bank where it would be kept for later analysis if anything went wrong.

"This transplant is both similar and different from the first one you had," explained Sandra. "Of course, these are unmanipulated cells, and that's different. Richard's marrow should be empty now and ready to accept the new cells, that is the same as before, and once the cells begin to grow, Graft vs. Host Disease can develop, that is also the same. But it's also different, because he didn't just complete a week of intensive chemotherapy, so he won't need to contend with mouth sores or a damaged marrow lining. And although he won't be making any red blood cells or platelets for a while, he had normal or even higher than normal numbers of those just yesterday. Those'll be around for a while. So, I expect that Richard will go through this post-transplant recovery process with less discomfort and less complications than the last one. Today is a new day zero, starting that count all over again. Since GvHD can still be a problem he'll receive small doses of cyclophosphamide on days +3 and +4 to reduce the complications of emerging T cells. Like before, he'll start Cellcept and tacrolimus on day +5. But since he's starting from a different baseline, he might be able to go home in less than two weeks. How does that sound?"

"Dr. Gardner, you forgot another way this one will be different," said Richie.

"What's that?" asked Sandra.

"No turtle tail!"

"Yes, this should be a turtle tail free transplant," smiled Sandra.

As Dr. Gardner walked out of the room, Richie was feeling pretty good about everything. Well there was still the burn care, the debridement would be difficult, for sure. But over time, as he healed, the dressing changes would be less frequent.

Richie reflected on everything that he'd been through. That first day in Dr. Pipkin's office, the blood tests and receiving the diagnosis. And all that followed, the procedures, the chemotherapy, multiple crises and the bone marrow transplant that had gone horribly wrong. He didn't know how close he'd come to dying as those nasty cells tried to strangle him, he thought it might have been pretty close. He thought of all the people that helped, the doctors and nurses, his donor, and so many others. And his mom, she was always there. And his special girl, Nancy, who had stuck with him through everything. All those scares, but somehow he had survived. He was on the other side and it had changed him. He closed his eyes and fell into a quiet, blissful sleep.

Richie transferred to the pediatric oncology unit the next afternoon. The following days passed uneventfully. The dressing changes spaced out, and then finally the last dressing came off, his skin was healing nicely. He underwent sessions of occupational therapy to prevent the development of joint contractures as his skin regrew. Sonya Tarrat and Dr. Pyre discharged him from their burn care.

Richie had visitors over the next few days. Newt, Saul and the Captain came one afternoon. They presented him with a model of the fishing boat. On the side at the bow was painted, '*Richard's Sea Hunt.*' The Captain also brought a lifetime pass for Richie and a guest, to come fishing with them any time, *weather permitting*.

Newt stayed a few minutes after Saul and the Captain left. He told Richie that he didn't remember much of that night on the boat, but Saul had told him what happened and that he certainly would have drowned and been lost at sea, if not for what Richie did. There were no words he said to adequately express his gratitude, but he was thankful. He had prayed for Richie's recovery, and he would continue to keep Richie in his prayers forevermore. Newt and Richie hugged, and Newt whispered, 'thank you." Richie watched a tear fall as he turned and left.

And, of course, Nancy came, and Betty found an excuse to leave the unit when she was there. Richie lit up when she was around. Nancy was a new girl now that Richie was recovering. She was carefree, happy, and wore a big smile on her face whenever they were together. They touched and leaned against each other, as they talked about anything, and everything except the cancer and its treatments. Young people in love, they chatted, texted, took selfies and sent them to each other. They made plans for when Richie would be home. They were not tentative or contingent plans, they were rock solid, definitive plans, with dates, times and locations. They would be together whenever they could. They would find ways to be alone, together, exploring and enjoying.

EPILOGUE

It was a brilliant, hot, sunny day at the end of August. Betty and Richie had been hunting for a parking space for the last 30 minutes. The lovely tree-lined streets of College Hill were swarming with parents and their kids, lugging boxes, carrying lamps and pulling their wheeled luggage on this crazy move-in day. Freshman orientation week at Brown University was starting and it was wild out there. He looked at all the new faces and wondered if they could possibly be as excited as he was.

Richie spotted a car at the curb with its directional signal blinking, and immediately alerted his mom about the spot that was about to become available. "Wow, that was lucky."

Once parked, Richie reached to his back pocket and pulled out the campus map he'd tucked away. He'd been studying it for the past few weeks, trying to commit it to memory. The building with his assigned dorm room was circled. He sat in the car, turning the map several times until he was able to match it to the real campus outside. Richie finally thought he knew where they were going and they could begin unloading his stuff.

He stretched out and breathed the air in as he got out of the car and gazed at his new world. Eager to get going, Richie walked around to the back of the car and peered through the car's opened rear gate, "it's really amazing how much stuff we were able to pack in there," said Richie. He'd spent the last two days trying to fit what he thought he might need, including the folding wagon, and some items his mom suggested. It was their first long trip in their brand new green Subaru Forester Hybrid.

Following the campus map, and after a couple of wrong turns, he finally found his room. Richie opened the door with the key he'd been given at check-in. He hadn't known what to expect. But it was an old dorm building on an old campus and the rooms were simple but spacious. He liked the exposed beams in the surprisingly high ceiling. As he looked around he could picture himself spending the coming year in this room. He seemed to have arrived before his roommate, who he had yet to meet, so he had an opportunity. There were two of everything, two twin beds, two desks, two lamps, two chairs, an armoire and not much else. After trying out both beds, he claimed the left side of the room for his own. With his mom's help, it didn't take long to fix the room up. He'd been able to move everything from the car in just two trips, using the folding wagon and the two large, wheeled suitcases. Besides all the usual stuff, he brought his drip coffee maker and a small fan essential for a room without A/C. He also remembered to bring a box of push pins to mount his Frankenstein, Count Dracula and the taped up Creature from the Black Lagoon posters on the wall around his bed. Betty found where the best lighting was for the easy to care for plants that she'd picked. She made sure they were nicely watered.

Richie could hardly believe that he was really in his own dorm room at Brown. He thought back to this time last year. He'd been recovering from his bone marrow transplant and trying to keep up with his classmates. He worked hard, determined to put all that horror behind him. It took a while. He struggled for the first months. But as he persisted, he not only managed, but he excelled through his senior year at Horace Mann High. He worked hard on his applications to colleges.

His grades, test scores and recommendations were good, but he believed that his humdinger of a personal essay is what put him over the top. When that thick envelope showed up with his acceptance to his first choice school, he jumped for joy. He ran to show his mom and they celebrated together. He smiled thinking about that day and how he felt. It was sweet reward that his mom didn't have to worry about college tuition or any other of his expenses. The settlement from PGL easily covered four years of college, the brand new Subaru, enough for Betty to start her own gallery and still have a chunk of change left to cover emergencies.

While his mom was tinkering with last minute details around the room, Richie took out his new laptop, accessed the school wi-fi and reviewed the classes he was planning to register for. He hoped they'd still have some places left by the time freshman got their chance to sign up. His first term would be heavy in science and math. Richie knew that he would need that background to work as an architect at NASA, hoping one day to be designing human colonies on Mars. His new spiral bound notebook was already filled with drawings of his ideas.

"OK, I think you are all set here," said Betty. She looked around his dorm room. "How about a big hug before I leave?"

Richie pulled off his sunglasses, pushed back his now long curly hair and smiled big as he gave his mom a squeeze.

"No matter how many times I see those eyes of yours," said his mom, "it still brings me back to that awful time."

"Yeah, it's kind of weird. Everything else is back to normal, but I guess these freaky pink eyes will always be here as a souvenir that will keep me from forgetting."

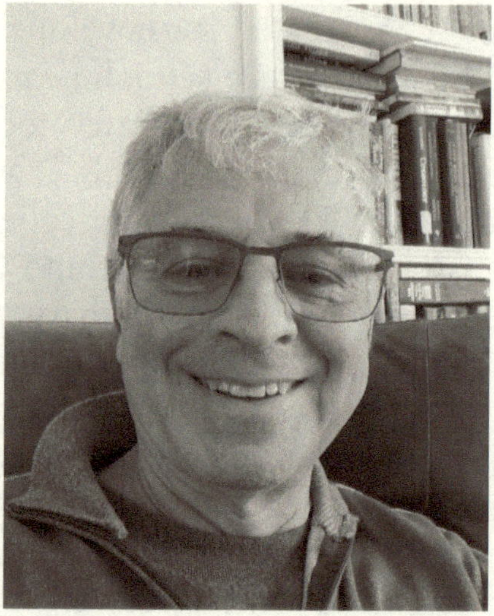

Howard is a retired pediatric oncologist, who started the pediatric bone marrow transplant program at Tufts Medical Center in Boston. He also created the Cycle for Life, a charity bicycle ride to raise money for Child Life Therapy at the Floating Hospital for Children. He was a co-founder of the ASPHO Special Interest Group in Hemoglobinopathy, with a focus on sickle cell disease.

The idea for this story, percolated through his thoughts for many years, and is now Dr. Grodman's first novel. He is a husband and father of two grown children. He spends his time reading, enjoying the water and teaching Basic Life Support. He makes his home back in Massachusetts.

www.ingramcontent.com/pod-product-compliance
Lightning Source LLC
LaVergne TN
LVHW090350240926
848801LV00011B/163/J
9798994137116